2013
YEAR BOOK OF
SPORTS MEDICINE®

The 2013 Year Book Series

Year Book of Critical Care Medicine®: Drs Dries, Zanotti-Cavazzoni, Latenser, Martinez, Rincon, and Zwank

Year Book of Emergency Medicine®: Drs Hamilton, Bruno, Handly, Minczak, Quintana, and Ramoska

Year Book of Endocrinology®: Drs Schott, Apovian, Clarke, Eugster, Meikle, Oetgen, Ovalle, Schteingart, and Toth

Year Book of Hand and Upper Limb Surgery®: Drs Yao, Adams, Isaacs, Lee, and Rizzo

Year Book of Medicine®: Drs Barker, Garrick, Gersh, Khardori, LeRoith, Panush, Talley, and Thigpen

Year Book of Neonatal and Perinatal Medicine®: Drs Fanaroff, Benitz, Donn, Neu, Papile, and Van Marter

Year Book of Neurology and Neurosurgery®: Drs Klimo, Minagar, Gandhi, House, Kevill, Liu, Mazia, Panagariya, Ragel, Riesenburger, Robottom, Schwendimann, Shafazand, Uhm, and Yang

Year Book of Obstetrics, Gynecology, and Women's Health®: Drs Dungan and Shulman

Year Book of Oncology®: Drs Arceci, Bauer, Chiorean, Gordon, Lawton, Murphy, Thigpen, and Tsao

Year Book of Ophthalmology®: Drs Rapuano, Cohen, Flanders, Hammersmith, Milman, Myers, Nagra, Nelson, Penne, Pyfer, Sergott, Shields, Talekar, and Vander

Year Book of Orthopedics®: Drs Morrey, Huddleston, Rose, Swiontkowski, and Trigg

Year Book of Otolaryngology-Head and Neck Surgery®: Drs Sindwani, Balough, Franco, Gapany, and Mitchell

Year Book of Pathology and Laboratory Medicine®: Drs Raab and Bissell

Year Book of Pediatrics®: Dr Stockman

Year Book of Plastic and Aesthetic Surgery™: Drs Miller, Boehmler, Gosman, Gutowski, Ruberg, Salisbury, and Smith

Year Book of Psychiatry and Applied Mental Health®: Drs Talbott, Ballenger, Buckley, Frances, Krupnick, and Mack

Year Book of Pulmonary Disease®: Drs Barker, Jones, Maurer, Spradley, Tanoue, and Willsie

Year Book of Sports Medicine®: Drs Shephard, Cantu, Desmeules, Galea, Jankowski, Janssen, Lebrun, and Nieman

Year Book of Surgery®: Drs Copeland, Behrns, Daly, Eberlein, Fahey, Huber, Klodell, Mozingo, and Pruett

Year Book of Urology®: Drs Andriole and Coplen

Year Book of Vascular Surgery®: Drs Moneta, Gillespie, Starnes, and Watkins

2013

The Year Book of
SPORTS MEDICINE®

Editor-in-Chief
Roy J. Shephard, MB, BS, MD (Lond), PhD, DPE, LLD (Hon Caus)
Faculty of Kinesiology & Physical Education, University of Toronto, Toronto, Ontario, Canada

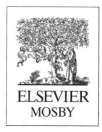

ELSEVIER
MOSBY

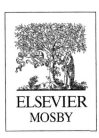

ELSEVIER
MOSBY

Vice President, Continuity Publishing: Kimberly Murphy
Editor: Patrick Manley
Production Supervisor, Electronic Year Books: Donna M. Skelton
Electronic Article Manager: Mike Sheets
Illustrations and Permissions Coordinator: Dawn Vohsen

Composition by TNQ Books and Journals Pvt Ltd, India

Printed and bound by CPI Group (UK) Ltd, Croydon, CR0 4YY

Transferred to digital print 2012

Editorial Office:
Elsevier, Inc.
Suite 1800
1600 John F. Kennedy Boulevard
Philadelphia, PA 19103-2899

International Standard Serial Number: 0162-0908
International Standard Book Number: 978-1-4557-7290-2

Associate Editors

Robert C. Cantu, MA, MD, FACS, FAANS, FACSM

Clinical Professor of Neurosurgery, Boston University School of Medicine; Co-Director, Neurological Sports Injury Center at Brigham and Women's Hospital; Neurosurgery Consultant, Boston College Eagles and Boston Cannons Lacrosse Teams; Co-Director, Center for the Study of Traumatic Encephalopathy (CSTE), Boston University Medical Center, Boston, Massachusetts; Co-Founder and Chairman, Medical Advisory Board Sports Legacy Institute (SLI), Waltham, Massachusetts; Chairman, Department of Surgery, Chief, Neurosurgery Service, and Director, Service Sports Medicine, Emerson Hospital, Concord, Massachusetts; Adjunct Professor, Exercise and Sport Science, University of North Carolina; Medical Director, National Center for Catastrophic Sports Injury, Research, Chapel Hill, North Carolina; Senior Advisor, National Football League (NFL) Head, Neck and Spine Committee, New York, New York

François Desmeules, pht, PhD/PT, PhD

Assistant Professor, School of Rehabilitation, Faculty of Medicine, University of Montreal, Montreal, Canada

Victoria Galea, PhD

Associate Professor, School of Rehabilitation Science, Department of Kinesiology and The Education Program in Anatomy, McMaster University, Hamilton, Ontario, Canada

Catherine M. Jankowski, PhD

Assistant Research Professor, Division of Geriatric Medicine, University of Colorado Denver, Aurora, Colorado

Ian Janssen, PhD

Associate Professor, School of Kinesiology and Health Studies, and Department of Community Health and Epidemiology, Queen's University, Kingston, Ontario, Canada

Connie Lebrun, MDCM, MPE, CCFP, Dip Sport Med, FACSM

Associate Professor, Faculty of Medicine and Dentistry, Department of Family Medicine, Consultant Sports Medicine Physician, Glen Sather Sports Medicine Clinic, University of Alberta, Edmonton, Alberta, Canada

David C. Nieman, DrPH

Professor, Appalachian State University, Boone, North Carolina; Director, The Human Performance Laboratory, North Carolina Research Campus, Kannapolis, North Carolina

Table of Contents

Journals Represented

Journals represented in this YEAR BOOK are listed below.

Acta Obstetricia et Gynecologica Scandinavica
Acta Paediatrica
AJR American Journal of Roentgenology
American Heart Journal
American Journal of Addictions
American Journal of Cardiology
American Journal of Clinical Nutrition
American Journal of Epidemiology
American Journal of Obstetrics and Gynecology
American Journal of Perinatology
American Journal of Physical Medicine & Rehabilitation
American Journal of Preventive Medicine
American Journal of Public Health
American Journal of Sports Medicine
American Journal of Transplantation
Annals of Emergency Medicine
Archives of Dermatology
Archives of Internal Medicine
Archives of Neurology
Archives of Physical Medicine and Rehabilitation
Arthroscopy
British Journal of Psychiatry
British Journal of Radiology
British Journal of Sports Medicine
British Medical Journal
Chest
Circulation
Clinical Journal of Sport Medicine
Clinical Neurology and Neurosurgery
Clinical Pediatrics
Contraception
Diabetes Care
European Heart Journal
European Journal of Applied Physiology
European Respiratory Journal
Exercise and Sport Sciences Reviews
Heart
Hypertension
International Journal of Obesity
International Journal of Sports Medicine
Journal of Applied Physiology
Journal of Athletic Training
Journal of Bone and Joint Surgery (American)
Journal of Bone Mineral Research
Journal of Clinical Endocrinology & Metabolism
Journal of Clinical Psychiatry

Journal of Hepatology
Journal of Neurological Sciences
Journal of Neurology, Neurosurgery, and Psychiatry
Journal of Neurosurgery
Journal of Neurosurgery Pediatrics
Journal of Orthopaedic and Sports Physical Therapy
Journal of Pain
Journal of Pain and Symptom Management
Journal of Pediatrics
Journal of Sports Medicine and Physical Fitness
Journal of the American College of Cardiology
Journal of the American Geriatrics Society
Journal of the American Medical Association
Journal of the American Medical Directors Association
Journal of the National Cancer Institute
Journal of Trauma and Acute Care Surgery
Journal of Ultrasound in Medicine
Journal of Vascular Surgery
Lancet
Maturitas
Medicine and Science in Sports and Exercise
Osteoporosis International
Pediatr Phys Ther
Pediatric Emergency Care
Pediatric Neurology
Pediatrics
Physical Therapy
Public Library of Science Medicine
Research in Developmental Disabilities
Spine Journal
Sports Medicine
Stroke
Wilderness & Environmental Medicine

Standard Abbreviations

The following terms are abbreviated in this edition: acquired immunodeficiency syndrome (AIDS), cardiopulmonary resuscitation (CPR), central nervous system (CNS), cerebrospinal fluid (CSF), computed tomography (CT), deoxyribonucleic acid (DNA), electrocardiography (ECG), health maintenance organization (HMO), human immunodeficiency virus (HIV), intensive care unit (ICU), intramuscular (IM), intravenous (IV), magnetic resonance (MR) imaging (MRI), ribonucleic acid (RNA), and ultrasound (US).

Note

To facilitate the use of the YEAR BOOK OF SPORTS MEDICINE as a reference tool, all illustrations and tables included in this publication are now identified as they appear in the original article. This change is meant to help the reader recognize that any illustration or table appearing in the YEAR BOOK OF SPORTS MEDICINE may be only one of many in the original article. For this reason, figure and table numbers will often appear to be out of sequence within the YEAR BOOK OF SPORTS MEDICINE.

Physical Activity and the Visceral Organs

Roy J. Shephard, MB, BS, MD (Lond), PhD, DPE, LLD (Hon Caus)

Faculty of Kinesiology & Physical Education, University of Toronto, Toronto, Ontario, Canada

Introduction

Sports medicine texts devote much space to physical injuries and the implications of acute and chronic physical activity for the health of the heart, lungs, and muscles, but the impact of physical activity upon the viscera receives much less attention. The organs concerned are less readily accessible, making it more difficult to evaluate their function. Moreover, the heart and lungs have a main function that can be summarized by a single variable, such as ejection fraction or forced vital capacity, but the viscera have multiple functions that are difficult to assess by any single test. We will thus take a brief look at our current knowledge of interactions between physical activity and visceral function. The introductory chapter this year discusses gastrointestinal responses to physical activity, and next year's chapter will address interactions between physical activity and the liver, gall bladder, kidneys, and urinary tract. In both lead articles, attention is directed firstly to the acute effects of a single bout of physical activity, and then to the consequences of repeated periods of physical activity, whether it's the impact of several months of deliberate training or the cumulative effects of repeated exhausting exercise.

Most of the findings apply equally to women and men. Regular moderate physical activity has a number of positive effects upon these various organs, but adverse consequences can follow very intensive bouts of exercise and/or training, particularly if the effort is sufficient to cause visceral hypoxia. It is thus important to recognize and monitor the potential dangers associated with excessive training and/or repeated participation in extreme events.

Many of the investigations to be discussed are based on clinical case reports or small-scale experimental studies of the metabolism and excretion of test substances. In contrast, epidemiological evaluations of the risks of cancer have typically involved large and carefully selected populations, although it has often been difficult to make full adjustment for important co-variates such as smoking history and alcohol consumption. Moreover, estimates of habitual physical activity (usually based on questionnaires) have had limited absolute accuracy. Our account includes animal studies that have allowed biopsy and postmortem examination of the viscera, as well as experimental evaluations of interactions between physical activity and deliberately administered carcinogens. However, caution is needed when extrapolating the observations on experimental tumors to the behavior of human cancers that have developed slowly over the course of many years. Moreover, an animal's physical activity is usually enforced (by electrical shock, or swimming to avoid drowning) rather than voluntarily chosen, and differences in body size and lifespan between laboratory animals and humans further hamper the clinical extrapolation of findings.

Gastro-intestinal tract: Acute physical activity

Acute concerns include altered esophageal mechanics, with a potential for gastric reflux, sensations of gastric nausea and fullness, increased colonic mobility, intestinal bleeding, and loss of the normal intestinal barrier function.

Esophageal mechanics and gastro-esophageal reflux

Regular, moderate physical activity seems to have a beneficial effect upon esophageal function, but both symptoms (heartburn, which must be distinguished carefully from angina,[1] and the monitoring of esophageal pH) suggest that some forms of intense exercise provoke acute episodes of gastric reflux, with a possible risk of esophagitis and neoplastic change.

Much of the immediate benefit of regular physical activity[2,3] is probably lifestyle-related.[3] Gastric reflux has been linked to smoking, and most active individuals are non-smokers. Obesity is also a substantial risk factor (an odds ratio of 1.94 with a body mass index > 30 kg/m^2), thus making the condition more probable among physically inactive individuals.[3-5] A further potential variable is stress, with moderate activity encouraging a reduction of stress, but intense competition augmenting the problem.

Evidence about the acute effects of physical activity upon esophageal mechanics is conflicting. One investigator found that in asymptomatic athletes, moderate intensity treadmill running induced a modest increase in pressure at the lower esophageal sphincter.[6] Other studies of trained athletes have noted that in untrained subjects there were decreases in esophageal contraction and sphincter pressures as the intensity of cycle ergometer exercise was increased from 45% to 90% of peak aerobic power.[7-10]

Some early studies reported little acute effect of exercise on the likelihood of esophageal reflux,[10,11] but others have found problems in a substantial proportion of competitors during intensive exercise, complaints being particularly likely in surf-boarding, the Valsalva maneuver during weight-lifting,[12] in cyclists (particularly if they report gastric symptoms),[13] and in rowers.[14] In one somewhat unlikely competitive scenario, exercise was performed at 70% of maximal heart rate 30 minutes after a meal, and in this situation physical activity led to disorganized esophageal contractions, with periods of reflux and an esophageal pH <4.0.[15] In patients with known combined or supine gastro-esophageal reflux, even moderate exercise may be sufficient to exacerbate symptoms.[16]

If a competitor is complaining of acute gastric reflux during exercise, the problem can sometimes be corrected by changes in the form of sport or the timing and composition of meals. Reflux seems more likely if athletes ingest hypertonic beverages containing carbohydrate or salt solutions rather than water.[3] However, if exercise-induced gastric pain is frequent and severe, pharmacological treatments such as antacids, histamine H$_2$ receptor blockers (cimetidine or ranitidine), dopamine antagonists or proton pump inhibitors such as omeprazole may be required.[17-19]

Gastric nausea, fullness, and epigastric pain

A study of 25 640 triathlon competitors found epigastric complaints (nausea, epigastric pain, or vomiting) in 8.9% of those questioned.[20] Some of these symptoms may reflect gastro-esophageal reflux (above). Other potential causes include an excessive ingestion of "replacement" fluids, a slowing of gastric emptying over the course of a prolonged event, and gastric ischemia.

Gastric emptying (particularly of solids) and small intestinal motility may be unchanged or even enhanced by moderate physical activity (to about 70% of maximal oxygen intake), but motility may be depressed by more intensive exercise.[21-24] Carrio et al found that basal gastric emptying was faster in marathon runners than in sedentary individuals (68 vs 85 min), but this basal rate was unaffected by 90 minutes of sustained running.[25] Runners should limit their fluid intake to 600 ml/hr, a volume that can empty from the stomach and be absorbed by the intestines during vigorous physical activity.[26]

During intensive exercise, there is a massive redistribution of blood flow from the viscera to the muscles[27]; this may be sufficient to cause gastric ischemia, with severe epigastric pain,[28,29] as well as changes in gut permeability (below).

Intestinal motility and absorption

A study of triathletes noted that 8% reported diarrhea or abdominal pain during or following an event.[20] A report on 606 endurance athletes found both gastric and intestinal symptoms in distance cyclists, but a predominance of intestinal symptoms (bloating, diarrhea, and flatulence) in runners.[17-30] Riddoch and Trinich[31] noted an urge to bowel movement in 53% of marathon participants, and Keeffe et al[32] observed a similar response in a third of marathon runners. The tendency for an exercise-induced increase of gastro-intestinal irritability may be exacerbated following abdominal irradiation (for example, as a continuing side effect of the treatment of prostatic cancer).

The impact of physical activity upon formal measurements of transit time seems to depend somewhat on the method of measurement. One author found an increased oral-cecal transit time when running at 70% of maximal power),[13] but in a study using pH telemetry neither small bowel nor colon transit times were changed significantly following exercise.[33] Scott[34] noted that the mouth-to-cecum transit time was unchanged by running 9.6 km (6 mi), and walking a distance of 4.5 km (2.8 mi) in one hour did not change the total transit time in previously sedentary laboratory workers. Moreover, 6 hours of intermittent cycle ergometer exercise speeded gastric emptying but had no effect upon the movement of food through the small intestines.[35] The absorption of water, electrolytes, and glucose also appears to be unaffected by physical activity.

A speeding of colonic activity by vigorous physical activity is more consistently reported,[21,22] and probably accounts for the diarrhea, urge to defecate, and cramps seen in runners.[36] Halvorson et al[37] found that 48% of marathon participants observed looser stools or more frequent defecation after they took up distance running. A carmine dye study of total gastro-intestinal transit found times decreased from 35 to 24 hours following 6 weeks of training.[38] A second study showed that an hour of exercise per day at 50% of maximal aerobic power reduced the transit time (as assessed by radio-opaque markers) from 51 hours to 37 hours (cycling) or 34 hours (jogging).[39] An exercise prescription may thus be helpful to a person who is suffering from chronic constipation. The athlete who suffers from diarrhea can often be helped by low residue diets, supplemented if necessary by medications such as Imodium.

Barrier function

Exhaustive exercise (running at 89% of peak aerobic power) has been shown to increase gastro-intestinal permeability, as shown by the urinary lactulose/rhamnose ratio,[40] well demonstrated in Alaskan sled dogs after participation in a 1770 km race.[41] Nevertheless, some of the change in permeability seen in human athletes may be due to a high consumption of NSAIDS.[42,43]

A prolonged and exhausting bout of physical activity can reduce blood flow to the gut, thus causing a variety of symptoms, and sometimes ischemic damage to the intestines.[44] One study demonstrated ischemia of the gastric mucosa with as little as 10 minutes of intensive exercise.[45] An important consequence is a drastic disruption of the gastro-intestinal barrier, bleeding being accompanied by a leakage of endotoxins from the gut into the bloodstream.[46,47] The affected individuals commonly complain of nausea, vomiting, and diarrhea.[47] Some have argued that the portal burden of endotoxin is increased by mechanical pressures during running, a vigorous descent of the diaphragm creating a "cecal slap."[48,49] On the other hand, regular training may induce some immunity to gut-derived endotoxin,[47-50] in part because this binds to HDL cholesterol.[51]

If circulating endotoxins are observed following a bout of exhausting exercise, these have come from the cell walls of gram-negative bacteria normally present in the gut. If hepatic function is also compromised, a portal vein endotoxemia can quickly progress to a systemic endotoxemia. The endotoxins stimulate release of the endogenous pyrogens tumor necrosis factor and interleukin-1; this sets in motion a chain of immunological disturbances that can progress to a form of endotoxic shock,[50] widely disseminated intravascular coagulation and many of the clinical manifestations of exercise-induced heat stroke.

The potential for an exercise-induced disturbance of inflammatory homeostasis[52,53] is exacerbated by adverse effects upon immune tissue within the gut (Peyer's patches).[54]

Intestinal bleeding

Minor gastrointestinal bleeding seems a relatively common phenomenon among long-distance runners, particularly if they make frequent use of nonsteroidal anti-inflammatory drugs such as aspirin. The reported incidence of stools with a positive occult blood test is quite variable (from as low as 1%, to as high as 85%, depending in part on the timing of stool sampling relative to competition and on the intensity of effort that has been undertaken.[9,21,22] Halvorson et al[55] examined fecal samples in 63 marathoners and found traces of blood in 8 of the 63 immediately after the event. After a 100-mile event, 30 of 35 runners showed occult blood in the stools.[56] Although bleeding was once blamed upon a mechanical shaking of the viscera, the dominant reason seems to be ischemia of the gut wall, whether induced by the redistribution of visceral blood flow,[57] or a subsequent septic reaction.[50] Another contributing factor may be the secretion of substances such as vasoactive intestinal peptide, secretin, and peptide-histidine-methionine.[44] Both occult and visible bleeding seem to peak 24 to 48 hours after a bout of exercise, and (probably because of differences in the intensity of effort) both are more prevalent following competition than after a practice run.

The stomach is usually the prime site of blood loss, although the colon is sometimes affected. One case report also described exercise-induced bleeding from esophageal varices in a body-builder who had been taking large doses of anabolic steroids[58]; however, it is unclear why anabolic agents should have such an effect except possibly through an association with the repeated performance of high-intensity resistance exercise.

The amount of blood loss in athletes is usually small. It may sometimes contribute to "athlete's anemia," but in most endurance competitors a low hemoglobin concentration reflects an expansion of plasma volume rather than blood loss. There have been suggestions that bleeding can be prevented by prophylactic administration of antihistamine medications or proton pump inhibitors[59,60]; however, this commonly has adverse effects on competitive performance and is not necessary in most competitors, since the blood loss generally resolves if the athlete takes 2 to 3 days of rest.

Chronic physical activity

There has been some discussion of the influence of habitual physical activity upon the risks of peptic ulcers and inflammatory bowel disease. However, the main effects of regular moderate physical activity upon the gastrointestinal tract seem to be a decrease in colonic transit time and/or an increase of intestinal segmentation, with a resulting decrease in the risk of certain forms of cancer. Patients with special dietary disease (such as those with celiac disease) may need careful advice on maintaining their diets during periods of intensive activity. However, there is little evidence that regular physical activity increases the risk of occult gastrointestinal hemorrhage.

Peptic ulcers

There is little evidence of a reduced risk of gastric ulcer in those who are physically active. However, it does appear to have some value in duodenal ulcers.[61] A cross-sectional study of 8529 men and 2884 women in the Cooper Clinic population found a reduced risk of duodenal ulcers in individuals who were physically active (relative hazard 0.38 in those who were "active" and 0.54 in those who were "moderately active."[62] Benefit does not appear to depend on changes in gastric secretion. Feldman and Nixon[63] found little effect of 45 minutes of cycle ergometer exercise (50% or 75% of maximal oxygen intake) upon gastric secretion. Others have seen some decrease in both basal and meal-stimulated secretions during or following exercise,[64,65] but on the other hand, one study reported that exercise increased stimulated gastric acid secretion in patients with duodenal ulcers.[66,67] Possibly, healing of the ulcer may be mediated in part through changes in immune function or a modulation of stress and an increase in overall well-being.[68]

Inflammatory bowel disease

Crohn disease is thought to reflect problems with the innate immune system,[69] particularly an imbalance between pro- and anti-inflammatory cytokines,[69,70] Evidence on the preventive and therapeutic merits of physical activity is limited, but there may be some preventive effects through the control of obesity and/or stress. In those with established disease, exercise certainly does not exacerbate the condition, and it may help to counteract a decrease of bone mineral density and weight loss, with improved immunological responses, better quality of life and overall psychological health, and a reduction of stress.[71,72] One recent report found an increase of neutrophil activation and an exacerbation of zinc deficiency when patients in remission from Crohn disease undertook a moderate exercise program. Since physical activity stimulates the production of heat shock proteins, this also could be helpful in the treatment of inflammatory bowel disorders such as diverticular disease and Crohn disease.[73]

Obesity is certainly associated with chronic systemic inflammation, in part because adipose tissue releases proinflammatory cytokines such as TNF and IL-6,[74] and a decreased incidence of chronic intestinal inflammation has been suggested as an important dividend of regular physical activity.[72-75] Two major mechanisms defending tissues against an excessive inflammatory response to stressors are the production of heat shock proteins (HSP) and mitogen-activation of protein kinases pathways (MAPK). The intestines seem particularly vulnerable to the effects of reactive oxygen species (ROS).[76] These effects are plainly modulated by physical activity, both in terms of an increased production of ROS during intensive effort and an increased activity of the enzymes that break down ROS in well-trained individuals. Studies of mice have shown an increased production of intestinal heat shock protein (HSP) in the 24 hours following exhaustive exercise (A.J. Gibson et al, unpublished data, 2011), and a down-regulation of mitogen-activated protein kinases (Breton-Honeyman et al, unpublished data, 2011). Conceivably, the increased levels of HSP could modulate MAPK pathways, leading to a greater activation of extracellular signal-regulated kinases (ERK), together with a decreased activation of the c-Jun N-terminal kinases (JNK) that cause expression of pro-inflammatory cytokines such as IL-6 and a suppression of anti-inflammatory cytokines such as IL-10.[77] Certainly, this type of response to exercise has been well documented in skeletal muscle.[78,79] In support of such a mechanism, trained rats no longer show JNK activation in response to acute exercise.[80]

One factor complicating some human studies is that athletes tend to take substantial amounts of anti-inflammatory drugs, and these are thought to act via MAPK pathways.[77] Further study is needed to examine the impact of regular physical activity on the risks of diverticulosis and inflammatory bowel disease.

Colonic motility

There is continued debate concerning the mechanical effects of exercise on the gastrointestinal tract; both acute and chronic changes in gastrointestinal motility may occur, although data on this question are inconsistent.[81] One uncertainty is whether running has a similar effect to seated exercise. Several reports have noted little effect on overall gastrointestinal transit.[8,33,34,82–85] Thus, the mouth-to-cecum transit time was unchanged by running 9.6 km (6 mi), and walking a distance of 4.5 km (2.8 mi) in one hour did not change the total transit time in previously sedentary laboratory workers.[13] Likewise, total colonic transit time was similar for laboratory technicians and soccer players who were training as much as 15 hours per week.[86] However, other studies have suggested a substantial effect of regular training. A 6-week endurance program reduced the total carmine transit time from 35 to 24 hours, whereas the transit for a control group remained at a sluggish 45 hours.[38] Likewise, one week of cycling or jogging at 50% of maximal oxygen intake almost doubled the speed of intestinal transit in healthy young adults,[39] and in a study of healthy and recreationally active elderly subjects, the deliberate two-week restriction of physical activity almost doubled the colonic transit time.[87] Other types of exercise may also be of benefit. Thus, 13 weeks of resistance training was sufficient enough to induce a 40% increase in the peak force developed by key muscle groups and more than doubled the speed of total intestinal transit, this change being due almost exclusively to faster movement through the large intestine.[88] Exercise-related changes in the type and quantity of food ingested may be an important issue. This idea is supported by the fact that no changes in bowel transit time were observed when training experiments were carried out in a metabolic laboratory, where subjects adhered to a controlled diet and sophisticated radioactive markers of fecal movement were used.[89]

Gastrointestinal polyps and cancers

The risk of gastrointestinal cancers is increased by chronic irritation (from gastric reflux and peptic ulcers) and by obesity (which, probably through an increased production of inflammatory cytokines, increases the risk of neoplastic lesions in the esophagus, gastric cardia, and colon). Chronic gastric reflux and obesity are thought to induce esophagitis,[90] and it has been suggested that this in turn can progress to Barrett esophagus (a metaplastic change in the cells lining the esophagus, with a risk of frank esophageal carcinoma).[91] Perhaps in part through effects on reflux and on obesity, the risks of both esophageal and gastric adenocarcinoma tend to be lower in those with a lifetime history of moderate physical activity. Vigen and associates[92] found respective odds ratios of 0.66 (0.38-0.99) and

0.67 (0.38-1.19) for active individuals. An 8-year follow-up of 487732 US citizens, comparing highest versus lowest physical activity ratings, confirmed that the active individuals had favorable risk ratios for esophageal (0.75), gastric non-cardial (0.62), and gastric cardial (0.83) adenocarcinomas; however, there was no association between habitual physical activity and esophageal squamous-cell carcinomas.[93]

Physical activity can have a significant effect in reducing the risk of colonic polyps. After 4 weeks of treadmill exercise, Colbert and associates[94] found a 48% reduction of polyps in male mice that ran consistently when compared with controls, but running apparently had no effect on female mice. This sex difference in response was confirmed by Mehl et al.[95] Mice also showed a negative relationship between the number of colonic polyps and the distance covered during voluntary wheel running, apparently linked to the development of a negative energy balance.[96] An important issue may be not only the amount of food ingested, but also its fat content. Thus, one study of mice found that regular moderate intensity treadmill exercise reduced the total number of polyps by 50%, and the number of large polyps by 67%, if the animals were fed a healthy diet (AIN-76A); however, if they were fed on a typical westernized (high-fat) diet, the number of polyps rose by 75%, and exercise was no longer effective in protecting the colon.[97]

Physical activity also protects against colonic cancers, particularly lesions in the descending colon (where the risk of cancers reduced by as much as 20-50% in a physically active person).[98-100] The intensity of effort has been no more than moderate in many of the epidemiological studies where benefit has been seen. One suggested protective mechanism is a speeding of passage of food, mechanical bouncing or changes in segmentation of the large intestine, perhaps mediated by prostaglandins, with a reduced exposure of the colon wall to toxins.[101] A second potential factor is the control of obesity.[102,103] Other hypothesized mechanisms include a decreased bile acid production, altered insulin levels, insulin-like growth factors, cholesterol and hormone profiles and prostaglandin levels,[81] reductions in gastrointestinal blood flow, and other neuroimmuno-endocrinological changes. The basis of protection certainly remains unclear, and there is a need for further careful observations on acute and chronic responses, looking at both changes in gastrointestinal motility and the risk of cancer with graded intensities of regular physical activity.

Following the treatment of colonic cancer, a program of regular physical activity is still beneficial, reducing both the risk of recurrence[104] and of colon-cancer-specific mortality.[105]

Celiac disease

Athletes who suffer from celiac disease often have problems with the absorption of iron, calcium, and vitamin D, and sports physicians should thus check such patients for anemia and poor bone health, as well as ensure that there is no disruption in their gluten-free diet during periods of intensive physical activity (this could exacerbate their poor absorption of nutrients).[106]

Occult hemorrhage

Elite distance runners often have not only exercise-induced hemolysis, but also some increase of intestinal blood loss.[9,21,73] This is usually compensated by an increased intake of dietary iron.[107] Specific supplements are needed only if serum ferritin levels are low.[108,109] But despite the occult hemorrhage observed during such bouts of intensive endurance exercise, a large scale 3-year prospective study of 8205 seniors aged > 68 years found that even after statistical adjustment for appropriate covariates, relative risks (RR) of severe gastrointestinal hemorrhage (sufficient to require hospital admission and/or transfusion) were substantially reduced in those individuals reporting regular walking (RR 0.5), gardening (R 0.8) or vigorous physical activity (RR 0.7).[110]

Conclusions

There is still surprisingly little information on either the minimum amount of physical activity needed to enhance gastrointestinal health or the threshold beyond which health deteriorates rather than improves. Many responses seem to depend upon the intensity of the effort that is undertaken rather than its volume, and it is thus important to define more clearly the level of physical activity where beneficial effects change to the threats posed by exhausting physical activity and/or excessive training; other variables also need careful control, including the fat and energy content of the diet. The search for accurate information on activity patterns may be helped by inferences of cumulative physical activity based upon either the individual's physical fitness or long-term objective assessments of physical activity using modern motion sensors. Given suggestions that overly strenuous exercise can cause local tissue necrosis, it may also be useful to make long-term comparisons of function between athletes who have engaged in repeated ultra-endurance competition and members of the general population who have limited their physical activity to current national recommendations.

References

1. Budzyński J. Exercise-provoked esophageal motility disorder in patients with recurrent chest pain. *World J Gastroenterol.* 2010;16:4428-4435.
2. Nilsson M, Johnsen R, Ye W, Hveem K, Lagergren J. Lifestyle related risk factors in the aetiology of gastro-oesophageal reflux. *Gut.* 2004;53:1730-1735.
3. Festi D, Scaioli E, Baldi F, et al. Body weight, lifestyle, dietary habits and gastroesophageal reflux disease. *World J Gastroenterol.* 2009;15:1690-1701.
4. Hampel H, Abraham NS, El-Serag HB. Meta-analysis: obesity and the risk for gastroesophageal reflux disease and its complications. *Ann Intern Med.* 2005; 143:199-211.
5. Anand G, Katz PO. Gastroesophageal reflux disease and obesity. *Rev Gastroenterol Disord.* 2008;8:233-239.
6. Worobetz LJ, Gerrard DF. Effect of moderate exercise on esophageal function in asymptomatic athletes. *Am J Gastroenterol.* 1986;81:1048-1051.
7. Peters O, Peters P, Clarys JT, et al. Esophageal motility and exercise. *Gastroenterology.* 1988;94. A351 (abstract).

8. Soffer EE, Wilson J, Duethman G, Launspach J, Adrian TE. Effect of graded exercise on esophageal motility and gastroesophageal reflux in nontrained subjects. *Dig Dis Sci*. 1994;39:193-198.
9. Peters HP, De Vries WR, Vanberge-Henegouwen GP, Akkermans LM. Potential benefits and hazards of physical activity and exercise on the gastrointestinal tract. *Gut*. 2001;48:435-439.
10. Jozkow P, Wasko-Czopnik D, Medras M, Paradowski L. Gastroesophageal reflux disease and physical activity. *Sports Med*. 2006;36:385-391.
11. van Nieuwenhoven MA, Brouns F, Brummer RJ. The effect of physical exercise on parameters of gastrointestinal function. *Neurogastroenterol Motil*. 1999;11:431-439.
12. Collings KL, Pierce Pratt F, Rodriguez-Stanley S, Bemben M, Miner PB. Esophageal reflux in conditioned runners, cyclists, and weightlifters. *Med Sci Sports Exerc*. 2003;35:730-735.
13. van Nieuwenhoven MA, Brouns F, Brummer RJ. Gastrointestinal profile of symptomatic athletes at rest and during physical exercise. *Eur J Appl Physiol*. 2004;91:429-434.
14. Yazaki E, Shawdon A, Beasley I, Evans DF. The effect of different types of exercise on gastro-oesophageal reflux. *Aust J Sci Med Sport*. 1996;28:93-96.
15. Choi SC, Yoo KH, Kim TH, Kim SH, Choi SJ, Nah YH. Effect of graded running on esophageal motility and gastroesophageal reflux in fed volunteers. *J Korean Med Sci*. 2001;16:183-187.
16. Ravi N, Stuart RC, Byrne PJ, Reynolds JV. Effect of physical exercise on esophageal motility in patients with esophageal disease. *Dis Esophagus*. 2005;18:374-377.
17. Peters HP, Bos M, Seebregts L, et al. Gastrointestinal symptoms in long-distance runners, cyclists, and triathletes: prevalence, medication, and etiology. *Am J Gastroenterol*. 1999;94:1570-1581.
18. Shawdon A. Gastro-oesophageal reflux and exercise. Important pathology to consider in the athletic population. *Sports Med*. 1995;20:109-116.
19. Simons SM, Kennedy RG. Gastrointestinal problems in runners. *Curr Sports Med Rep*. 2004;3:112-116.
20. Lopez AA, Preziosi JP, Chateau P, Auguste P, Plique O. Digestive disorders and self medication observed during a competition in endurance athletes. Prospective epidemiological study during a championship of triathlon [Article in French]. *Gastroenterol Clin Biol*. 1994;18:317-322.
21. Moses FM. The effect of exercise on the gastrointestinal tract. *Sports Med*. 1990;9:159-172.
22. Moses FM. Physical activity and the digestive processes. In: Bouchard C, Shephard RJ, Stephens T, eds. *Physical Activity, Fitness, and Health*. Champaign, IL: Human Kinetics; 1994:383-400.
23. Marzio L, Formica P, Fabiani F, LaPenna D, Vecchiett L, Cuccurullo F. Influence of physical activity on gastric emptying of liquids in normal human subjects. *Am J Gastroenterol*. 1991;86:1433-1436.
24. Neufer PD, Young AJ, Sawka MN. Gastric emptying during walking and running: effects of varied exercise intensity. *Eur J Appl Physiol Occup Physiol*. 1989;58:440-445.
25. Carrió I, Estorch M, Serra-Grima R, et al. Gastric emptying in marathon runners. *Gut*. 1989;30:152-155.
26. Kavanagh T, Shephard RJ. Maintenance of hydration in post-coronary marathon runners. *Br J Sports Med*. 1975;9:130-135.
27. Rowell LB. Visceral blood flow and metabolism during exercise. In: Shephard RJ, ed. *Frontiers of Fitness*. Springfield, IL.: C.C. Thomas; 1971:210-232.
28. Michel H, Larrey D, Blanc P. Hepato-digestive disorders in athletic practice [Article in French]. *Presse Med*. 1994;23:479-484.
29. ter Steege RW, Kolkman JJ, Huisman AB, Geelkerken RH. Gastrointestinal ischaemia during physical exertion as a cause of gastrointestinal symptoms [Article in Dutch]. *Ned Tijdschr Geneeskd*. 2008;152:1805-1808.

30. Peters HP, De Kort AF, Van Krevelen H, et al. The effect of omeprazole on gastro-oesophageal reflux and symptoms during strenuous exercise. *Aliment Pharmacol Ther.* 1999;13:1015-1022.
31. Riddoch C, Trinick T. Gastrointestinal disturbances in marathon runners. *Br J Sports Med.* 1988;22:71-74.
32. Keeffe EB, Lowe DK, Goss JR, Wayne R. Gastrointestinal symptoms of marathon runners. *West J Med.* 1984;141:481-484.
33. Rao KA, Yazaki E, Evans DF, Carbon R. Objective evaluation of small bowel and colonic transit time using pH telemetry in athletes with gastrointestinal symptoms. *Br J Sports Med.* 2004;38:482-487.
34. Scott D, Scott B. Should an athlete eat straight after training?–A study of intestinal transit time and its relationship to prior exercise. *Br J Sports Med.* 1994; 28:22-24.
35. Cammack J, Read NW, Cann PA, Greenwood B, Holgate AM. Effect of prolonged exercise on the passage of a solid meal through the stomach and small intestine. *Gut.* 1982;23:957-961.
36. Sullivan SN, Wong C. Runners' diarrhea. Different patterns and associated factors. *J Clin Gastroenterol.* 1992;14:101-104.
37. Halvorsen FA, Lyng J, Glomsaker T, Ritland S. Gastrointestinal disturbances in marathon runners. *Br J Sports Med.* 1990;24:266-268.
38. Cordain L, Latin RW, Behnke JJ. The effects of an aerobic running program on bowel transit time. *J Sports Med Phys Fitness.* 1986;26:101-104.
39. Oettlé GJ. Effect of moderate exercise on bowel habit. *Gut.* 1991;32:941-944.
40. Pals KL, Chang RT, Ryan AJ, Gisolfi CV. Effect of running intensity on intestinal permeability. *J Appl Physiol.* 1997;82:571-576.
41. Royer CM, Willard M, Williamson K, et al. Exercise stress, intestinal permeability and gastric ulceration in racing Alaskan sled dogs. *Equine Comp Exerc Physiol.* 2005;2:53-59.
42. Smetanka RD, Lambert GP, Murray R, Eddy D, Horn M, Gisolfi CV. Intestinal permeability in runners in the 1996 Chicago marathon. *Int J Sport Nutr.* 1999; 9:426-433.
43. Lambert GP, Boylan M, Laventure JP, Bull A, Lanspa S. Effect of aspirin and ibuprofen on GI permeability during exercise. *Int J Sports Med.* 2007;28: 722-726.
44. Brouns F, Beckers E. Is the gut an athletic organ? Digestion, absorption and exercise. *Sports Med.* 1993;15:242-257.
45. Otte JA, Oostveen E, Geelkerken RH, Groeneveld AB, Kolkman JJ. Exercise induces gastric ischemia in healthy volunteers: a tonometry study. *J Appl Physiol.* 2001;91:866-871.
46. Berg A, Müller HM, Rathmann S, Deibert P. The gastrointestinal system–an essential target organ of the athlete's health and physical performance. *Exerc Immunol Rev.* 1999;5:78-95.
47. Bosenberg AT, Brock-Utne JG, Gaffin SL, Wells MT, Blake GT. Strenuous exercise causes systemic endotoxemia. *J Appl Physiol.* 1988;65:106-108.
48. Porter AM. Marathon running and the caecal slap syndrome. *Br J Sports Med.* 1982;16:178.
49. Rehrer NJ, Meijer GA. Biomechanical vibration of the abdominal region during running and bicycling. *J Sports Med Phys Fitness.* 1991;31:231-234.
50. Marshall JC. The gut as a potential trigger of exercise-induced inflammatory responses. *Can J Physiol Pharmacol.* 1998;76:479-484.
51. Flegel WA, Baumstark MW, Weinstock C, Berg A, Northoff H. Prevention of endotoxin-induced monokine release by human low- and high-density lipoproteins and by apolipoprotein A-I. *Infect Immun.* 1993;61:5140-5146.
52. Kregel KC. Heat shock proteins: modifying factors in physiological stress responses and acquired thermotolerance. *J Appl Physiol.* 2002;92:2177-2186.
53. Pasparakis M. Regulation of tissue homeostasis by NF-kappaB signalling: implications for inflammatory diseases. *Nat Rev Immunol.* 2009;9:778-788.

54. Börsch G. The gastrointestinal tract as an immunologic organ: the gut-associated immune system. *Klin Wochenschr.* 1984;62:699-709.
55. Halvorsen FA, Lyng J, Ritland S. Gastrointestinal bleeding in marathon runners. *Scand J Gastroenterol.* 1986;21:493-497.
56. Baska RS, Moses FM, Graeber G, Kearney G. Gastrointestinal bleeding during an ultramarathon. *Dig Dis Sci.* 1990;35:276-279.
57. Wade OL, Bishop JM. *Cardiac Output and Regional Blood Flow.* Oxford, UK: Blackwell Scientific; 1962.
58. Winwood PJ, Robertson DA, Wright R. Bleeding oesophageal varices associated with anabolic steroid use in an athlete. *Postgrad Med J.* 1990;66:864-865.
59. Montgomery LC, Deuster PA. Effects of antihistamine medications on exercise performance. Implications for sportspeople. *Sports Med.* 1993;15:179-195.
60. Thalmann M, Sodeck GH, Kavouras S, et al. Proton pump inhibition prevents gastrointestinal bleeding in ultramarathon runners: a randomised, double blinded, placebo controlled study. *Br J Sports Med.* 2006;40:359-362.
61. Meeroff JC. Aerobic training: an esoteric treatment for ulcer disease? *Am J Gastroenterol.* 1985;80. A843.
62. Cheng Y, Macera CA, Davis DR, Blair SN. Does physical activity reduce the risk of developing peptic ulcers? *Br J Sports Med.* 2000;34:116-121.
63. Feldman M, Nixon JV. Effect of exercise on postprandial gastric secretion and emptying in humans. *J Appl Physiol.* 1982;53:851-854.
64. Markiewicz K, Cholewa M, Górski L, Chmura J. Effect of physical exercise on gastric basal secretion in healthy men. *Acta Hepatogastroenterol (Stuttg).* 1977; 24:377-380.
65. Ramsbottom N, Hunt JN. Effect of exercise on gastric emptying and gastric secretion. *Digestion.* 1974;10:1-8.
66. Markiewicz K, Lukin M. The effect of physical exercise on gastric secretion and chronic duodenal ulcer patients. *Dig Dis Sci.* 1986;31:344S.
67. Markiewicz K, Lukin M. Maximal gastric secretion during physical exertion and restitution in patients with chronic duodenal ulcer [Article in Polish]. *Pol Arch Med Wewn.* 1988;79:13-19.
68. Landers DM, Petruzello SJ. Physical activity, fitness and anxiety. In: Bouchard C, Shephard RJ, Stephens T, eds. *Physical Activity, Fitness and Health.* Champaign, IL.: Human Kinetics; 1994:868-882.
69. Hume GE, Fowler EV, Lincoln D, et al. Angiotensinogen and transforming growth factor beta1: novel genes in the pathogenesis of Crohn's disease. *J Med Genet.* 2006;43:e51.
70. Benazzato L, Varnier M, Dal Pont E, et al. Effect of moderate acute aerobic exercise in patients with Crohn's disease in clinical remission. *Dig Liver Dis.* 2006; 38:S121-S122.
71. Narula N, Fedorak RN. Exercise and inflammatory bowel disease. *Can J Gastroenterol.* 2008;22:497-504.
72. Ng V, Millard W, Lebrun C, Howard J. Exercise and Crohn's disease: speculations on potential benefits. *Can J Gastroenterol.* 2006;20:657-660.
73. de Oliveira EP, Burini RC. The impact of physical exercise on the gastrointestinal tract. *Curr Opin Clin Nutr Metab Care.* 2009;12:533-538.
74. Halle M, Korsten-Reck U, Wolfarth B, Berg A. Low-grade systemic inflammation in overweight children: impact of physical fitness. *Exerc Immunol Rev.* 2004;10:66-74.
75. Loudon CP, Corroll V, Butcher J, Rawsthorne P, Bernstein CN. The effects of physical exercise on patients with Crohn's disease. *Am J Gastroenterol.* 1999; 94:697-703.
76. Kokura S, Yoshikawa T. Large intestine heat shock proteins. *J Clin Biochem Nutr.* 2006;38:156-160.
77. Malago JJ, Koninkx JF, van Dijk JE. The heat shock response and cytoprotection of the intestinal epithelium. *Cell Stress Chaperones.* 2002;7:191-199.

78. Lee JS, Bruce CR, Spurrell BE, Hawley JA. Effect of training on activation of extracellular signal-regulated kinase 1/2 and p38 mitogen-activated protein kinase pathways in rat soleus muscle. *Clin Exp Pharmacol Physiol.* 2002;29:655-660.

79. Ryder JW, Fahlman R, Wallberg-Henriksson H, Alessi DR, Krook A, Zierath JR. Effect of contraction on mitogen-activated protein kinase signal transduction in skeletal muscle. Involvement of the mitogen- and stress-activated protein kinase 1. *J Biol Chem.* 2000;275:1457-1462.

80. Boluyt MO, Loyd AM, Roth MH, Randall MJ, Song EY. Activation of JNK in rat heart by exercise: effect of training. *Am J Physiol Heart Circ Physiol.* 2003; 285:H2639-H2647.

81. Quadrilatero J, Hoffman-Goetz L. Physical activity and colon cancer. A systematic review of potential mechanisms. *J Sports Med Phys Fitness.* 2003;43: 121-138.

82. Bingham SA, Cummings JH. Effect of exercise and physical fitness on large intestinal function. *Gastroenterology.* 1989;97:1389-1399.

83. Kayaleh RA, Meshkinpour H, Avinashi A, Tamadon A. Effect of exercise on mouth-to-cecum transit in trained athletes: a case against the role of runners' abdominal bouncing. *J Sports Med Phys Fitness.* 1996;36:271-274.

84. Soffer EE, Merchant RK, Deuthman G, et al. The effect of graded exercise on esophageal motility and gastroesophageal reflux in trained athletes. *Gastroenterol.* 1991;100. A497 (abstract).

85. Robertson G, Meshkinpour H, Vandenberg K, James N, Cohen A, Wilson A. Effects of exercise on total and segmental colon transit. *J Clin Gastroenterol.* 1993;16:300-303.

86. Sesboüé B, Arhan P, Devroede G, et al. Colonic transit in soccer players. *J Clin Gastroenterol.* 1995;20:211-214.

87. Liu F, Kondo T, Toda Y. Brief physical inactivity prolongs colonic transit time in elderly active men. *Int J Sports Med.* 1993;14:465-467.

88. Koffler KH, Menkes A, Redmond RA, Whitehead WE, Pratley RE, Hurley BF. Strength training accelerates gastrointestinal transit in middle-aged and older men. *Med Sci Sports Exerc.* 1992;24:415-419.

89. Coenen C, Wegener M, Wedmann B, Schmidt G, Hoffmann S. Does physical exercise influence bowel transit time in healthy young men? *Am J Gastroenterol.* 1992;87:292-295.

90. Kraus BB, Sinclair JW, Castell DO. Gastroesophageal reflux in runners. Characteristics and treatment. *Ann Intern Med.* 1990;112:429-433.

91. Winzer BM, Paratz JD, Reeves MM, Whiteman DC. Exercise and the Prevention of Oesophageal Cancer (EPOC) study protocol: a randomized controlled trial of exercise versus stretching in males with Barrett's oesophagus. *BMC Cancer.* 2010;10:292.

92. Vigen C, Bernstein L, Wu AH. Occupational physical activity and risk of adenocarcinomas of the esophagus and stomach. *Int J Cancer.* 2006;118:1004-1009.

93. Leitzmann MF, Koebnick C, Freedman ND, et al. Physical activity and esophageal and gastric carcinoma in a large prospective study. *Am J Prev Med.* 2009; 36:112-119.

94. Colbert LH, Mai V, Perkins SN, et al. Exercise and intestinal polyp development in APCMin mice. *Med Sci Sports Exerc.* 2003;35:1662-1669.

95. Mehl KA, Davis JM, Clements JM, Berger FG, Pena MM, Carson JA. Decreased intestinal polyp multiplicity is related to exercise mode and gender in ApcMin/+ mice. *J Appl Physiol.* 2005;98:2219-2225.

96. Colbert LH, Mai V, Tooze JA, Perkins SN, Berrigan D, Hursting SD. Negative energy balance induced by voluntary wheel running inhibits polyp development in APCMin mice. *Carcinogenesis.* 2006;27:2103-2107.

97. Baltgalvis KA, Berger FG, Peña MM, Davis JM, Carson JA. The interaction of a high-fat diet and regular moderate intensity exercise on intestinal polyp development in Apc Min/+ mice. *Cancer Prev Res (Phila).* 2009;2:641-649.

98. Shephard RJ, Futcher R. Physical activity and cancer: how may protection be maximized? *Crit Rev Oncog.* 1997;8:219-272.

99. Samad AK, Taylor RS, Marshall T, Chapman MA. A meta-analysis of the association of physical activity with reduced risk of colorectal cancer. *Colorectal Dis.* 2005;7:204-213.

100. Meyerhardt JA, Ogino S, Kirkner GJ, et al. Interaction of molecular markers and physical activity on mortality in patients with colon cancer. *Clin Cancer Res.* 2009;15:5931-5936.

101. Kamaleeswari M, Deeptha K, Sengottuvelan M, Nalini N. Effect of dietary caraway (Carum carvi L.) on aberrant crypt foci development, fecal steroids, and intestinal alkaline phosphatase activities in 1,2-dimethylhydrazine-induced colon carcinogenesis. *Toxicol Appl Pharmacol.* 2006;214:290-296.

102. Ahmed RL, Thomas W, Schmitz KH. Interactions between insulin, body fat, and insulin-like growth factor axis proteins. *Cancer Epidemiol Biomarkers Prev.* 2007;16:593-597.

103. Russo A, Franceschi S, La Vecchia C, et al. Body size and colorectal-cancer risk. *Int J Cancer.* 1998;78:161-165.

104. Meyerhardt JA, Heseltine D, Niedzwiecki D, et al. Impact of physical activity on cancer recurrence and survival in patients with stage III colon cancer: findings from CALGB 89803. *J Clin Oncol.* 2006;24:3535-3541.

105. Meyerhardt JA, Giovannucci EL, Holmes MD, et al. Physical activity and survival after colorectal cancer diagnosis. *J Clin Oncol.* 2006;24:3527-3534.

106. Mancini LA, Trojian T, Mancini AC. Celiac disease and the athlete. *Curr Sports Med Rep.* 2011;10:105-108.

107. Zoller H, Vogel W. Iron supplementation in athletes–first do no harm. *Nutrition.* 2004;20:615-619.

108. Nielsen P, Nachtigall D. Iron supplementation in athletes. Current recommendations. *Sports Med.* 1998;26:207-216.

109. Garza D, Shrier I, Kohl HW 3rd, Ford P, Brown M, Matheson GO. The clinical value of serum ferritin tests in endurance athletes. *Clin J Sport Med.* 1997;7:46-53.

110. Pahor M, Guralnik JM, Salive ME, Chrischilles EA, Brown SL, Wallace RB. Physical activity and risk of severe gastrointestinal hemorrhage in older persons. *JAMA.* 1994;272:595-599.

1 Epidemiology, Prevention of Injuries, Lesions of Head and Neck

Epidemiology of Injuries

The Effect of Smoking on Ligament and Cartilage Surgery in the Knee: A Systematic Review

Kanneganti P, Harris JD, Brophy RH, et al (The Ohio State Univ Sports Medicine Ctr, Columbus; Washington Univ School of Medicine, St Louis, MO; et al)
Am J Sports Med 40:2872-2878, 2012

Background.—The adverse effects of smoking on various health conditions such as cancer, diabetes, and cardiovascular disease have been well documented. Many orthopaedic conditions, such as fracture healing, wound repair, and bone mineral density, have been reported to be adversely affected by smoking. However, no known systematic reviews have investigated the effects of smoking on ligament and cartilage knee surgery.

Purpose.—We hypothesized that smoking would have a negative influence from both a basic science and clinical outcome perspective on these types of knee surgeries.

Study Design.—Systematic review.

Methods.—A systematic review of multiple medical databases was performed evaluating clinical and basic science studies to determine the effects of smoking on ligament and cartilage knee surgery.

Results.—Fourteen studies were found for inclusion and analysis. Eight of these studies addressed the relationship between smoking and knee ligaments, and 6 investigated the relationship between smoking and articular cartilage. With the exception of 1, all of the basic science and clinical studies exploring the relationship between smoking and knee ligaments found a negative association of smoking, either molecularly, biomechanically, or clinically. One basic science and 3 clinical studies found a negative influence of smoking on articular cartilage of the knee. No studies were found that investigated the relationship of smoking and menisci.

Conclusion.—The current literature reveals a negative influence of smoking on the results of knee ligament surgery, both from a basic science and clinical perspective, implying that smoking cessation would benefit patients undergoing these procedures. The association between smoking and knee articular cartilage was less clear, although the literature still suggests an overall negative influence and highlights the need for further investigation.

▶ The adverse effects of smoking have been extensively demonstrated for various systemic conditions. For musculoskeletal disorders, the adverse effects are not as well understood, but evidence has linked smoking to various disorders or delays in healing of injured musculoskeletal structures. Nicotine is potentially 1 of the important components of cigarette smoke implicated in the pathogenesis of these problems. Commonly cited deleterious effects of nicotine include impeded inflammatory response, chronic vasoconstriction, hypoperfusion, and ischemia. Because the literature on knee ligament and cartilage surgery and the potential negative effects of smoking is scarce, this review tries to synthesize evidence on the effect of smoking and these 2 types of surgery. The authors included 14 studies from basic and clinical science. Of note the authors did not assess the methodological quality of included studies. Nonetheless, the results are interesting for the clinician because they have implications for the outcomes and rehabilitation of patients undergoing these surgeries. The authors conclude on the negative effects of smoking: molecularly, biomechanically, and clinically at the patient level, mainly in terms of pain and function. Although the authors did not make any specific clinical recommendations regarding the effects of smoking, it is important to point out that in light of the current evidence, surgical and perisurgical protocols and rehabilitation protocols may need to be modified to try to address the present findings. Protocols may need to be modified for smokers. For example, rehabilitation protocols may need to be less aggressive and longer in duration before full return to activities.

F. Desmeules, PT, PhD

Sex and Age Differences in Depression and Baseline Sport-Related Concussion Neurocognitive Performance and Symptoms
Covassin T, Elbin RJ III, Larson E, et al (Michigan State Univ, East Lansing; Univ of Pittsburgh, PA; Humboldt State Univ, Arcata, CA)
Clin J Sport Med 22:98-104, 2012

Objective.—To examine depression and baseline neurocognitive function and concussion symptoms in male and female high school and college athletes.

Design.—Cross sectional.

Setting.—Athletes completed testing at a designated computer laboratory at high schools and colleges.

Participants.—Participants included 1616 collegiate (n = 837) and high school (n = 779) athletes from 3 states participating in a variety of competitive sports.

Interventions.—Participants completed the baseline Immediate Postconcussion Assessment and Cognitive Test (ImPACT), symptom inventory, and Beck Depression Inventory II (BDI-II).

Main Outcome Measures.—Between-group comparisons for depression groups on ImPACT composite scores (verbal and visual memory, reaction time, motor processing speed), total symptoms, and symptom cluster (sleep, cognitive, emotional, somatic/migraine) scores. Between-group comparisons for age and sex on BDI-II, ImPACT, total symptoms, and symptom cluster scores.

Results.—The severe depression group scored worse on visual memory and reported more total, somatic/migraine, cognitive, emotional, and sleep symptoms than less depressed groups. High school athletes reported more somatic/migraine symptoms than collegiate athletes, whereas collegiate athletes reported more emotional and sleep symptoms than high school athletes. Women had higher verbal memory and reported more cognitive, emotional, and sleep symptom clusters compared with men. Women outperformed men on verbal memory, whereas collegiate athletes outperformed high school athletes on processing speed.

Conclusions.—Athletes with severe depression scored lower on visual memory than those with minimal depression. Athletes with severe depression report more concussion symptoms than athletes with minimal and moderate depression scores. Symptoms of depression should be included in baseline assessments to help disentangle depression from concussion symptoms.

▶ This study pointed out the importance of screening for depression on baseline concussion assessment tools. The authors found athletes with severe depression scoring lower on visual memory and having more postconcussion symptoms than athletes with minimal or no depression. In addition to screening for symptoms at baseline, this reviewer feels strongly that other conditions that can negatively influence recovery from concussion should be screened for at baseline as well. Conditions that would be included in this group would include attention deficit disorder/attention deficit hyperactivity disorder or other learning disabilities, panic attacks, anxiety disorders, migraines, and seizure disorders.

These researchers also found, as they have reported previously, that female athletes performed better than male athletes on verbal memory and processing speed. In contrast to what they have previously reported in the literature, they found men and women demonstrating similar performance to visual memory and reaction times whereas previously men performed better on these tasks. Also in contrast to previous publications, there were no sex differences on depression scores or total concussion symptoms. They speculated that the reasons for these differences from previous publications may have been the increased number of high school athletes in the current study. To this reviewer, it simply means more research in these areas is necessary by other research teams.

R. C. Cantu, MD, MA

Sex and Age Differences in Depression and Baseline Sport-Related Concussion Neurocognitive Performance and Symptoms

Covassin T, Elbin RJ III, Larson E, et al (Michigan State Univ, East Lansing; Univ of Pittsburgh, PA; Humboldt State Univ, Arcata, CA)
Clin J Sport Med 22:98-104, 2012

Objective.—To examine depression and baseline neurocognitive function and concussion symptoms in male and female high school and college athletes.

Design.—Cross sectional.

Setting.—Athletes completed testing at a designated computer laboratory at high schools and colleges.

Participants.—Participants included 1616 collegiate (n = 837) and high school (n = 779) athletes from 3 states participating in a variety of competitive sports.

Interventions.—Participants completed the baseline Immediate Postconcussion Assessment and Cognitive Test (ImPACT), symptom inventory, and Beck Depression Inventory II (BDI-II).

Main Outcome Measures.—Between-group comparisons for depression groups on ImPACT composite scores (verbal and visual memory, reaction time, motor processing speed), total symptoms, and symptom cluster (sleep, cognitive, emotional, somatic/migraine) scores. Between-group comparisons for age and sex on BDI-II, ImPACT, total symptoms, and symptom cluster scores.

Results.—The severe depression group scored worse on visual memory and reported more total, somatic/migraine, cognitive, emotional, and sleep symptoms than less depressed groups. High school athletes reported more somatic/migraine symptoms than collegiate athletes, whereas collegiate athletes reported more emotional and sleep symptoms than high school athletes. Women had higher verbal memory and reported more cognitive, emotional, and sleep symptom clusters compared with men. Women outperformed men on verbal memory, whereas collegiate athletes outperformed high school athletes on processing speed.

Conclusions.—Athletes with severe depression scored lower on visual memory than those with minimal depression. Athletes with severe depression report more concussion symptoms than athletes with minimal and moderate depression scores. Symptoms of depression should be included

TABLE 2.—Summary Statistics for Depression Scores by Minimal, Mild, Moderate, and Severe Depression

	Male (n = 1090), n (%)	Female (n = 512), n (%)	High School (n = 779), n (%)	College (n = 837), n (%)
Minimal (0-13)	1040 (95.4)	483 (94.3)	711 (91.3)	829 (99)
Mild (14-19)	32 (3)	16 (3.1)	48 (6.2)	0 (0)
Moderate (20-28)	13 (1.2)	7 (1.4)	20 (2.6)	0 (0)
Severe (28-63)	5 (.45)	6 (1.2)	3 (0.39)	8 (1)

in baseline assessments to help disentangle depression from concussion symptoms (Table 2).

▶ Recommendations for diagnosis and management of sport-related concussion call for a multifaceted approach that includes symptom reports, vestibular assessments, clinical evaluations, and computerized neurocognitive testing. The role of baseline testing has been emphasized, particularly with regard to neurocognitive testing, in order to account for individual differences in baseline performance. Many variables, such as age, sex, and concussion history, can influence baseline neurocognitive performance and symptoms, but an important component is also mood (ie, depression). This cross-sectional study of 1616 collegiate (n = 837) and high school athletes (n = 779) examined the relationships between baseline depressive symptoms and performance on the computerized Immediate Postconcussion Assessment and Cognitive Test (ImPACT) and symptom inventory. Using the Beck Depression Inventory II (BDI-II), which is an instrument containing 21 self-report symptoms that report on a scale of 1 to 3 (maximum score 63), athletes' total scores could be characterized into minimal (0—13), mild (14—19), moderate (20—28), and severe (29—63) depression categories (Table 2). Athletes with severe depression scored worse (lower) on some of the specific composite scores on ImPACT and reported more symptoms (total, as well as migraine and cognitive concussion symptoms) than athletes with minimal and moderate depression scores. The authors conclude that baseline assessment of depression and mood be conducted in conjunction with existing protocols for preparticipation physicals and postconcussion neurocognitive, symptom, and balance testing. Additionally, a mental health professional should be involved to supervise the use and interpretation of results including depression and other mood instruments. From a clinical perspective, student-athletes with or at risk for depression and its effects (eg, suicide) could be identified early and referred on for appropriate further diagnosis and treatment.

C. Lebrun, MDCM, MPE, CCFP, Dip Sport Med, FACSM

Nine-Year Risk of Depression Diagnosis Increases With Increasing Self-Reported Concussions in Retired Professional Football Players
Kerr ZY, Marshall SW, Harding HP Jr, et al (Univ of North Carolina at Chapel Hill; Florida State Univ, Tallahassee)
Am J Sports Med 40:2206-2212, 2012

Background.—Concussions may accelerate the progression to long-term mental health outcomes such as depression in athletes.

Purpose.—To prospectively determine the effects of recurrent concussions on the clinical diagnosis of depression in a group of retired football players.

Study Design.—Cohort study; Level of evidence, 2.

Methods.—Members of the National Football League Retired Players Association responded to a baseline General Health Survey (GHS) in 2001. They also completed a follow-up survey in 2010. Both surveys asked about demographic information, number of concussions sustained during their professional football career, physical/mental health, and prevalence of diagnosed medical conditions. A physical component summary (Short Form 36 Measurement Model for Functional Assessment of Health and Well-Being [SF-36 PCS]) was calculated from responses for physical health. The main exposure, the history of concussions during the professional playing career (self-report recalled in 2010), was stratified into 5 categories: 0 (referent), 1 to 2, 3 to 4, 5 to 9, and 10+ concussions. The main outcome was a clinical diagnosis of depression between the baseline and follow-up GHS. Classic tabular methods computed crude risk ratios. Binomial regression with a Poisson residual and robust variance estimation to stabilize the fitting algorithm estimated adjusted risk ratios. χ^2 analyses identified associations and trends between concussion history and the 9-year risk of a depression diagnosis.

Results.—Of the 1044 respondents with complete data from the baseline and follow-up GHS, 106 (10.2%) reported being clinically diagnosed as depressed between the baseline and follow-up GHS. Approximately 65% of all respondents self-reported sustaining at least 1 concussion during their professional careers. The 9-year risk of a depression diagnosis increased with an increasing number of self-reported concussions, ranging from 3.0% in the "no concussions" group to 26.8% in the "10+" group (linear trend: $P < .001$). A strong dose-response relationship was observed even after controlling for confounders (years retired from professional football and 2001 SF-36 PCS). Retired athletes with a depression diagnosis also had a lower SF-36 PCS before diagnosis. The association between concussions and depression was independent of the relationship between decreased physical health and depression.

Conclusion.—Professional football players self-reporting concussions are at greater risk for having depressive episodes later in life compared with those retired players self-reporting no concussions.

► Nearly a decade ago, Guskiewicz and colleagues studying retired National Football League players reported those who self-reported 3 or more concussions during their professional career were 3 times more likely to report being diagnosed with depression than athletes with no self-reported concussions. This study 9 years later resampled the same database. Individuals who had been diagnosed with depression at the time of the initial study were eliminated. Thus, this database represents individuals who were diagnosed with depression in the 9-year window since the initial study was carried out. More than a thousand respondents comprised the data, and 10% reported being diagnosed with concussion in the 9-year window of the study. There was a linear significant trend between the number of self-reported concussions and a clinical diagnosis of depression. Those reporting no concussions had a 3% incidence, whereas those with more than 10 reported concussions had a 27% incidence of depression. This study thus adds further proof of the association between reported concussions and later life clinical diagnosis of depression in retired professional football players.

R. C. Cantu, MD, MA

Prevention of Injuries, Equipment

Analysis of Baseball-to-Helmet Impacts in Major League Baseball

Athiviraham A, Bartsch A, Mageswaran P, et al (Cleveland Clinic, OH)
Am J Sports Med 40:2808-2814, 2012

Background.—In Major League Baseball (MLB), helmet hit-by-pitch (H-HBP) incidents are a leading cause of concussion. However, not all H-HBPs result in diagnosed concussion.

Purpose.—This study was designed to (1) quantify batter concussion risk as a function of H-HBP pitch velocity, time duration batter spent on the ground post–H-HBP, first responder assessment time duration, and number of days missed post–H-HBP and (2) estimate H-HBP impact locations on the helmet with respect to current National Operating Committee on Standards for Athletic Equipment (NOCSAE) helmet test standards and correlate impact locations with concussion diagnosis.

Study Design.—Case-control study; Level of evidence, 3.

Methods.—A retrospective case-control study of 18 MLB players with H-HBP incidents in the 2009 and 2010 seasons was undertaken. A database was compiled via quantitative and qualitative analysis using video coverage obtained from MLB. Quantitative factors included batter concussion diagnosis, pitch velocity, number of days missed post–H-HBP, time duration batter spent on the ground post–H-HBP, and first responder assessment time duration. The H-HBP impact location was among several qualitative factors developed via video analysis of each H-HBP from 4 raters.

Results.—In our study, 9 players (50%) were diagnosed with concussion. Concussion diagnoses were more frequent for posterior versus anterior impacts. The majority of H-HBP impact locations were different from those in the current NOCSAE standard tests. First responders took an average of approximately 65 seconds (time to reach batter plus assessment time) to decide on batter removal/return to play. The 25% logistic regression concussion risk threshold for pitch velocity and days missed was 86.2 mph and 1.3 days, respectively. The number of days missed after H-HBP showed a significant correlation ($P = .02$) among concussed and nonconcussed batters.

Conclusion.—In professional baseball H-HBP incidents, first responders should (1) be aware of pitch velocity in excess of 86 mph and (2) be provided ample time when assessing batters removal/return to play.

Clinical Relevance.—First responders should not rely solely on visual indicators such as batter reaction, holding head, or amount of time spent on the ground after H-HBP when assessing batters for concussion. Batting helmets in the MLB should maximize protection and mitigate impact dosage for H-HBP impact locations and velocity in addition to NOCSAE standard test locations and velocities.

▶ This is the first review of Major League Baseball (MLB) helmet hit-by-pitch incidents in terms of the risk of causing a concussion. The control study was of small sample size, 18 MLB players, but the findings were rather clear. That which correlated best with risk of concussion was a batter being hit in the helmet by a pitch in excess of 86 mph. Other visual indicators, such as the amount of time the batter stayed on the ground or whether he held his head with his hands, did not correlate with the risk of concussion. The authors correctly stress the need for first responders to thoroughly assess for concussion and be provided ample time when determining whether a batter should be removed or allowed to continue playing.

R. C. Cantu, MD, MA

Effectiveness of the SLICE Program for Youth Concussion Education

Bagley AF, Daneshvar DH, Schanker BD, et al (Harvard Med School, Boston, MA; Boston Univ School of Medicine, MA; Harvard Univ, Boston, MA; et al)
Clin J Sport Med 22:385-389, 2012

Objective.—To analyze the effectiveness of the Sports Legacy Institute Community Educators (SLICE) curriculum for student-athletes on recognition and appropriate responses to concussions.

Design.—Prospective cohort study, level II.

Setting.—The SLICE concussion workshop.

Participants.—All students ranging from 9 to 18 years (n = 636) taking the SLICE concussion education program.

Intervention.—The SLICE concussion education program featuring interactive demonstrations, discussion, and case studies of athletes delivered by medical students and others in health-related fields.

Main Outcome Measures.—Evaluations assessing knowledge of concussion recognition and appropriate response were administered before and after participating in the SLICE concussion education program.

Results.—Students displayed significant improvements in absolute mean score on the concussion knowledge quiz between prepresentation and postpresentation ($P < 0.0001$). Significant improvements in mean score were observed among both male and female students within each age group. The proportion of students who passed the quiz increased from 34% prepresentation to 80% postpresentation ($P < 0.0001$). However, the percentage who passed the quiz postpresentation was significantly higher among female students compared with male students ($P < 0.0001$) and among students 13 years of age or older compared with students less than 13 years ($P < 0.0001$). Using multivariable logistic regression, we identified age group and gender as the most significant factors associated with passing the quiz postpresentation.

Conclusion.—The SLICE program promotes effective learning and knowledge about concussion recognition and response among students ranging from 9 to 18 years. Lessons from the SLICE program may be broadly applicable to youth concussion education.

▶ In 2007, Chris Nowinski and this reviewer founded the Sports Legacy Institute to promote concussion awareness, including prevention, treatment, and research. To enhance the student athlete's recognition and appropriate responses to concussion, the Sports Legacy Institute Community Educators (SLICE) program for student athletes was initiated. The SLICE concussion education program uses interactive demonstrations, discussion, and case studies of athletes with concussion, delivered by medical students and others in health-related fields. This article reflects the effectiveness of the SLICE program with regard to knowledge about concussion recognition and response in the student athlete. A dramatic increase in ability to pass a concussion quiz from 34% prepresentation to 80% postpresentation ($P < .001$) was seen. Females as well as those older than the age of 13 performed significantly better. The SLICE program dramatically demonstrates the value of youth concussion education and the ability of this population to assimilate the information. Lessons from the SLICE program are broadly applicable to youth concussion education. Such education is currently being mandated by 40 states at the high school level and it is certainly hoped by this reviewer that it will be mandated for all youth participating in contact/collision sports.

R. C. Cantu, MD, MA

An evidence-based review: Efficacy of safety helmets in the reduction of head injuries in recreational skiers and snowboarders
Haider AH, on behalf of the Eastern Association for the Surgery of Trauma Injury Control/Violence Prevention Committee (Johns Hopkins School of Medicine, Baltimore, MD; et al)
J Trauma Acute Care Surg 73:1340-1347, 2012

Background.—Approximately 600,000 ski- and snowboarding-related injuries occur in North America each year, with head injuries accounting for up to 20% of all injuries. Currently, there are no major institutional recommendations regarding helmet use for skiers and snowboaders in the United States, in part owing to previous conflicting evidence regarding their efficacy. The objective of this review was to evaluate existing evidence on the efficacy of safety helmets during skiing and snowboarding, particularly in regard to head injuries, neck and cervical spine injuries, and risk compensation behaviors. These data will then be used for potential recommendations regarding helmet use during alpine winter sports.

Methods.—The PubMed, Cochrane Library, and EMBASE databases were searched using the search string *helmet* OR *head protective devices* AND (*skiing* OR *snowboarding* OR *skier* OR *snowboarder*) for articles on human participants of all ages published between January 1980 and April 2011. The search yielded 83, 0, and 96 results in PubMed, Cochrane Library, and EMBASE, respectively. Studies published in English describing

TABLE 1.—Summary of Class II Studies Included in Evidence-Based Review on the Efficacy of Safety Helmets in Recreational Skiing and Snowboarding (1980–2011)

Authors	Title	Citation	Summary
Case-control, case-crossover studies			
Hagel BE, Pless IB, Goulet C, et al.[38]	Effectiveness of helmets in skiers and snowboarders: Case-control and case crossover study.	BMJ. 2005;330:281	A study including 4,377 participants was conducted between 2001 and 2002. Helmets reduced the risk of any head injury (adjusted OR, 0.71; 95% CI, 0.55–0.92; 29% risk reduction) and head injury requiring evacuation via ambulance (adjusted OR, 0.44; 95% CI, 0.24–0.81; 56% reduction in risk).
Case-control studies			
Hagel BE, Russell K, Goulet C, et al.[44]	Helmet use and risk of neck injury in skiers and snowboarders.	Am J Epidemiol. 2010; 171:1134–1143.	Data from 100,394 participants between 1995 and 2005 was analyzed. Helmets did not increase the risk of neck or cervical spine injuries in skiers and snowboarders (adjusted OR: 1.09 [95% CI, 0.95–1.25] for any neck injury, 1.28 [95% CI, 0.96–1.71] for isolated ambulance-evacuated neck injuries, and 1.02 [95% CI, 0.79–1.31] for cervical spine fractures or dislocations).
Hasler RM, Berov S, Benneker L, et al.[37]	Are there risk factors for snowboard injuries? A casecontrol multicentre study of 559 snowboarders.	Br J Sports Med. 2010;44:816–821.	A survey of 559 snowboarders was conducted using a questionnaire in 2007–2008. A trend to an association with injury was observed for not wearing a helmet (OR, 4.65; 95% CI, 0.94–23.05; $p = 0.0595$). Using conditional inference trees, the following group was found to be at risk for injury: not wearing a helmet and riding on icy slopes.
Hasler RM, Dubler S, Benneker LM, et al.[36]	Are there risk factors in alpine skiing? A controlled multicentre survey of 1278 skiers.	Br J Sports Med. 2009; 43:1020–1025.	A survey of 1,278 skiers was conducted using a questionnaire in 2007–2008. Use of helmet didn't emerge as a significant parameter for the patient group (OR, 1.44; 95% CI, 0.69–3.02; $p = 0.331$). Using conditional inference tree, following group was identified to be at risk for injury: VAS_{speed} of 4–7, icy slopes, and not wearing a helmet.
Mueller BA, Cummings P, Rivara FP, et al.[12]	Injuries of the head, face, and neck in relation to ski helmet use.	Epidemiology. 2008;19:270–276.	A study including 21,898 skiers and snowboarders at three ski resorts during six seasons was conducted. Helmets had a protective effect with regard to head injury (adjusted OR, 0.85; 95% CI, 0.76–0.95; 15% reduction in risk).
Sulheim S, Holme I, Ekeland A, et al.[39]	Helmet use and risk of head injuries in alpine skiers and snowboarders.	JAMA. 2006;295: 919–924.	A study with 6,269 participants was conducted in 2002. Helmet use reduced the risk of head contusions by 60% (adjusted OR, 0.40; 95% CI, 0.30–0.55), fractures by 53% (adjusted OR, 0.47; 95% CI, 0.33–0.66), and severe head injury by 57% (adjusted OR, 0.43; 95% CI, 0.25–0.77). Risk-taking skiers and snowboarders were more likely to wear a helmet (OR, 1.48; 95% CI, 1.21–1.81).

Authors	Title	Reference	Findings
Hagel B, Pless IB, Goulet C, et al.[47]	The effect of helmet use on injury severity and crash circumstances in skiers and snowboarders.	*Accid Anal Prev.* 2005; 37:103–108.	A study including 3,295 participants from 19 areas of Quebec was conducted in 2001–2002. The study found no evidence of an increase in the severity of non–head-face-neck injury with helmet use in terms of the requirement of evacuation by ambulance (adjusted OR, 1.17; 95% CI, 0.79–1.73) and need for admission to hospital (adjusted OR, 0.79; 95% CI, 0.53–1.18). Similarly, no evidence was seen regarding the association of helmet use and fast selfreported speed (adjusted OR, 1.06; 95% CI, 0.68–1.66) and participation on a more difficult run (adjusted OR, 1.28; 95% CI, 0.79–20.8).
Macnab AJ, Smith T, Gagnon FA, et al.[54]	Effect of helmet wear on the incidence of head/face and cervical spine injuries in young skiers and snowboarders.	*Inj Prev.* 2002;8:324–327.	A study in children G13 years (n = 70) between 1998 and 1999 showed that failure to wear a helmet increased the risk of head, neck, or face injury (RR, 2.24; 95% CI, 1.23–4.12; corrected RR for activity, 1.77; 95% CI, 0.98–3.19) during skiing and snowboarding. The trend of the risk of cervical spine injury was seen to be toward the higher side when not wearing a helmet (RR, 2.0; 95% CI, 0.8–5.65; $p = 0.15$).
Cross-sectional studies Ruedl G, Pocecco E, Sommersacher R, et al.[50]	Factors associated with self-reported risk-taking behaviour on ski slopes.	*Br J Sports Med.* 2010; 44:204–206.	527 skiers and snowboarders in –20082009 subjectively classified themselves as cautious (n = 369) or risk taking (n = 168). Objective measurements of maximum speed attained on the slope by a radar speed gun were also made. The two groups were not significantly different with regard to helmet use ($p > 0.1$).
Scott MD, Buller DB, Andersen PA, et al.[49]	Testing the risk compensation hypothesis for safety helmets in alpine skiing and snowboarding.	*Inj Prev.* 2007;13:173–177	1,779 participants were interviewed at 34 ski resorts in western United States and Canada in 2003. Helmet wearers skied/snowboarded at lower speeds (adjusted OR, 0.51; 95% CI, 0.38–0.68) and challenged themselves compared with nonhelmet wearers (adjusted OR, 0.67; 95% CI, 0.50–0.88).
Machold W, Kwasny O, Gässler P, et al.[41]	Risk of injury through snowboarding.	*J Trauma.* 2000;48: 1109–1114.	2,579 students in 1996–1997 in Austria, who engaged in snowboarding, filled out questionnaires. Results were suggestive of the protective effect of helmets in head injury (7.6% of snowboarders with helmet [196] had no head injury, while 0.7% of snowboarders without a helmet experienced head injury). No ORs were reported.
Retrospective cohort studies Rughani AI, Lin CT, Ares WJ, et al.[43]	Helmet use and reduction in skull fractures in skiers and snowboarders admitted to the hospital.	*J Neurosurg Pediatr.* 2011;7:268–271.	In a sample of 57 children with head injuries sustained during skiing or snowboarding, helmet use was associated with lower incidence of skull fractures (5.3% vs. 36.8%, $p = 0.009$) and overall craniofacial fractures (15.8 vs. 44.7%, $p = 0.03$). The OR of a skull fracture in nonhelmeted skiers and snowboarders presenting to the hospital was 10.5 (95% CI 1.26–87.4) as compared with helmet users. There was no significant difference in the incidence of cervical spine injury among helmeted and nonhelmeted patients ($p = 0.74$).
Greve MW, Young DJ, Goss AL, et al.[40]	Skiing and snowboarding head injuries in 2 areas of the United States.	*Wilderness Environ Med.* 2009;20: 234–238.	A study between 2002 and 2004 including 1,013 participants from nine medical facilities in Colorado, New York, and Vermont was conducted. There was a decreased incidence of loss of consciousness in case of striking a fixed object while wearing a safety helmet ($\chi^2 = 5.8$; $p < 0.05$).

(Continued)

Table 1.—(*Continued*)

Authors	Title	Citation	Summary
Case series			
Cundy TP, Systermans BJ, Cundy WJ, et al.[48]	Helmets for snow sports: prevalence, trends, predictors and attitudes to use.	*J Trauma.* 2010;69: 1486–1490.	A retrospective case series of 3,984 ski patrol accident reports from 2003 to 2008 was performed in Australia. Helmet use was more likely in those who thought that helmets reduce their chance of severe injury (OR, 3.6; 95% CI, 2.1–6.4) and among those who thought that helmet use should be mandatory (OR, 4.8; 95% CI, 2.7–8.5).
Fukuda O, Hirashima Y, Origasa H, et al.[35]	Characteristics of helmet or knit cap use in head injury of snowboarders.	*Neurol Med Chir (Tokyo).* 2007;47: 491–494	Questionnaire-based data was collected from 1,190 snowboarders between 1999 and 2003. Patients were divided into three groups: helmet group (n = 92), knit cap group (n = 913), and no cap group (n = 185). Serious head injury was overall observed in 46.1% patients (549 of 1,190). 59 serious head injuries occurred in the helmet group (64.1%, 59 of 92), 421 in knit cap group (46.1%, 421 of 913) and 69 in the no cap group (37.3%, 69 of 185). After adjusting for jumping, a nonsignificant protective effect of helmet use on severe head injuries was seen (OR, 0.66, CI 0.32–1.35).
Bridges EJ, Rouah F, Johnston KM.[45]	Snowblading injuries in Eastern Canada.	*Br J Sports Med.* 2003; 37:511–515.	A prospective case series was conducted in 1999–2000 including 1,332 participants with traumatic injury related to winter sports. There was no increased incidence of neck injuries in injured participants wearing a helmet, even when adjusted for age and activity.

Editor's Note: Please refer to original journal article for full references.

the analysis of original data on helmet use in relation to outcomes of interest, including death, head injury, severity of head injury, neck or cervical spine injury, and risk compensation behavior, were selected. Sixteen published studies met a priori inclusion criteria and were reviewed in detail by authors.

Results.—Level I recommendation is that all recreational skiers and snow-boarders should wear safety helmets to reduce the incidence and severity of head injury during these sports. Level II recommendation/observation is that helmets do not seem to increase risk compensation behavior, neck injuries, or cervical spine injuries among skiers and snowboarders. Policies and interventions to increase helmet use should be promoted to reduce mortality and head injury among skiers and snowboarders.

Conclusion.—Safety helmets clearly decrease the risk and severity of head injuries in skiing and snowboarding and do not seem to increase the risk of neck injury, cervical spine injury, or risk compensation behavior. Helmets are strongly recommended during recreational skiing and snowboarding (Table 1).

▶ This evidence-based review critically appraises the literature regarding the efficacy of safety helmets in reduction of head injuries in recreational skiers and snowboarders. After a thorough search strategy, only 16 published studies reviewed met the stringent a priori inclusion criteria, and were reviewed in detail by the authors of this publication (Table 1). Questions addressed were as follows:

A. Does helmet use increase or decrease the rate of fatal and nonfatal head injury among skiers and snowboarders?

B. Does helmet use increase or decrease the rates of neck or cervical spine injury in skiers and snowboarders?

C. Is helmet use associated with higher or lower risk compensation behavior among skiers and snowboarders?

Current legislative practices in some states and several European countries were also briefly mentioned.

Despite the lack of Class I evidence (randomized controlled trials), the authors felt that the studies reviewed provided enough evidence to make a Level I recommendation that all recreational skiers and snowboarders should wear safety helmets to reduce the incidence and severity of head injury during these sports. This is a very strong and powerful statement and requires wider dissemination and implementation. Level II recommendations/observations were that helmets do not seem to increase risk compensation behaviors or the risk of neck and cervical spine injuries among skiers and snowboarders, and that policies and interventions directed toward increasing and promoting helmet use should be promoted to reduce mortality and head injury in recreational skiers and snowboarders. The issues of helmet design, fit, and efficacy were not addressed, but these are also important considerations.

C. Lebrun, MDCM, MPE, CCFP, Dip Sport Med, FACSM

The Epidemiology of Mountain Bike Park Injuries at the Whistler Bike Park, British Columbia (BC), Canada

Ashwell Z, McKay MP, Brubacher JR, et al (The George Washington Univ, DC; The Univ of British Columbia, Vancouver, Canada; et al)
Wilderness Environ Med 23:140-145, 2012

Objective.—To describe the epidemiology of injuries sustained during the 2009 season at Whistler Mountain Bike Park.

Methods.—A retrospective chart review was performed of injured bike park cyclists presenting to the Whistler Health Clinic between May 16 and October 12, 2009.

Results.—Of 898 cases, 86% were male (median age, 26 years), 68.7% were Canadian, 19.4% required transport by the Whistler Bike Patrol, and 8.4% arrived by emergency medical services. Identification of 1759 specific injury diagnoses was made, including 420 fractures in 382 patients (42.5%). Upper extremity fractures predominated (75.4%), 11.2% had a traumatic brain injury, and 8.5% were transferred to a higher level of care: 7 by helicopter, 62 by ground, and 5 by personal vehicle. Two patients refused transfer.

Conclusions.—Mountain bikers incurred many injuries with significant morbidity while riding in the Whistler Mountain Bike Park in 2009. Although exposure information is unavailable, these findings demonstrate serious risks associated with this sport and highlight the need for continued research into appropriate safety equipment and risk avoidance measures (Table 2).

▶ In recent years, teenagers and young men have apparently been seeking ever more hazardous recreational sports. Mountain biking is one such example. Ski

TABLE 2.—Fractures by Body Region and Location

Body Region (N, %)	Location	Number
Face (8, 1.8%)	Face	8
Vertebrae (21, 4.7%)	Neck	2
	Spine	21
Torso (38, 8.5%)	Ribs	32
	Pelvis	6
Upper extremity (330, 74.2%)	Shoulder (includes clavicle)	122
	Humerus	12
	Elbow	37
	Forearm	8
	Wrist	109
	Hand/fingers	42
Lower extremity (48, 10.8%)	Hip	4
	Femur	1
	Knee	4
	Lower leg	1
	Ankle	25
	Foot	13
Sum		445

resorts that desire to remain profitable during the summer months have been allowing mountain bikers to use the resorts' gondolas to take mountain bikes to quite high elevations, and the cyclists have then descended rock-strewn hills at incredible speed. This article provides injury data for 1 such resort (Whistler, British Columbia), where a single gondola takes bicycles to its upper terminus. Over a 5-month period, 898 mountain bikers sought treatment at the Whistler Health Centre, the only primary treatment facility for the ski run, with a large amount of both fractures and traumatic brain injuries (Table 2). These authors were unfortunately unable to obtain data on the number of bicycle passes sold, so they could not calculate a formal injury rate. Given the limited nature of the medical facilities in Whistler, there may also have been other serious cases that were transferred directly to hospitals in Squamish and Vancouver. But even if 898 were the total number of casualties, it seems an unreasonably high number for a 5-month period. In a newspaper interview, one of the authors commented that danger seemed an important motivator for the bikers, and many patients were anxious to have their gory injuries photographed before treatment, in order to post them on their Facebook page. Moreover, the resort offered safety training at low cost, and whereas female bikers usually availed themselves of this instruction, most of the young males refused it. Given this attitude, injury prevention seems difficult except by the drastic measure of closing the trails to those who have not reached a certified level of competence.

R. J. Shephard, MD (Lond), PhD, DPE

Thoracic kyphosis comparisons in adolescent female competitive field hockey players and untrained controls
Rajabi R, Mobarakabadi L, Alizadhen HM, et al (Univ of Tehran, Iran)
J Sports Med Phys Fitness 52:545-550, 2012

Aim.—The aim of this study was to compare the thoracic kyphosis angles of adolescent female field hockey players and non-athletes and to examine the relationship between the thoracic kyphosis and training regimes in hockey.

Methods.—Seventy-four female participants including 37 field hockey players (mean age 19.03 ± 1.24 years) and 37 non-athletes (mean age 18.21 ± 1.22) were recruited in this cross-sectional study. The hockey players met a minimum criterion of 3 years of experience in the Iranian first division female hockey league. The thoracic kyphosis degree was measured between T1-T12 using a non-invasive flexible ruler.

Results.—A significant difference in the thoracic kyphosis degree between athletes ($M = 41.71°$, $SD = 5.38°$) and non-athletes ($M = 36.72°$, $SD = 6.01°$); $t(72) = 3.76$, $P = 0.001$ was revealed. The magnitude of these differences in the means was very large (eta squared $= 0.016$). There was a moderately positive correlation between the athletic history (number of years of hockey participation) and thoracic kyphosis, $r = 0.36$, $N. = 37$, $P = 0.031$. However, the relationship between the cumulative training exposure (yearly training hours) and the degree of thoracic kyphosis was not significant.

Conclusion.—Thoracic kyphosis was significantly increased in adolescent female field hockey players and was found to be associated with the cumulative number of years of hockey participation. These results suggest a possible association between the semi-crouched posture in field hockey and thoracic kyphosis in elite adolescent athletes. The results also suggest that number of years of field hockey participation is a determinant in the increased kyphosis.

▶ Thoracic kyphosis detracts from personal appearance and, if extreme, can lead to respiratory problems. Previous authors have noted a tendency to kyphosis in various other sports that involve the adoption of a crouched position,[1] including cycling[1,2] and kayaking,[3] but this is the first report relative to female field hockey. The increased angle relative to nonathletes from the same milieu (5°) is appreciable, particularly as the individuals concerned were training for less than 300 hours per year. The degree of curvature was also correlated with the number of years that the girl had been seriously involved in the sport. It suggests the need for corrective measures. Although spinal curvature has sometimes been reported also in ice hockey players, I have often been impressed by the erect posture of top players when they are not actively engaged with the puck. Possibly, the remedy is for coaches to stress the need to take a deliberately erect stance when not actively engaged in a playing maneuver.

R. J. Shephard, MD (Lond), PhD, DPE

References

1. Usabiaga J, Crespo R, Iza I, Aramendi J, Terrados N, Poza JJ. Adaptation of the lumbar spine to different positions in bicycle racing. *Spine.* 1997;22:1965-1999.
2. Rajabi R, Freemont T, Doherty P. The investigation of thoracic kyphosis in cyclists and non-cyclists. In: Marfell-Jones M, Reilly T, eds. *Kinanthropometry VIII: Proceedings of the International Society for the Advancement of Kinanthropometry.* London, UK: Routledge; 2003:263-273.
3. Lopez-Minarro PA, Muyor JM, Alacid F. Saggital spinal curvature and pelvic tilt in elite young kayakers. *Med Del Sportr.* 2010;63:509-519.

Prevention of acute knee injuries in adolescent female football players: cluster randomised controlled trial
Waldén M, Atroshi I, Magnusson H, et al (Linköping Univ, Sweden; Hässleholm-Kristianstad-Ystad Hosps, Sweden; et al)
BMJ 344:e3042, 2012

Objective.—To evaluate the effectiveness of neuromuscular training in reducing the rate of acute knee injury in adolescent female football players.

Design.—Stratified cluster randomised controlled trial with clubs as the unit of randomisation.

TABLE 4.—Effectiveness of Neuromuscular Warm-Up Programme in Adolescent Female Football Players According to Intention to Treat. Values are Numbers (Percentages) of injured Players Unless Stated Otherwise

Injuries	Intervention Group (n=2479 Injuries Players)	Control Group (n=2085 Players)	Rate Ratio (95% CI)*	P Value
Anterior cruciate ligament injury	7 (0.28)	14 (0.67)	0.36 (0.15 to 0.85)	0.02
Severe knee injury	26 (1.05)	31 (1.49)	0.70 (0.42 to 1.18)	0.18
Any acute knee injury	48 (1.94)	44 (2.11)	0.92 (0.61 to 1.40)	0.71

Editor's Note: Please refer to original journal article for full references.
*Rate ratios from unadjusted analyses, stratified by district, using Cox regression with robust variance estimation to account for correlation of outcomes within each club.[26]

Setting.—230 Swedish football clubs (121 in the intervention group, 109 in the control group) were followed for one season (2009, seven months).

Participants.—4564 players aged 12-17 years (2479 in the intervention group, 2085 in the control group) completed the study.

Intervention.—15 minute neuromuscular warm-up programme (targeting core stability, balance, and proper knee alignment) to be carried out twice a week throughout the season.

Main outcome measures.—The primary outcome was rate of anterior cruciate ligament injury; secondary outcomes were rates of severe knee injury (>4 weeks' absence) and any acute knee injury.

Results.—Seven players (0.28%) in the intervention group, and 14 (0.67%) in the control group had an anterior cruciate ligament injury. By Cox regression analysis according to intention to treat, a 64% reduction in the rate of anterior cruciate ligament injury was seen in the intervention group (rate ratio 0.36, 95% confidence interval 0.15 to 0.85). The absolute rate difference was −0.07 (95% confidence interval −0.13 to 0.001) per 1000 playing hours in favour of the intervention group. No significant rate reductions were seen for secondary outcomes.

Conclusions.—A neuromuscular warm-up programme significantly reduced the rate of anterior cruciate ligament injury in adolescent female football players. However, the absolute rate difference did not reach statistical significance, possibly owing to the small number of events.

Trial registration.—Clinical trials NCT00894595 (Table 4).

▶ Sports physicians have long debated the issue of warmup as a means of preventing sports injuries, although it has always seemed logical that warm and less viscous tissues would be less susceptible to injury. The issue of the need for a warmup is by no means trivial, given the frequency of anterior cruciate ligament injuries in soccer players, the current prevalence of the sport among both men and women, and the serious long-term consequences of such injuries. It is thus surprising that there have been no previous high-quality randomized trials of the question.[1] This study was conducted in adolescent females, who are particularly vulnerable for injury.[2,3] The study was massive and carefully conducted, involving 4900 players and almost 280 000 hours of soccer, with cluster random-ization of clubs to avoid contamination between intervention and control groups, and evaluation of injuries by well-qualified, blinded sports physicians. Unfortu-nately, from the viewpoint of scientific proof, the number of severe knee injuries was smaller than anticipated (57 knee injuries, 21 of these involving the anterior cruciate ligaments). Although the injury rate was substantially lower with warmup than without (0.28% vs 0.67%, Table 4), the probability of benefit as assessed by various statistical tests was modest (in the range $P = .02$ to .03). Nevertheless, the results are sufficiently encouraging that trials of this type of warmup should be extended to male subjects and to other types of sports.

R. J. Shephard, MD (Lond), PhD, DPE

References

1. Hägglund M, Waldén M, Atroshi I. Preventing knee injuries in adolescent female football players—design of a cluster randomized controlled trial [NCT00894595]. *BMC Musculoskelet Disord.* 2009;10:75.
2. Waldén M, Hägglund M, Werner J, Ekstrand J. The epidemiology of anterior cruciate ligament injury in football (soccer): a review of the literature from a gender-related perspective. *Knee Surg Sports Traumatol Arthrosc.* 2011;19:3-10.
3. Shea KG, Pfeiffer R, Wang JH, Curtin M, Apel PJ. Anterior cruciate ligament injury in pediatric and adolescent soccer players: an analysis of insurance data. *J Pediatr Orthop.* 2004;24:623-628.

Lesions of Head and Neck

Dementia Resulting From Traumatic Brain Injury: What Is the Pathology?

Shively S, Scher AI, Perl DP, et al (Uniformed Services Univ of the Health Sciences, Bethesda, MD)
Arch Neurol 69:1245-1251, 2012

Traumatic brain injury (TBI) is among the earliest illnesses described in human history and remains a major source of morbidity and mortality in the modern era. It is estimated that 2% of the US population lives with long-term disabilities due to a prior TBI, and incidence and prevalence rates are even higher in developing countries. One of the most feared long-term consequences of TBIs is dementia, as multiple epidemiologic studies show that experiencing a TBI in early or midlife is associated with an increased risk of dementia in late life. The best data indicate that moderate and severe TBIs increase risk of dementia between 2- and 4-fold. It is less clear whether mild TBIs such as brief concussions result in increased dementia risk, in part because mild head injuries are often not well documented and retrospective studies have recall bias. However, it has been observed for many years that multiple mild TBIs as experienced by professional boxers are associated with a high risk of chronic traumatic encephalopathy (CTE), a type of dementia with distinctive clinical and pathologic features. The recent recognition that CTE is common in retired professional football and hockey players has rekindled interest in this condition, as has the recognition that military personnel also experience high rates of mild

TBIs and may have a similar syndrome. It is presently unknown whether dementia in TBI survivors is pathophysiologically similar to Alzheimer disease, CTE, or some other entity. Such information is critical for developing preventive and treatment strategies for a common cause of acquired dementia. Herein, we will review the epidemiologic data linking TBI and dementia, existing clinical and pathologic data, and will identify areas where future research is needed.

▶ This article is a fine review of the link between repetitive brain injury and chronic traumatic encephalopathy (CTE). It also gives a fine illustration of the similarities and differences between CTE and Alzheimer disease. The neuropathology of CTE in this article has been obtained from Dr Ann McKee, internationally recognized neuropathologist and codirector of our Center for the Study of Traumatic Encephalopathy at Boston University School of Medicine. The article reviews the 51 cases of CTE in the world's literature as of 2009. Unfortunately, this publication occurred 2 months before McKee's December 2012 *Brain* publication of 68 additional cases of CTE. In that publication, McKee outlines her grading scale of CTE 1—4. Of the 68 cases of CTE, 6 were in the high school population. This reviewer supports the conclusions of this article, that certain members of our society, such as our military service members and professional athletes, are at particular risk for CTE, which should stimulate research on preventive strategies focused on these individuals.

R. C. Cantu, MD, MA

Compliance with return-to-play regulations following concussion in Australian schoolboy and community rugby union players
Hollis SJ, Stevenson MR, McIntosh AS, et al (The Univ of Sydney, New South Wales, Australia; The Univ of New South Wales, Sydney, Australia; et al)
Br J Sports Med 46:735-740, 2012

Background.—There is a risk of concussion when playing rugby union. Appropriate management of concussion includes compliance with the return-to-play regulations of the sports body for reducing the likelihood of premature return-to-play by injured players.

Purpose.—To describe the proportion of rugby union players who comply with the sports body's regulations on returning to play postconcussion.

Study Design.—Prospective cohort study.

Methods.—1958 community rugby union players (aged 15—48 years) in Sydney (Australia) were recruited from schoolboy, grade and suburban competitions and followed over ≥1 playing seasons. Club doctors/ physiotherapists/coaches or trained injury recorders who attended the game reported players who sustained a concussion. Concussed players were followed up over a 3-month period and the dates when they returned to play (including either a game or training session) were recorded, as well as any return-to-play advice they received.

TABLE 2.—Return-to-Play Advice and Player Behaviour in Comparison with Return-to-Play Regulation

Return-to-Play Advice and Behaviour Postconcussion	Players' Actual Compliance with Return-to-Play Regulation		
	No, n (%)	Yes, n (%)	Total, n (%)
Self-reported return-to-play advice postconcussion			
Advice received			
No	79 (78)	2 (100)	81 (78)
Yes	23 (22)	0 (0)	23 (22)
Type of advice			
Play next week	5 (22)	0 (0)	5 (22)
1 week off	5 (22)	0 (0)	5 (22)
2 weeks off	8 (35)	0 (0)	8 (35)
3 weeks off	0 (0)	0 (0)	0 (0)
International Rugby Board regulation stand-down period (3 weeks) indicated by dotted line.			
Get medical advice before play	4 (17)	0 (0)	4 (17)
4—6 weeks off	1 (4)	0 (0)	1 (4)
Did advice follow return-to-play regulation			
No	18 (78)	0 (0)	18 (78)
Yes	5 (22)	0 (0)	5 (22)
Advice provider			
Physiotherapist	7 (30)	0 (0)	7 (30)
General practitioner	7 (30)	0 (0)	7 (30)
Sports doctor	3 (13)	0 (0)	3 (13)
Coach, family etc	2 (9)	0 (0)	2 (9)
Chiropractor	1 (4)	0 (0)	1 (4)
Missing data	3 (13)	0 (0)	3 (13)
Return-to-play behaviour postconcussion			
Returned to play			
Without coming off	35 (95)	2 (5)	37 (34)
After blood bin	11 (100)	0 (0)	11 (10)
Retired from game because of			
Concussion	43 (39)	0 (0)	43 (40)
Other injury	10 (9)	0 (0)	10 (9)
Other*	8 (7)	0 (0)	8 (7)

*'Other' case examples may be player substitution, a player coming off the field but returning to play later.

Results.—187 players sustained ≥1 concussion throughout the follow-up. The median number of days before players returned to play (competition game play or training) following concussion was 3 (range 1—84). Most players (78%) did not receive return-to-play advice postconcussion, and of those who received correct advice, all failed to comply with the 3-week stand-down regulation.

Conclusions.—The paucity of return-to-play advice received by community rugby union players postconcussion and the high level of non-compliance with return-to-play regulations highlight the need for better dissemination and implementation of the return-to-play regulations and improved understanding of the underlying causes of why players do not adhere to return-to-play practices (Table 2).

▶ A quick review of back issues of the YEAR BOOK for the past 5 years shows that there have been many articles on the appropriate treatment of concussion following sports injury. However, this is not a big advance if such information is ignored by the practitioner, trainers, and players (Table 2). It is discouraging to read that a study of US certified trainers found that only 3% were fully compliant with concussion management guidelines,[1] and other studies at various levels of competition in Canada,[2,3] the United States,[4] and New Zealand[5] have shown a substantial prevalence of both poor compliance and ignorance of appropriate management. There is plainly a need to improve understanding and communication; hopefully, this will occur without a medical adviser facing a major lawsuit for negligence.

R. J. Shephard, MD (Lond), PhD, DPE

References

1. Notebaert AJ, Guskiewicz KM. Current trends in athletic training practice for concussion assessment and management. *J Athl Train*. 2005;40:320-325.
2. Cusimano MD. Canadian minor hockey participants' knowledge about concussion. *Can J Neurol Sci*. 2009;36:315-320.
3. American Academy of Neurology. Practice parameter: the management of concussion in sports (summary statement). Report of the Quality Standards Subcommittee. *Neurology*. 1997;48:581-585.
4. Yard EE, Comstock RD. Compliance with return to play guidelines following concussion in US high school athletes, 2005-2008. *Brain Inj*. 2009;23:888-898.
5. Sye G, Sullivan SJ, McCrory P. High school rugby players' understanding of concussion and return to play guidelines. *Br J Sports Med*. 2006;40:1003-1005.

Depression and Neurocognitive Performance After Concussion Among Male and Female High School and Collegiate Athletes

Kontos AP, Covassin T, Elbin RJ, et al (Univ of Pittsburgh School of Medicine, PA; Michigan State Univ, East Lansing; et al)
Arch Phys Med Rehabil 93:1751-1756, 2012

Objectives.—To prospectively examine the relationship of sport-related concussion with depression and neurocognitive performance and symptoms among male and female high school and college athletes. A secondary objective was to explore age and sex differences.

Design.—Pretest, multiple posttest, repeated-measures design.

Setting.—Laboratory.

Participants.—High school and collegiate athletes (N = 75) with a diagnosed concussion.

Interventions.—Not applicable.

Main Outcome Measures.—Beck Depression Inventory-II and computerized neurocognitive test battery (Immediate Post-concussion Assessment and Cognitive Test), which includes concussion symptoms (Post-concussion Symptom Scale) at baseline and at 2, 7, and 14 days postinjury.

Results.—Concussed athletes exhibited significantly higher levels of depression from baseline at 2 days ($P \leq .001$), 7 days ($P = .006$), and 14 days postconcussion ($P = .04$). Collegiate athletes demonstrated a significant increase in depression at 14 days postconcussion than did high school athletes ($P = .03$). There were no sex differences in depression levels.

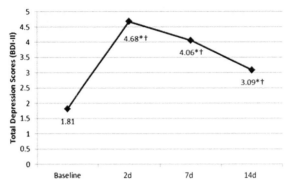

FIGURE 1.—Depression scores on the BDI-II after sport-related concussion (N = 75). *$P < .05$. †Significantly higher than baseline. (Reprinted from Kontos AP, Covassin T, Elbin RJ, et al. Depression and neurocognitive performance after concussion among male and female high school and collegiate athletes. *Arch Phys Med Rehabil.* 2012;93:1751-1756, with permission from the American Congress of Rehabilitation Medicine.)

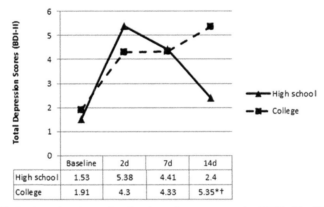

FIGURE 2.—Age × time interaction for depression scores on the BDI-II (N = 75). *$P < .05$. †Significantly higher than high school athletes at 14d. (Reprinted from Kontos AP, Covassin T, Elbin RJ, et al. Depression and neurocognitive performance after concussion among male and female high school and collegiate athletes. *Arch Phys Med Rehabil.* 2012;93:1751-1756, with permission from the American Congress of Rehabilitation Medicine.)

Neurocognitive decrements at 14 days were supported for reaction time ($P = .001$) and visual memory ($P = .001$). Somatic depression at 7 days post-concussion was related to slower reaction time at 7 days postconcussion. Somatic depression at 14 days postinjury was related to lower visual memory scores at 14 days postinjury.

Conclusions.—Although not clinically significant, athletes experienced increased depression scores up to 14 days after concussion that coincided with neurocognitive decrements in reaction time and visual memory. Somatic depression appears to be most salient with regard to lower neurocognitive performance. Mood assessments after concussion are warranted to help monitor and enhance recovery (Figs 1 and 2).

▶ Sport-related concussion can cause a number of somatic, cognitive, and emotional symptoms, which may persist up to several weeks following injury. The diagnostic symptoms of depression often overlap with those of concussion (eg, sadness, irritability, fatigue, and sleep problems), sometimes making it difficult to discern the cause of these symptoms. Additional issues, such as the uncertainly of prognosis (ie, lack of an active rehabilitation), removal from sport, isolation, and lack of social support in dealing with concussion may influence mood in athletes who have sustained a concussion. This prospective study of depression and neurocognitive performance used interesting methodology to attempt to disentangle these 2 conditions. A total of 75 high school and collegiate athletes who had all undergone baseline testing with the Beck Depression Inventory-II and a computerized neurocognitive test battery (Immediate Post-concussion Assessment and Cognitive Test or ImPACT) were followed with repeat testing at 2 days, 5 to 7 days, and 10 to 14 days or so postinjury, or until they were cleared to return to play by a sports medicine professional. Ten symptoms (headache, nausea, vomiting, balance problems, dizziness, sensitivity to light, sensitivity to noise, numbness/tingling, visual problems, and fogginess) listed on the 22-item Post-concussion Symptom Scale (contained within the ImPACT test), were identified as "nondepressive" symptoms, totaled, and used as a covariate in the subsequent analyses to account for the potential confounding effect of other concussion symptoms on depression.

Previous smaller studies have used the Profile of Mood States to prospectively examine emotional function in collegiate athletes with concussion, uninjured collegiate athletes, and nonathletes[1,2], documenting elevated levels of depression and mood disturbances in athletes with concussion. The current study confirmed these findings and, furthermore, demonstrated a time-dependent elevation in depressive symptoms from baseline, followed by some resolution at 10-14 days postinjury (Fig 1). Interestingly, although the high school athletes displayed an inverted U type of response, the collegiate athletes actually exhibited more depressive symptoms with time (Fig 2). The authors postulated that this might be due to higher competition levels, stress, and scholarships in the collegiate athletes, whereas the high school athletes may have stronger support systems (eg, family members and friends) to help them cope with their injury.

There were significant associations between the neurocognitive decrements in reaction time and visual memory and somatic depression. Unexpectedly, there were no sex differences found in depression levels, but this might have been related to the relatively smaller number of females studied. In any case, further research is warranted on the role of depression in specific neurocognitive deficits and potential prolonged recovery from concussion.

C. Lebrun

References

1. Mainwaring LM, Bisschop SM, Green REA, et al. Emotional reaction of varsity athletes to sport-related concussion. *J Sport Exerc Psychol.* 2004;26:119-135.

2. Mainwaring LM, Hutchison M, Bisschop SM, Comper P, Richards DW. Emotional response to sport concussion compared to ACL injury. *Brain Inj.* 2010;24:589-597.

Video Incident Analysis of Head Injuries in High School Girls' Lacrosse

Caswell SV, Lincoln AE, Almquist JL, et al (George Mason Univ, Fairfax, VA; MedStar Sports Medicine Res Ctr, Baltimore, MD; et al)
Am J Sports Med 40:756-762, 2012

Background.—Knowledge of injury mechanisms and game situations associated with head injuries in girls' high school lacrosse is necessary to target prevention efforts.

Purpose.—To use video analysis and injury data to provide an objective and comprehensive visual record to identify mechanisms of injury, game characteristics, and penalties associated with head injury in girls' high school lacrosse.

Study Design.—Descriptive epidemiology study.

Methods.—In the 25 public high schools of 1 school system, 529 varsity and junior varsity girls' lacrosse games were videotaped by trained videographers during the 2008 and 2009 seasons. Video of head injury incidents was examined to identify associated mechanisms and game characteristics using a lacrosse-specific coding instrument.

Results.—Of the 25 head injuries (21 concussions and 4 contusions) recorded as game-related incidents by athletic trainers during the 2 seasons, 20 head injuries were captured on video, and 14 incidents had sufficient image quality for analysis. All 14 incidents of head injury (11 concussions, 3 contusions) involved varsity-level athletes. Most head injuries resulted from stick-to-head contact (n = 8), followed by body-to-head contact (n = 4). The most frequent player activities were defending a shot (n = 4) and competing for a loose ball (n = 4). Ten of the 14 head injuries occurred inside the 12-m arc and in front of the goal, and no penalty was called in 12 injury incidents. All injuries involved 2 players, and most resulted from unintentional actions. Turf versus grass did not appear to influence number of head injuries.

Conclusion.—Comprehensive video analysis suggests that play near the goal at the varsity high school level is associated with head injuries. Absence of penalty calls on most of these plays suggests an area for exploration, such as the extent to which current rules are enforced and the effectiveness of existing rules for the prevention of head injury.

▶ It has been documented in multiple studies that the most common mechanism for sustaining a concussion in women's lacrosse is being hit in the face or head with a lacrosse stick. This article found that to be the case as well. Furthermore, it found that penalties were not called in more than 90% of injuries and that most occurred inside the 12-meter arc in front of the goal. Video analysis was used to record the injury mechanism in this study. The absence of penalty calls suggests that further exploration as to the extent current rules are being enforced and the effectiveness of existing rules for the prevention of head injuries is needed. This reviewer has gone on record as strongly recommending helmets for girls lacrosse to prevent the stick-to-the-head blow leading to concussions. It is important to realize that almost all stick-to-head contact was unintentional.

R. C. Cantu, MD, MA

High School Soccer Players With Concussion Education Are More Likely to Notify Their Coach of a Suspected Concussion

Bramley H, Patrick K, Lehman E, et al (Penn State Milton S. Hershey Med Ctr, Hershey, PA; Penn State College of Medicine, Hershey, PA)
Clin Pediatr 51:332-336, 2012

Previously published studies have found that concussion symptoms are underreported in youth athletics. This study evaluated the likelihood high school soccer players would identify themselves as having concussion related symptoms during game situations. A questionnaire inquiring about past concussion education and the likelihood of notifying their coach of concussion symptoms was administered to 183 high school soccer players. Of the 60 (33%) who completed the survey, 18 (72%) athletes who had acknowledged receiving concussion training responded that they would always notify their coach of concussion symptoms, as compared with 12 (36%) of the players who reported having no such training ($P = .01$). The results of this study suggest that athletes with past concussion training are more likely to notify their coach of concussion symptoms, potentially reducing their risk for further injury. Concussion education should be considered for all high school soccer players.

▶ Currently there are 40 states that require Lystedt concussion laws, which mandate concussion education for players, parents, and coaches. This article is proof of the need and importance of such legislation. It found athletes who had received prior concussion education to be twice as likely to report concussions to their coach as compared with players who had not received concussion education. In our personal experience, we have also found that individuals who have received concussion education—in particular education concerning the symptoms of concussion —to be much more likely to report concussions than those who did not have such education. This is not a surprise as 1 of the reasons most commonly given by athletes for not reporting a concussion is that they did not know they had sustained a concussion. Nonetheless, athletes in this study were noted to be more reluctant to notify the coach or trainer of a concussion during a championship game as compared with a regular season game. This study was a retrospective questionnaire in design and therefore subject to the weaknesses of that design.

R. C. Cantu, MD, MA

Sport Concussion Assessment Tool–2: Baseline Values for High School Athletes

Jinguji TM, Bompadre V, Harmon KG, et al (Seattle Children's Hosp, WA; Univ of Washington, Seattle)

Br J Sports Med 46:365-370, 2012

Background.—Concussion head injuries are common in high school athletes. The Sport Concussion Assessment Tool–2 (SCAT2) has been recommended and widely adopted as a standardised method of evaluating an injured athlete with a suspected concussion. Sideline return to play decisions can hinge on the results of a SCAT2 score. However, most athletes will not have had baseline testing performed for comparison if injury occurs. Therefore, establishing of age-, sex- and sport-matched normative data for the high school athlete population is critical.

Purpose.—To determine baseline scores in all SCAT2 domains among high school athletes with no prior history of a concussion and to examine subgroup differences for girls and boys, age and sport to establish normative ranges.

Materials and Methods.—The SCAT2 was administered to 214 high school athletes (155 males and 59 females) who participated in football, women's soccer, men's basketball, gymnastics, baseball, softball and track with no prior history of concussion. There were 111 athletes in the 13–15-year-old cohort and 103 in the 16–19-year-old group with a mean age of 15.7 years of age. In all SCAT2 domains the mean and SD of the results were determined. The domains were analysed using age, sex and sport as covariates. Component parts of the cognitive (concentration) domain (digit sequencing and months of year in reverse order) were also analysed by age, sex and sport. The percentage of high school athletes able to perform each digit-sequencing test was calculated as was the percentage of participants who could recite the months of the year in reverse order.

Results.—The average SCAT2 score for these high school athletes was 89 of a possible 100 with a SD of 6 units. Athletes reported two or three symptoms at baseline with older students reporting more symptoms than younger ones. The average balance score was 25.82 (of 30), and all athletes were able to complete the double-leg stance. Females scored significantly higher on the balance, immediate memory and concentration scores. Concentration scores in non-concussed high school athletes were low. Only 67% of high school athletes could recite the months of the year backward and only 41% could correctly sequence 5 digits backward. Only 55% of high school football players could correctly recite the months of the year backward and 32% could sequence 5 digits.

Conclusions.—Non-concussed high school athletes scored near the total possible in most domains of the SCAT2 with the exception of concentration testing and balance testing. All athletes were able to complete the double-leg stance at baseline; however, there was significant variability of tandem and single-leg stance. Baseline testing is important when considering balance tests. Concentration testing in high school athletes is unreliable because of high baseline error and is likely to result in a high rate of false positives and false negatives. Return to play decisions should not rely on concentration testing without a baseline test for comparison.

▶ Increasingly, tests are being used in helping to guide return-to-play decisions after a concussion. Perhaps the most widely used is the Immediate Post-Concussion Assessment and Cognitive Testing (ImPACT) test. Since the Zurich International Concussion Consensus Statement of 2009, the Sport Concussion Assessment Tool—2 (SCAT—2) has been increasingly used. Any test of cognition or other neurologic function such as vision or balance is most precise when one is compared with his or her own baseline. For this reason, many of us will not use ImPACT or other neuropsychological tests for making return-to-play decisions without a baseline. This study essentially attempted to establish normative data for the SCAT—2 test. It found there was such variability in concentration testing and balance testing that normative data were unreliable. To be compared with normative data resulted in a high rate of false positives and false negatives. It was therefore determined that return-to-play decisions should not rely on concentration or balance testing without a baseline for comparison.

R. C. Cantu, MD, MA

Identifying Impairments after Concussion: Normative Data versus Individualized Baselines

Schmidt JD, Register-Mihalik JK, Mihalik JP, et al (The Univ of North Carolina at Chapel Hill)

Med Sci Sports Exerc 44:1621-1628, 2012

Purpose.—This study aimed to determine whether agreement exists between baseline comparison (comparison of postconcussion scores to individualized baseline scores) and normative comparison (comparison of postconcussion scores to a normative mean) in identifying impairments after concussion.

Methods.—A total of 1060 collegiate student-athletes completed baseline testing as part of an ongoing clinical program. Gender-specific normative means were obtained from a subset of 673 athletes with no history of self-reported concussion, learning disabilities, or attention-deficit disorders. Concussions were later diagnosed in 258 athletes who had completed baseline testing. The athletes completed their first assessment within 10 d after injury. Athletes completed a computerized neurocognitive test (Automated Neuropsychological Assessment Metrics), postural control assessment (Sensory Organization Test), and a 15-item graded symptom checklist at baseline and again after injury. We computed two postconcussion difference scores for each outcome measure: 1) baseline difference = postconcussion score − individualized baseline score and 2) normative difference = postconcussion score − normative mean. Athletes were considered impaired if postconcussion difference exceeded the reliable change parameters. McNemar tests were used to assess agreement on impairment status (impaired and unimpaired) between comparison methods for each outcome measure.

Results.—The baseline comparison method identified 2.6 times more impairments than the normative comparison method for the Simple Reaction Time Test 1 ($P = 0.043$). The normative comparison method identified 7.6 times more impairments than the baseline comparison method for Mathematical Processing ($P < 0.001$). No other disagreements were observed for postural control or symptom severity.

Conclusions.—Our findings suggest that, when using these concussion assessment tools, clinicians may consider using normative data in lieu of individualized baseline measures. This may be especially useful to clinicians with limited resources and an inability to capture valid baselines on all athletes.

▶ In an ideal situation, comparison of one's concussion profile with his or her own baseline should be superior to comparisons with normative data. The reality, though, is that one's neurocognitive performance and concussion profile often varies with multiple testing. Nothing is more important than the effort put forward, yet such effort can be modified by many human factors. Besides the obvious of not trying one's hardest to falsely obtain a lower baseline score, other factors can include sleep deprivation, lack of an adequate quiet setting for the examination, and emotional circumstances that may preclude a maximum effort. Although comparison to one's own baseline should theoretically be superior to comparison with age- and sex-matched normative data, is it? This is the first comparative study between normative and baseline evaluation methods to have been carried out to this reviewer's knowledge. It suggests that, although there are some minor variances, overall there is quite good correlation such that clinicians can consider using normative data in lieu of individualized baseline measures. In this reviewer's experience, though, baseline measures ideally obtained are always preferable to normalized data.

R. C. Cantu, MD, MA

A Revised Factor Structure for the Post-Concussion Symptom Scale: Baseline and Postconcussion Factors
Kontos AP, Elbin RJ, Schatz P, et al (Univ of Pittsburgh Med Ctr, PA; Univ of Pittsburgh, PA; Saint Joseph's Univ, Philadelphia, PA; et al)
Am J Sports Med 40:2375-2384, 2012

Background.—Symptom reports play a critical role in the assessment and management of concussions. Symptoms are often conceptualized as factors comprising several related symptoms (eg, somatic factor = headache, nausea, vomiting). Previous research examining the factor structure of the 22-item Post-Concussion Symptom Scale (PCSS) has been limited to small samples and has not adequately evaluated factor loadings at both baseline and postconcussion for male and female athletes at the high school and collegiate levels.

Purpose.—To examine the factor structure of the 22-item PCSS in independent samples of high school and collegiate athletes reported at baseline and postconcussion, and to evaluate sex and age differences in the resulting baseline and postconcussion symptom factor scores.

Study Design.—Case series; Level of evidence, 4.

Methods.—Exploratory factor analytic (EFA) methods were applied to 2 separate samples of athletes who completed the PCSS at baseline (n = 30,455) and 1 to 7 days after a sport-related concussion (n = 1438). The baseline sample (mean ± standard deviation) was 15.74 ± 1.78 years, with a range of 13 to 22 years, and the postconcussion sample was 17.14 ± 2.25 years, with a range of 13 to 24 years.

Results.—A 4-factor solution accounting for 49.1% of the variance at baseline included a cognitive-sensory, sleep-arousal, vestibular-somatic, and affective factor structure. A 4-factor solution that included cognitive-fatigue-migraine, affective, somatic, and sleep was revealed for the postconcussion EFA. High school athletes reported higher baseline levels of the cognitive-sensory and vestibular-somatic symptom factors and lower levels of the sleep-arousal factor than college athletes. Female participants reported higher symptoms on all postconcussion factors than male participants.

Conclusion.—The current findings reveal different symptom factors at baseline and postinjury and several age and sex differences on the symptom factors. At postconcussion, symptoms aggregated into a global concussion factor including cognitive, fatigue, and migraine symptoms. Symptoms reported at baseline are not the same as those reported after injury. The presence of a global postconcussion symptom comprising the fatigue factor highlights the importance of physical and cognitive rest during the first week after a concussion. Although headache was the most commonly reported symptom, it was not the greatest contributor to the global postconcussion symptom factor.

▶ The postconcussion symptom checklist is still the gold standard for the clinical recognition of concussion. Generally, the 22-to-26 symptom checklist that can be used groups symptoms in the cognitive, somatic, emotional, and sleep categories. These authors chose to look at the symptoms in high school and college athletes at baseline and following a concussion, grouping the symptoms into 4 categories: cognitive-sensory, sleep-arousal, vestibular-somatic, and affective. They found distinctly different baseline profiles in the high school and college athletes, with the high school athletes reporting higher baseline levels of cognitive-sensory and vestibular-somatic symptoms and lower levels of sleep-arousal symptoms. This very likely reflects the later nights and less sleep obtained by the college athletes. These authors found a higher level of postconcussion symptoms in female athletes as compared with male athletes. More than 15 different sports were included in this study, so the findings were clearly not sport-specific. The female athletes in this study also had more postconcussion symptoms at baseline than male athletes. Thus, studies, with one exception to this reviewer's knowledge, continue to support age and gender differences at baseline and following athletic concussions.

R. C. Cantu, MD, MA

Use of a rapid visual screening tool for the assessment of concussion in amateur rugby league: A pilot study
King D, Clark T, Gissane C (Auckland Univ of Technology, New Zealand; Massey Univ, Wellington, New Zealand; St Mary's Univ College, Twickenham, Middlesex, UK)
J Neurol Sci 320:16-21, 2012

Aim.—This study undertook to use the K-D sideline test with the SCAT2 to see if concussions could be identified in amateur rugby league players over a representative competition period.

Method.—A prospective cohort study was conducted on two teams participating in an amateur rugby league. All players were tested for signs of concussion utilising the K-D test and players with longer times than their baseline scores undertook a further concussion assessment with the SCAT2.

Results.—Five athletes with suspected concussion were evaluated by K-D testing. Three concussions were associated with witnessed events during the matches and two athletes were identified by the team medic as having longer K-D time scores incidentally post-match compared to baseline. Post-match K-D scores for all concussed athletes were worse than baseline for those with reported or witnessed concussion events (7 s; 5.0–7.1; $p = 0.025$) and for those identified incidentally (>5 s; 8.9–9.1 s). Both groups also reported more symptoms on the PCSS (a part of the SCAT2) post-match.

Discussion.—In this rugby cohort, the K-D test was not only useful in identifying changes in players with witnessed head trauma, but in identifying changes in players with an un-witnessed suspected concussion.

▶ It is estimated that roughly 50% of brain pathways involve visual/oculomotor and learning functions. It is thus not surprising that after traumatic brain injuries, visual symptoms and oculomotor and learning functions are impaired. The King-Devick (K-D) test uses a series of charts of numbers that progressively become more difficult to read in a flowing manner and thus discern impaired oculomotor functions. It has been proposed as a rapid sideline screening tool for concussion that is quicker to administer than the Standard Assessment of Concussion or the Sports Concussion Assessment Tool. This study in a small number of participants confirmed the efficacy of this tool. All athletes with concussions were noted to have K-D scores worse than baseline. In 2 instances, athletes with unwitnessed head trauma but with impaired K-D scores postmatch were indeed found to have suffered a concussion. This supports the K-D test as being a useful tool for decision-making with regard to ruling in or out a player's further participation in a contest.

R. C. Cantu, MD, MA

Choice of Reliable Change Model Can Alter Decisions Regarding Neuropsychological Impairment After Sports-Related Concussion
Hinton-Bayre AD (Univ of Queensland, Brisbane, Australia)
Clin J Sport Med 22:105-108, 2012

Objective.—Impaired neuropsychological test performance after concussion has been used to guide restraint from play, in particular using reliable change indices (RCI). It remains unclear which of the RCI is most appropriate.

Design.—Athletes were assessed prospectively before and after cerebral concussion and compared with control athletes.

Setting.—Athletes were assessed in a clinical office environment after referral from a Sports Physician.

Participants.—One hundred ninety-four Australian rugby league athletes were assessed preseason (time 1).

Interventions.—Twenty-seven concussed athletes were assessed 2 days after trauma (time 2) and compared with 26 distribution-matched volunteer uninjured controls.

Main Outcome Measures.—Cognitive performance was assessed on 5 neuropsychological measures of speed of information processing, psychomotor speed, and response inhibition. Four previously reported RCI models used in sports concussion were contrasted, as described by Barr and McCrea (2001) and Maassen et al (2006).

Results.—Reliable change index models were marginally comparable in classifying the control sample. In the concussed sample, no one model seemed to be consistently more or less sensitive. Moreover, the same model could be most sensitive for one individual and least sensitive for another, even on the same test.

Conclusions.—Reliable change index models can yield different outcomes regarding whether an athlete has experienced cognitive impairment after concussion. Reliable change index model sensitivity to impairment depends on multiple test and situational factors, including test-retest reliability, differences in test and retest variances, and the individual's relative position on initial testing. In the absence of consensus, the clinician must use highly reliable measures with suitably matched controls if using an RCI.

▶ The use of paper-and-pencil neuropsychological test batteries in concussion without a baseline preconcussion evaluation uses normative data and the "Reliable Change Index" (RCI). The RCI has been based on normative data from comparable controls tested on 2 occasions in time. This researcher found that RCI models can yield very different outcomes if the athlete has experienced cognitive impairment. Furthermore, no one RCI model was felt to be consistently superior to another. Thus, it was the conclusion of these researchers and is supported by this reviewer that when paper-and-pencil neuropsychological testing is carried out that a suitably trained neuropsychologist should be involved in the interpretation of changed scores after concussion. This has long been the opinion of neuropsychologists such as William Barr, Michael McCrea, and Rubin Echemendia and is certainly supported by this reviewer. Only a trained neuropsychologist can fully interpret the RCI, which is susceptible to multiple test situational factors, including test–retest reliability, variances, and the individual's relative position on initial testing.

R. C. Cantu, MD, MA

Efficacy of Immediate and Delayed Cognitive and Physical Rest for Treatment of Sports-Related Concussion
Moser RS, Glatts C, Schatz P (Sports Concussion Ctr of New Jersey, Lawrenceville)
J Pediatr 161:922-926, 2012

Objectives.—To evaluate the efficacy of cognitive and physical rest for the treatment of concussion.

Study Design.—High school and collegiate athletes (N = 49) underwent post-concussion evaluations between April 2010 and September 2011 and were prescribed at least 1 week of cognitive and physical rest. Participants were assigned to groups on the basis of the time elapsed between sustaining a concussion and the onset of rest (1-7 days, 8-30 days, 31 + days). Main outcome measures included Concussion Symptom Scale ratings and scores on the 4 composite indices of the Immediate Post-Concussion Assessment and Cognitive Testing measure, both before and following rest. Mixed-factorial design ANOVA were used to compare changes on the dependent measures within and between groups.

Results.—Participants showed significantly improved performance on Immediate Post-Concussion Assessment and Cognitive Testing and decreased symptom reporting following prescribed cognitive and physical rest ($P < .001$), regardless of the time between concussion and onset of rest ($P = .44$).

Conclusion.—These preliminary data suggest that a period of cognitive and physical rest may be a useful means of treating concussion-related symptoms, whether applied soon after a concussion or weeks to months later.

▶ The participants in this study were 49 college-aged individuals who sustained an athletic concussion. Immediate Post-Concussion Assessment and Cognitive Testing was the tool used to evaluate cognitive functioning and symptoms. It is well known and documented that physical and cognitive rest is the hallmark of clinical management of an acute concussion. This is the first study to this reviewer's knowledge that documents a similar benefit from physical and cognitive rest in individuals with postconcussion syndrome more than a month after they sustained their acute concussion. Clearly further research and careful evaluation is needed, especially in light of the increasing documentation regarding the emotional benefit of low-level physical exertion below levels that provoke any concussion symptoms in postconcussion syndrome patients.

R. C. Cantu, MD, MA

Content Validity of the Rodeo-SCAT

Lafave MR, Butterwick DJ, Murray RP, et al (Mount Royal Univ, Calgary, Canada; Univ of Calgary, Canada; Mountain Orthopedics, Bountiful, UT; et al)
Int J Sports Med 34:170-175, 2013

The purpose of this study was to establish the content validity of the Rodeo SCAT for the sport of rodeo and bull riding. The study design was comprised of expert consensus and content validation. A modified Ebel procedure was employed to content validate the rodeo SCAT. Content validation using this method includes experts agreeing on the importance of each item that comprises the rodeo SCAT. This 3-stage process involved: 1) face validation by a local committee: 2) initial expert consensus measurement via distance; and 3) a face-to-face discussion for items that did not originally achieve 80% consensus of the group. Experts were chosen from the Canadian Professional Rodeo Sport Medicine Team (Canada) and the Justin Sports Medicine Team (USA). 27 out of a total possible 68 items achieved 80% consensus in the second stage. In the third stage, 4 of the 68 items were removed with consensus from the expert group. All remaining items achieved 80% consensus for inclusion. In summary, the rodeo SCAT is content valid and thus, appropriate for use in the sport of rodeo context or environment.

▶ The Concussion in Sport (CIS) group has recently created the Sport Concussion Assessment Tool (SCAT) 3 and the Child SCAT, which was published in the March 2013 issue of the *International Journal of Sports Medicine*. These authors, using portions of the SCAT 1 and SCAT 2, developed a consensus tool to be used in rodeo and bull riding-specific environments. This reviewer is impressed with the sport-specific nature of the rodeo SCAT that, because it has undergone the consensus review process, will undoubtedly have a higher use by medical professionals working in the rodeo sports medicine injury area than if it had not undergone this process to make it sports-specific. It thus can serve as a model for other sports at high risk of concussion that are outside of the mainstream of school sports.

R. C. Cantu, MD, MA

Age-Related Differences and Reliability on Computerized and Paper-and-Pencil Neurocognitive Assessment Batteries

Register-Mihalik JK, Kontos DL, Guskiewicz KM, et al (WakeMed Health & Hosps, Raleigh, NC; The Univ of North Carolina at Chapel Hill; Matthew Gfeller Sport-Related Traumatic Brain Injury Res Ctr, Raleigh, NC; et al)
J Athl Train 47:297-305, 2012

Context.—Neurocognitive testing is a recommended component in a concussion assessment. Clinicians should be aware of age and practice effects on these measures to ensure appropriate understanding of results.

Objective.—To assess age and practice effects on computerized and paper-and-pencil neurocognitive testing batteries in collegiate and high school athletes.

Design.—Cohort study.

Setting.—Classroom and laboratory.

Patients or Other Participants.—Participants consisted of 20 collegiate student-athletes (age = 20.00 ± 0.79 years) and 20 high school student-athletes (age = 16.00 ± 0.86 years).

Main Outcome Measure(s).—Hopkins Verbal Learning Test scores, Brief Visual-Spatial Memory Test scores, Trail Making Test B total time, Symbol Digit Modalities Test score, Stroop Test total score, and 5 composite scores from the Immediate Post-Concussion Assessment and Cognitive Testing (ImPACT) served as outcome measures. Mixed-model analyses of variance were used to examine each measure.

Results.—Collegiate student-athletes performed better than high school student-athletes on ImPACT processing speed composite score ($F_{1,38} = 5.03$, $P = .031$) at all time points. No other age effects were observed. The Trail Making Test B total time ($F_{2,66} = 73.432$, $P < .001$), Stroop Test total score ($F_{2,76} = 96.85$, $P = < .001$) and ImPACT processing speed composite score ($F_{2,76} = 5.81$, $P = .005$) improved in test sessions 2 and 3 compared with test session 1. Intraclass correlation coefficient calculations demonstrated values ranging from 0.12 to 0.72.

Conclusions.—An athlete's neurocognitive performance may vary across sessions. It is important for clinicians to know the reliability and precision of these tests in order to properly interpret test scores.

▶ These authors concluded what has been found by others—that an athlete's neurocognitive performance, whether it be measured with paper-and-pencil testing such as the Hopkins Verbal Learning Test, Brief Visual-Spatial Memory Test, Trail Making Test B, Symbol Digit Modality Test, Stroop Test, or neurocognitive computer-based testing such as ImPACT—varies widely from one test session to another. Therefore, it is imperative that clinicians understand the reliability and precision of these tests to properly interpret test scores. This reviewer feels strongly that paper-and-pencil neuropsychological tests should only be administered and interpreted by suitably trained neuropsychologists. This has long been the feeling of eminent neuropsychologists but has been felt by some to reflect protection of their turf. To this reviewer, however, it reflects the complexity of the test's interpretation, which can be so highly influenced by the motivation of the individual at the time the test is taken.

R. C. Cantu, MD, MA

Sports-Related Concussion: Assessment and Management
Ma R, Miller CD, Hogan MV, et al (Univ of Virginia, Charlottesville)
J Bone Joint Surg Am 94:1618-1627, 2012

▶ Most major U.S. professional sports and the National Collegiate Athletic Association (NCAA) have adopted concussion policies. Current National Football League and NCAA guidelines do not permit an athlete with a concussion to return to play on the same day as the injury. No adolescent or high-school athletes with a concussion should be allowed to return to play on the same day regardless of severity.

▶ Loss of consciousness is uncommon with concussion.

▶ Acute concussion symptoms are generally self-limited, and most symptoms typically resolve within two weeks. Concussion risk and severity may be affected by age, sex, and genetic predisposition.

▶ Athletes with a concussion should rest physically and cognitively until symptoms have resolved at rest and with exertion. Rehabilitation following concussion progresses through a stepwise graded fashion.

▶ Neuropsychological testing can provide objective data on an athlete after a concussion. However, it alone cannot be used to diagnose a concussion or determine when an athlete is allowed to return to play.

▶ Retirement from contact or collision sports may be necessary for an athlete who has sustained multiple concussions or has a history of prolonged symptoms after concussions.

▶ Long-term effects of concussions are still relatively unknown, and further research is required to offer guidance for athletes of all levels.

▶ This is a relatively good review of sports-related concussion, especially as to recognition and management. I would take issue with several comments in the article in which the authors say "helmets have been shown to decrease head injuries and concussion risks by reducing the acceleration of the head on impact." Whereas helmets clearly do reduce the risk of head injuries such as skull fractures and intracranial bleeding, they do not significantly reduce the risk of concussion from rotational forces. A helmet can reduce focal linear impacts such as a stick to the head, but it does little in reducing the rotational accelerations, such as those sustained when one is hit on the side of the face mask in football. The Riddell study that these authors cite has notable design flaws, not the least of which was comparing new helmets with older helmets. I do agree with their conclusions that mouth guards have not been shown to reduce sports-related concussion.

The other part of this article, on chronic traumatic encephalopathy (CTE), is weak, but these are not CTE researchers. For a most up-to-date review of this subject, I suggest the 2012 *Brain* paper first authored by Ann McKee on 68 cases of CTE.

R. C. Cantu, MD, MA

Response to acute concussive injury in soccer players: is gender a modifying factor?
Zuckerman SL, Solomon GS, Forbes JA, et al (Vanderbilt Univ School of Medicine, Nashville, TN; Vanderbilt Sports Concussion Ctr, Nashville, TN; et al)
J Neursurg Pediatr 10:504-510, 2012

Object.—Several studies have suggested a gender difference in response to sports-related concussion (SRC). The Concussion in Sport group did not include gender as a modifying factor in SRC, concluding that the evidence at that point was equivocal. In the present study the authors endeavored to assess acute neurocognitive and symptom responses to an SRC in equivalent cohorts of male and female soccer players. The authors hypothesized that female athletes would experience greater levels of acute symptoms and neurocognitive impairment than males.

Methods.—Baseline symptom and neurocognitive scores were determined in 40 male and 40 female soccer players by using the Immediate Postconcussion Assessment and Cognitive Testing (ImPACT) scale prior to any SRC. After sustaining an SRC, each athlete completed postconcussion ImPACT tests and was carefully matched on a wide array of biopsychosocial variables. Baseline symptom and neurocognitive test scores were compared, and their acute symptoms and neurocognitive responses to concussive injury were assessed.

Results.—Specific a priori hypotheses about differences between males and females at baseline and at postconcussion measurements of verbal and visual memory ImPACT scores were evaluated according to simple main effects of the gender variable and according to baseline-to-postconcussion main effect and interaction of 2×2 split-plot ANOVA. Neither the interaction nor the main effects nor the simple main effects for either ImPACT variable were found to be statistically significant. Exploratory ANOVAs applied to the remaining ImPACT variables of visualmotor speed, reaction time, impulse control, and symptom total scores revealed only a single statistically significant baseline-to-postconcussion main effect for the symptom total.

Conclusions.—The results failed to replicate prior findings of gender-specific baseline neurocognitive differences in verbal and visual memory. The findings also indicated no differential gender-based acute response to concussion (symptoms or neurocognitive scores) among high school soccer players. The implications of these findings for the inclusion of gender as a modifying factor in this tightly matched cohort are addressed. Potential explanations for the null findings are discussed.

▶ In the past several years, there have been a number of publications that found an increased risk of concussions in female athletes playing the same sports as males (soccer, basketball, ice hockey). It has been speculated that the major reasons for this finding may be that females are more honest in reporting concussion symptoms and that their weaker necks place them at increased risk of sustaining a concussion. This reviewer is part of a submitted article studying high school athletes that did find those with weaker necks at greater risk of sustaining a concussion than those with stronger necks. Multiple studies have also found that females tend to recover from concussion more slowly than males. There also have been reports of gender-based symptom reporting differences in the acute postconcussive phase. These authors, using the Immediate Post-Concussion Assessment and Cognitive Testing (ImPACT) tool, found no gender differences. This underscores the need for further research regarding gender-based differences in the acute concussion response in high school athletes. It is possible the lack of differences in this study is explained by the modest sample size.

R. C. Cantu, MD, MA

Spectrum of acute clinical characteristics of diagnosed concussions in college athletes wearing instrumented helmets

Duhaime A-C, Beckwith JG, Maerlender AC, et al (Harvard Univ, Boston, MA; Simbex, Lebanon, NH; Dartmouth Med School, Lebanon, NH; et al)
J Neurosurg 117:1092-1099, 2012

Object.—Concussive head injuries have received much attention in the medical and public arenas, as concerns have been raised about the potential short- and long-term consequences of injuries sustained in sports and other activities. While many student athletes have required evaluation after concussion, the exact definition of concussion has varied among disciplines and over time. The authors used data gathered as part of a multiinstitutional longitudinal study of the biomechanics of head impacts in helmeted collegiate athletes to characterize what signs, symptoms, and clinical histories were used to designate players as having sustained concussions.

Methods.—Players on 3 college football teams and 4 ice hockey teams (male and female) wore helmets instrumented with Head Impact Telemetry (HIT) technology during practices and games over 2–4 seasons of play. Preseason clinical screening batteries assessed baseline cognition and reported symptoms. If a concussion was diagnosed by the team medical staff, basic descriptive information was collected at presentation, and concussed players were reevaluated serially. The specific symptoms or findings associated with the diagnosis of acute concussion, relation to specific impact events, timing of symptom onset and diagnosis, and recorded biomechanical parameters were analyzed.

Results.—Data were collected from 450 athletes with 486,594 recorded head impacts. Forty-eight separate concussions were diagnosed in 44 individual players. Mental clouding, headache, and dizziness were the most common presenting symptoms. Thirty-one diagnosed cases were associated with an identified impact event; in 17 cases no specific impact event was identified. Onset of symptoms was immediate in 24 players, delayed in 11, and unspecified in 13. In 8 cases the diagnosis was made immediately after a head impact, but in most cases the diagnosis was delayed (median 17 hours). One diagnosed concussion involved a 30-second loss of consciousness; all other players retained alertness. Most diagnoses were based on self-reported symptoms. The mean peak angular and rotational acceleration values for those cases associated with a specific identified impact were 86.1 ± 42.6 g (range $16.5-177.9$ g) and 3620 ± 2166 rad/sec^2 (range $183-7589$ rad/sec^2), respectively.

Conclusions.—Approximately two-thirds of diagnosed concussions were associated with a specific contact event. Half of all players diagnosed with concussions had delayed or unclear timing of onset of symptoms. Most had no externally observed findings. Diagnosis was usually based on a range of self-reported symptoms after a variable delay. Accelerations clustered in the higher percentiles for all impact events, but encompassed a wide range. These data highlight the heterogeneity of criteria for concussion diagnosis, and in this sports context, its heavy reliance on self-reported symptoms. More specific and standardized definitions of clinical and objective correlates of a "concussion spectrum" may be needed in future research efforts, as well as in the clinical diagnostic arena.

▶ It is well known that many mild concussions are not recognized at the time of injury and that concussion symptoms can be delayed in their onset. This study involving male and female college football and ice hockey teams found that nearly half of the players diagnosed with concussions had delayed or unclear timing of the onset of symptoms. In reality, that group either escaped concussion recognition on the day of the game or perhaps truly did not have symptoms until several days later.

This group was all instrumented with Head Impact Telemetry (HIT) technology. Those with concussions had an incredibly wide range of recorded linear accelerations (16.5 g—177.9 g) and rotational accelerations (range 183—7589 rads/sec^2). This wide range raises the question of the accuracy of the HIT technology in off-center of gravity head hits in which the helmet may be spun on the head and the accelerometers uncoupled from the scalp, resulting in spuriously low recordings of linear and rotational accelerations.

R. C. Cantu, MD, MA

American Medical Society for Sports Medicine position statement: concussion in sport
Harmon KG, Drezner JA, Gammons M, et al (Univ of Washington, Seattle; Vermont Orthopaedic Clinic, Rutland; et al)
Br J Sports Med 47:15-26, 2013

Purpose of the Statement.— ▶ To provide an evidence-based, best practises summary to assist physicians with the evaluation and management of sports concussion.

▶ To establish the level of evidence, knowledge gaps and areas requiring additional research.

Importance of an AMSSM Statement.—▶ Sports medicine physicians are frequently involved in the care of patients with sports concussion.

▶ Sports medicine physicians are specifically trained to provide care along the continuum of sports concussion from the acute injury to return-to-play (RTP) decisions.

▶ The care of athletes with sports concussion is ideally performed by healthcare professionals with specific training and experience in the assessment and management of concussion. Competence should be determined by training and experience, not dictated by specialty.

▶ While this statement is directed towards sports medicine physicians, it may also assist other physicians and healthcare professionals in the care of patients with sports concussion.

Definition.—▶ Concussion is defined as a traumatically induced transient disturbance of brain function and involves a complex pathophysiological process. Concussion is a subset of mild traumatic brain injury (MTBI) which is generally self-limited and at the less-severe end of the brain injury spectrum.

Pathophysiology.—▶ Animal and human studies support the concept of postconcussive vulnerability, showing that a second blow before the brain has recovered results in worsening metabolic changes within the cell.

▶ Experimental evidence suggests the concussed brain is less responsive to usual neural activation and when premature cognitive or physical activity occurs before complete recovery the brain may be vulnerable to prolonged dysfunction.

Incidence.—▶ It is estimated that as many as 3.8 million concussions occur in the USA per year during competitive sports and recreational activities; however, as many as 50% of the concussions may go unreported.

▶ Concussions occur in all sports with the highest incidence in football, hockey, rugby, soccer and basketball.

Risk factors for Sport-Related Concussion.—▶ A history of concussion is associated with a higher risk of sustaining another concussion.

▶ A greater number, severity and duration of symptoms after a concussion are predictors of a prolonged recovery.

▶ In sports with similar playing rules, the reported incidence of concussion is higher in female athletes than in male athletes.

▶ Certain sports, positions and individual playing styles have a greater risk of concussion.

▶ Youth athletes may have a more prolonged recovery and are more susceptible to a concussion accompanied by a catastrophic injury.

▶ Preinjury mood disorders, learning disorders, attentiondeficit disorders (ADD/ADHD) and migraine headaches complicate diagnosis and management of a concussion.

Diagnosis of Concussion.—▶ Concussion remains a clinical diagnosis ideally made by a healthcare provider familiar with the athlete and knowledgeable in the recognition and evaluation of concussion.

▶ Graded symptom checklists provide an objective tool for assessing a variety of symptoms related to concussions, while also tracking the severity of those symptoms over serial evaluations.

▶ Standardised assessment tools provide a helpful structure for the evaluation of concussion, although limited validation of these assessment tools is available.

'Sideline' Evaluation and Management.—▶ Any athlete suspected of having a concussion should be stopped from playing and assessed by a licenced healthcare provider trained in the evaluation and management of concussions.

▶ Recognition and initial assessment of a concussion should be guided by a symptoms checklist, cognitive evaluation (including orientation, past and immediate memory, new learning and concentration), balance tests and further neurological physical examination.

▶ While standardised sideline tests are a useful framework for examination, the sensitivity, specificity, validity and reliability of these tests among different age groups, cultural groups and settings is largely undefined. Their practical usefulness with or without an individual baseline test is also largely unknown.

▶ Balance disturbance is a specific indicator of a concussion, but not very sensitive. Balance testing on the sideline may be substantially different than baseline tests because of differences in shoe/cleat-type or surface, use of ankle tape or braces, or the presence of other lower extremity injury.

▶ Imaging is reserved for athletes where intracerebral bleeding is suspected.

▶ There is no same day RTP for an athlete diagnosed with a concussion.

▶ Athletes suspected or diagnosed with a concussion should be monitored for deteriorating physical or mental status.

Neuropsychological Testing.—▶ Neuropsychological (NP) tests are an objective measure of brain—behaviour relationships and are more sensitive for subtle cognitive impairment than clinical exam.

▶ Most concussions can be managed appropriately without the use of NP testing.

▶ Computerised neuropsychological (CNP) testing should be interpreted by healthcare professionals trained and familiar with the type of test and the individual test limitations, including a knowledgeable assessment of the reliable change index, baseline variability and false-positive and falsenegative rates.

▶ Paper and pencil NP tests can be more comprehensive, test different domains and assess for other conditions which may masquerade as or complicate assessment of concussion.

▶ NP testing should be used only as part of a comprehensive concussion management strategy and should not be used in isolation.

▶ The ideal timing, frequency and type of NP testing have not been determined.

▶ In some cases, properly administered and interpreted NP testing provides an added value to assess cognitive function and recovery in the management of sports concussions.

▶ It is unknown if use of NP testing in the management of sports concussion helps prevent recurrent concussion, catastrophic injury or longterm complications.

▶ Comprehensive NP evaluation is helpful in the post-concussion management of athletes with persistent symptoms or complicated courses.

Return to Class.—▶ Students will require cognitive rest and may require academic accommodations such as reduced workload and extended time for tests while recovering from a concussion.

Return to Play.—▶ Concussion symptoms should be resolved before returning to exercise.

▶ A RTP progression involves a gradual, step-wise increase in physical demands, sports-specific activities and the risk for contact.

▶ If symptoms occur with activity, the progression should be halted and restarted at the preceding symptom-free step.

▶ RTP after concussion should occur only with medical clearance from a licenced healthcare provider trained in the evaluation and management of concussions.

Short-Term Risks of Premature RTP.—▶ The primary concern with early RTP is decreased reaction time leading to an increased risk of a repeat concussion or other injury and prolongation of symptoms.

Long-Term Effects.—▶ There is an increasing concern that head impact exposure and recurrent concussions contribute to long-term neurological sequelae.

▶ Some studies have suggested an association between prior concussions and chronic cognitive dysfunction. Large-scale epidemiological studies are needed to more clearly define risk factors and causation of any long-term neurological impairment.

Disqualification from Sport.—▶ There are no evidence-based guidelines for disqualifying/retiring an athlete from a sport after a concussion. Each case should be carefully deliberated and an individualised approach to determining disqualification taken.

Education.—▶ Greater efforts are needed to educate involved parties, including athletes, parents, coaches, officials, school administrators and healthcare providers to improve concussion recognition, management and prevention.

▶ Physicians should be prepared to provide counselling regarding potential long-term consequences of a concussion and recurrent concussions.

Prevention.—▶ Primary prevention of some injuries may be possible with modification and enforcement of the rules and fair play.

▶ Helmets, both hard (football, lacrosse and hockey) and soft (soccer, rugby) are best suited to prevent impact injuries (fracture, bleeding, laceration, etc.) but have not been shown to reduce the incidence and severity of concussions.

▶ There is no current evidence that mouth guards can reduce the severity of or prevent concussions.

▶ Secondary prevention may be possible by appropriate RTP management.

Legislation.—▶ Legislative efforts provide a uniform standard for scholastic and nonscholastic sports organisations regarding concussion safety and management.

Future Directions.—▶ Additional research is needed to validate current assessment tools, delineate the role of NP testing and improve identification of those at risk of prolonged post-concussive symptoms or other long-term complications.

▶ Evolving technologies for the diagnosis of concussion, such as newer neuroimaging techniques or biological markers, may provide new insights into the evaluation and management of sports concussion.

▶ This overall is a well-written position statement, especially with regard to the sideline evaluation and management of concussion. It also has an insightful section on prevention and a quite useful review of concussion-related legislation efforts at the state level. The one area of concern to this reviewer is their definition of concussion as a "traumatically induced transient disturbance of brain function." The term "transient" is contradictory to biological findings in animal models of injury, and neurophysiological and neuroimaging findings in humans, which suggest high risk for long-lasting, both ultrastructural and functional, brain alteration induced by even a single concussive blow. Using susceptibility-weighted imaging, functional magnetic imaging, diffusion tensor imaging, magnetic resonance spectroscopy, and positron emission tomography, advanced neuroimaging techniques have demonstrated structural and metabolic alterations after single and multiple concussions. Thus, a concussion is not purely metabolic in all instances and is often not transient but with long-lasting effects if advanced neurophysiological and neuroimaging modalities are used.

R. C. Cantu, MD, MA

2 Other Musculoskeletal Injuries

Shoulder, Arm, and Hand

Effect of specific exercise strategy on need for surgery in patients with subacromial impingement syndrome: randomised controlled study

Holmgren T, Björnsson Hallgren H, Öberg B, et al (Linköping Univ, Sweden; Univ Hosp, Sweden)

BMJ 344:e787, 2012

Objective.—To evaluate if a specific exercise strategy, targeting the rotator cuff and scapula stabilisers, improves shoulder function and pain more than unspecific exercises in patients with subacromial impingement syndrome, thereby decreasing the need for arthroscopic subacromial decompression.

Design.—Randomised, participant and single assessor blinded, controlled study.

Setting.—Department of orthopaedics in a Swedish university hospital.

Participants.—102 patients with long standing (over six months) persistent subacromial impingement syndrome in whom earlier conservative treatment had failed, recruited through orthopaedic specialists.

Interventions.—The specific exercise strategy consisted of strengthening eccentric exercises for the rotator cuff and concentric/eccentric exercises for the scapula stabilisers in combination with manual mobilisation. The control exercise programme consisted of unspecific movement exercises for the neck and shoulder. Patients in both groups received five to six individual guided treatment sessions during 12 weeks. In between these supervised sessions the participants performed home exercises once or twice a day for 12 weeks.

Main Outcome Measures.—The primary outcome was the Constant-Murley shoulder assessment score evaluating shoulder function and pain. Secondary outcomes were patients' global impression of change because of treatment and decision regarding surgery.

Results.—Most (97, 95%) participants completed the 12 week study. There was a significantly greater improvement in the Constant-Murley score in the specific exercise group than in the control exercise group (24 points (95% confidence interval 19 to 28.0) *v* 9 points (5 to 13); mean difference between group: 15 points (8.5 to 20.6)). Significantly more patients in the specific exercise group reported successful outcome (defined as large improvement or recovered) in the patients' global assessment of change because of treatment: 69% (35/51) *v* 24% (11/46); odds ratio 7.6, 3.1 to 18.9; *P* < 0.001. A significantly lower proportion of patients in the specific exercise group subsequently chose to undergo surgery: 20% (10/51) *v* 63% (29/46); odds ratio 7.7, 3.1 to 19.4; *P* < 0.001.

Conclusion.—A specific exercise strategy, focusing on strengthening eccentric exercises for the rotator cuff and concentric/eccentric exercises for the scapula stabilisers, is effective in reducing pain and improving shoulder function in patients with persistent subacromial impingement syndrome. By extension, this exercise strategy reduces the need for arthroscopic subacromial decompression within the three month timeframe used in the study.

Trial Registration.—Clinical trials NCT01037673.

▶ This is an interesting randomized, controlled trial with a fairly large sample of participants on the effects of exercise as a treatment for shoulder impingement syndrome. Although there is mounting evidence suggesting that supervised exercises and manual therapy delivered by physiotherapists are effective, the objective of this study is somewhat different, as one of the outcomes measured is the risk to undergo subacromial decompression after the initial exercise approach. Often, in clinic, when the initial conservative approach fails, patients are offered this surgery. The study included patients who were waiting for a subacromial decompression, some of whom were chronic cases with symptoms duration of more than 6 months and had a first rehabilitation protocol failure. This study shows that in conjunction with an initial steroid injection, a 3-month exercise program with an emphasis on eccentric strengthening and with a manual therapy intervention can significantly improve pain level and function. In terms of risk to undergo surgery, a significantly lower proportion of patients in the exercise group subsequently chose to undergo surgery: 20% (10 of 51) versus 63% (29 of 46); odds ratio 7.7, 3.1 to 19.4. The implications of such results are important and suggest that surgical options for this population should not be offered too quickly. Finally, while the study did not address this, it would have been interesting to see what the outcomes were in terms of pain and function in the 20% that decided to undergo subacromial decompression after the exercise regimen. It is possible that these patients did not do so well with surgery either.

F. Desmeules, PT, PhD

Manual Physical Therapy for Injection–Confirmed Nonacute Acromioclavicular Joint Pain

Harris KD, Deyle GD, Gill NW, et al (Brooke Army Med Ctr, Fort Sam Houston, TX)
J Orthop Sports Phys Ther 42:66-80, 2012

Study Design.—Prospective single-cohort study.

Objectives.—To determine and document changes in pain and disability in patients with primary, nonacute acromioclavicular joint (ACJ) pain treated with a manual therapy approach.

Background.—To our knowledge, there are no published studies on the physical therapy management of nonacute ACJ pain. Manual physical therapy has been successful in the treatment of other shoulder conditions.

Methods.—The chief inclusion criterion was greater than 50% pain relief with an ACJ diagnostic injection. Patients were excluded if they had sustained an ACJ injury within the previous 12 months. Treatment was conducted utilizing a manual physical therapy approach that addressed all associated impairments in the shoulder girdle and cervicothoracic spine. The primary outcome measure was the Shoulder Pain and Disability Index. Secondary measures were the American Shoulder and Elbow Surgeon and global rating of change scales. Outcomes were collected at baseline, 4 weeks, and 6 months. The Shoulder Pain and Disability Index and American Shoulder and Elbow Surgeon scale values were analyzed with a repeated-measures analysis of variance.

Results.—Thirteen patients (11 male; mean ± SD age, 41.1 ± 9.6 years) completed treatment consisting of an average of 6.4 sessions. Compared to baseline, there was a statistically significant and clinically meaningful improvement for the Shoulder Pain and Disability Index at 4 weeks ($P = .001$; mean, 25.9 points; 95% confidence interval [CI]: 11.9, 39.8) and 6 months ($P < .001$; mean, 29.8 points; 95% CI: 16.5, 43.0), and the American Shoulder and Elbow Surgeon scale at 4 weeks ($P < .001$; mean, 27.9 points; 95% CI: 14.7, 41.1) and 6 months ($P < .001$; mean, 32.6 points; 95% CI: 21.2, 43.9).

Conclusion.—Statistically significant and clinically meaningful improvements were observed in all outcome measures at 4 weeks and 6 months, following a short series of manual therapy interventions. These results, in a small cohort of patients, suggest the efficacy of this treatment approach but need to be verified by a randomized controlled trial.

Level of Evidence.—Therapy, level 4.

▶ Acromioclavicular joint (ACJ) pathology is not necessarily that frequent, but effective management of these patients remains a challenge. Therefore this is an interesting study, because there are very few trials looking at the effectiveness of conservative treatments for ACJ pain. Although physiotherapists report using manual therapy regularly to treat ACJ pain in nonacute and nontraumatic cases, this is the first published study with preliminary results on the effectiveness of this kind of approach. This is a single-cohort prospective study with a small sample size and therefore a formal conclusion regarding the effectiveness of this manual therapy intervention cannot be made at this point, but it does provide preliminary evidence that may guide the clinician when selecting treatment options for this population of patients. The authors have shown that a well-defined, efficient manual therapy intervention, mainly including passive mobilizations of the acromioclavicular joint, may be effective in reducing pain and improving function in this population. The improvements shown from validated outcome measures were all statistically and clinically important in the short term at 4 weeks and persisted 6 months after treatment. The methodological quality of the study is very good as eligibility criteria were well-defined and relevant to identify correctly patients suffering from ACJ pain, treatment regimen was standardized and relevant to current clinical practice, and the outcomes measures used were validated.

F. Desmeules, PT, PhD

Back and Hip

Evaluation of the Painful Athletic Hip: Imaging Options and Imaging-Guided Injections

Jacobson JA, Bedi A, Sekiya JK, et al (Univ of Michigan, Ann Arbor; et al)
AJR Am J Roentgenol 199:516-524, 2012

Objective.—This article reviews diagnostic imaging tests and injections that provide important information for clinical management of patients with sports-related hip pain.

Conclusion.—In the evaluation of sports-related hip symptoms, MR arthrography is often used to evaluate intraarticular pathology of the hip. The addition of short- and long-acting anesthetic agents with the MR arthrography injection adds additional information that can distinguish between symptomatic and asymptomatic imaging findings. Osseous abnormalities can be characterized with radiography, MRI, or CT. Ultrasound is important in the assessment of iliopsoas abnormalities, including tendon snapping, and to guide diagnostic anesthetic injection.

▶ This article reviews various differential diagnoses for sports-related hip pain, from the point of view of several radiologists. It covers imaging and imaging-guided anesthetic injections that are helpful and important in the workup and for potential surgical planning. General anatomy and common pathologies are reviewed, including injuries to the acetabular labrum and articular hyaline cartilage of the hip, femoroacetabular impingement of both the cam-type and the pincer-type, osteoarthritis, iliopsoas tendinosis/bursitis, and "snapping hip syndrome." Imaging options are plain radiographs (different views), ultrasound, magnetic resonance imaging (with intraarticular gadolinium), and computed tomography. The role of imaging-guided injections is also discussed. The accompanying figures (eg, Figs 2, 6, 7, 9, and 11 in the original article) provide excellent illustrations of specific conditions.

C. Lebrun, MDCM, MPE, CCFP, Dip Sport Med, FACSM

Does antenatal physical therapy for pregnant women with low back pain or pelvic pain improve functional outcomes? A systematic review
Richards E, van Kessel G, Virgara R, et al (Univ of South Australia, Adelaide, Australia; The Lyell McEwin Hosp, Adelaide, South Australia, Australia)
Acta Obstet Gynecol Scand 91:1038-1045, 2012

Objective.—A systematic review was undertaken to update the understanding of the available evidence for antenatal physical therapy interventions for low back or pelvic pain in pregnant women to improve functional outcomes when compared with other treatments or no treatment.

Data Sources.—Seven electronic databases were systematically searched and supplemented by hand searching through reference lists.

Methods of Study Selection.—Two reviewers independently selected trials for inclusion and independently assessed the internal validity of the included trials using the Clinical Appraisal Skills Program tool.

Results.—Four trials with 566 participants were identified that met the inclusion criteria. The validity of the trials was moderate. Exercise, pelvic support garments and acupuncture were found to improve functional outcomes in pregnant women with low back or pelvic pain. No meta-analysis was performed because of the heterogeneity of functional outcome measures.

Conclusions.—While there is some evidence that physical therapy using exercise, acupuncture and pelvic supports may be useful, further research needs to consider other treatment modalities used by physical therapists and establish an appropriate, reliable and valid functional outcome measure to assess low back and pelvic pain in pregnancy.

▶ Low back and pelvic pain in pregnant women are very prevalent and may lead to significant disability. Because of their condition and concern for fetal health, women may seek nonpharmacological treatment options, including physiotherapy. However, a significant proportion will seek the help of other unregulated practitioners, which may raise concerns regarding the safety and efficacy of the interventions then performed. Manual therapy interventions such as mobilizations and manipulations have been reported to be used by various unregulated practitioners, but experts support that they are contraindicated because of hormonal changes and hyperlaxity in pregnant woman. This review is interesting as it brings much-needed evidence to inform physicians, health care practitioners, and pregnant women of the benefits and safety of antenatal physiotherapy for low back or pelvic pain. This review concludes, although the evidence is scarce, that exercise such as core muscle training, pelvic floor muscle training, and stretching is effective in reducing disability in pregnant women. Moreover, a home exercise program under the supervision of a physiotherapist may be all that is needed to treat efficaciously this population. The addition of a support brace or belt may further improve the outcomes for these women.

F. Desmeules, PT, PhD

Leg, Knee, Ankle, and Foot

Anterior Cruciate Ligament Reconstruction in Skeletally Immature Patients With Transphyseal Tunnels
Redler LH, Brafman RT, Trentacosta N, et al (Columbia Univ Med Ctr, NY)
Arthroscopy 28:1710-1717, 2012

Purpose.—Our purpose was to evaluate the results of transphyseal anterior cruciate ligament (ACL) reconstruction with hamstring autograft in skeletally immature patients.

Methods.—Eighteen knees in 18 skeletally immature pubescent patients with a mean chronologic age of 14.2 years underwent transphyseal ACL reconstruction with hamstring autograft between 2002 and 2007. Concurrent meniscal surgery was performed in 9 knees. The final patient evaluation occurred at a mean of 43.4 months (range, 24.0 to 86.6 months) and included physical examination, KT-1000 arthrometry testing (MEDmetric, San Diego, CA), and functional outcome instruments, including the International Knee Documentation Committee subjective knee form, the Lysholm knee score, and the Tegner knee activity scale.

Results.—At the latest follow-up, the mean International Knee Documentation Committee subjective knee score was 92.4 ± 10, the mean Lysholm knee score was 94.3 ± 8.8, and the mean Tegner activity scale score was 8.5 ± 1.4. Lachman and pivot-shift testing were negative in all knees. No restriction in knee range of motion of 5° or greater when compared with the contralateral knee was observed in any patient. The mean manual maximum side-to-side difference with KT-1000 testing was 0.29 ± 1.07 mm, and no patients had a difference greater than 3 mm. No angular deformities were noted, and all leg-length measurements were symmetric bilaterally on clinical examination. No patients had traumatic graft disruption or underwent revision ACL reconstruction, whereas 3 patients sustained an ACL injury in the contralateral leg while participating in sports.

Conclusions.—Transphyseal ACL reconstruction with autogenous quadrupled hamstring graft with metaphyseal fixation in skeletally immature pubescent patients yielded excellent functional outcomes in a high percentage of patients without perceived clinical growth disturbance.

Level of Evidence.—Level IV, therapeutic case series.

▶ This is a relatively small (18 patients) retrospective case series of transphyseal anterior cruciate ligament (ACL) reconstruction in skeletally immature patients (mean chronological age, 14.2 years), using autogenous quadrupled hamstring graft with metaphyseal fixation. All procedures were performed by the principle investigator between 2002 and 2007, and there was a minimum follow-up time of 2 years. Theoretical concerns in such patients, with significant remaining growth potential, include partial or complete physeal arrest, resulting in subsequent limb-length discrepancy or angular deformity. However, nonoperative treatment has shown traditionally poor outcomes, especially in children who return to sport, with a substantial risk of further injury and progressive intra-articular damage, including secondary meniscal or chondral injuries. Physeal-sparing combined intra- and extra-articular reconstruction with an autogenous iliotibial band is neither anatomic nor isometric and requires excessive dissection. Therefore, it is reassuring to note the excellent functional outcome in this group of pubescent patients, based on validated objective functional outcome analyses (International Knee Documentation Committee or International Knee Documentation Committee subjective knee form, Lysholm knee score and Tegner activity scale), clinical examination, and KT-1000 arthrometer testing as well as clinical assessment of growth disturbances.

C. Lebrun, MDCM, MPE, CCFP, Dip Sport Med, FACSM

A Pair-Matched Comparison of Return to Pivoting Sports at 1 Year in Anterior Cruciate Ligament—Injured Patients After a Nonoperative Versus an Operative Treatment Course

Grindem H, Eitzen I, Moksnes H, et al (NIMI/NAR, Oslo, Norway; Oslo Univ Hosp, Norway; et al)
Am J Sports Med 40:2509-2516, 2012

Background.—Patients usually return to pivoting sports between 6 months and 1 year after anterior cruciate ligament (ACL) reconstruction, but no matched study has so far examined 1-year return to sport rates in nonoperatively and operatively treated ACL injured patients.

Hypothesis.—Anterior cruciate ligament-injured patients following a nonoperative treatment course, including recommendation of activity modification, will have lower return to pivoting sport rates than operatively treated patients 1 year after baseline testing/ surgery, when matched by preinjury sports activity, age, and sex.

Study Design.—Cohort study; level of evidence, 3.

Methods.—Sixty-nine nonoperatively treated ACL-injured patients were pair-matched with 69 operatively treated patients (n = 138), based on specific preinjury sport, age, and sex. Nonoperatively treated patients were recommended not to return to level I sports. Patients were defined as nonoperatively or operatively treated according to their status at follow-up. The baseline and follow-up testing included registration of sports participation, KT-1000 arthrometer measurements, 4 hop tests, and patient-reported outcome measures. McNemars test and paired t tests or Wilcoxon test were used to compare outcomes of nonoperatively and operatively treated patients.

Results.—No significant baseline differences were found. At 12.9 ± 1.2 months (mean ± standard deviation) after baseline testing (nonoperative) and 12.7 ± 1.2 months after surgery (operative), there was no significant difference in overall return to sport rates (nonoperative: 68.1%, operative: 68.1%, $P = 1.00$), or in return to level I sport rates (nonoperative: 54.8%, operative: 61.9%, $P = .66$). Nonoperatively treated patients who participated in level I sports before injury had a significantly

TABLE 3.—Outcomes at 1-Year Follow-up[a]

	Nonoperative (n = 69)	Operative (n = 69)	P
Overall return to sport[b]	47/69 (68.1%)	47/69 (68.1%)	1.00
Return to level I sport[b]	23/42 (54.8%)	26/42 (61.9%)	.66
Return to level II sport[b]	24/27 (88.9%)	21/27 (77.8%)	.51
Sports frequency, times per week	3.3 (1.6)	3.3 (1.8)	.83
KT-1000 side-to-side difference, mm	5.6 (2.8)	2.7 (1.8)	<.001
Single hop for distance, LSI	96.3 (6.4)	90.5 (14.0)	.009
Crossover hop, LSI	95.9 (6.2)	91.3 (11.2)	.02
Triple hop for distance, LSI	97.1 (5.5)	92.6 (11.4)	.01
6-m timed hop, LSI	97.7 (5.5)	93.5 (9.8)	.005
KOS-ADLS	95.4 (4.9)	91.0 (7.7)	<.001
GRS for knee function	88.8 (12.0)	88.7 (10.7)	.95
IKDC 2000	88.5 (9.2)	85.0 (11.6)	.05

[a]Values are presented as mean (standard deviation) unless otherwise inidicated. GRS, global rating scale; IKDC, International Knee Documentation Committee Subjective Knee Form; KOS-ADLS, Knee Outcome Survey Activities of Daily Living; LSI, limb symmetry index.
[b]Patients returned/patients who participated in the respective level of sport preinjury (%).

lower return to sport rate (54.8%) than nonoperatively treated patients who participated in level II sports (88.9%, P = .003). The nonoperatively treated patients had significantly higher knee joint laxity, but significantly better hop test limb symmetry indexes, Knee Outcome Survey Activities of Daily Living scores, and International Knee Documentation Committee Subjective Knee Form 2000 scores. None of the functional differences was larger than the smallest detectable difference.

Conclusion.—Anterior cruciate ligament-injured patients following a nonoperative treatment course, including recommendations of activity modifications, and operatively treated patients did not have significantly different rates of returning to pivoting sports after 1 year in this pair-matched cohort study. Clinicians should be aware of a potentially high level of noncompliance to recommendations of activity modifications. Although these results show that it is possible for nonoperatively treated patients to return to sport after rehabilitation, future follow-ups are needed to examine whether these patients maintain sports participation over time, and what long-term consequences they may suffer regarding subsequent injuries and knee osteoarthritis (Table 3).

▶ This pair-matched comparison of operatively and nonoperatively treated patients with anterior cruciate ligament injury is the first and the largest study to examine return to pivoting sport activities at 1 year. The strengths of this study lie in the careful matching of specific preinjury sport, sex, and age as well as the rigorous collection of data measuring physical (KT-1000 side-to-side difference), functional (limb symmetry index for 4 hop tests), and quality-of-life (and sport) outcomes in each group at baseline and after 1 year. Pivoting sports were divided into level I (frequent pivoting—soccer, team handball, floorball, basketball) and level II (less frequent pivoting—racket sports, alpine skiing, snowboarding, gymnastics, aerobics). A surprising finding was that there was no significant difference between groups in the rate of return to pivoting sports after 1 year (Table 3), despite the recommendations for activity modifications for the nonoperatively treated patients. Nonoperatively treated patients who participated in level I sports had a significantly lower return to sports rate (54.8%) than patients who participated in level II sports prior to injury (88.9%). However, as the factors influencing surgical decision making included a wish to return to level I sports, dynamic instability, age, and the preferred treatment of the patient, it is possible that this may have introduced a confounding bias. In addition, few centers would be able to achieve the same degree of successful rehabilitation of patients as this institution. Their program included heavy resistance strength training, neuromuscular training, and plyometric exercises, with stringent return to sport criteria of at least 90% hamstring and quadriceps strength, and limb symmetry indexes of at least 90% on 4 hop tests. Nevertheless, these results show that it is possible for nonoperatively treated patients to return to pivoting sports after rehabilitation; the question remains unanswered as to what long-term consequences they may suffer, such as subsequent injuries and knee osteoarthritis.

C. Lebrun, MDCM, MPE, CCFP, Dip Sport Med, FACSM

Anterior Cruciate Ligament Injuries: Anatomy, Physiology, Biomechanics, and Management
Siegel L, Vandenakker-Albanese C, Siegel D (Occidental College, Los Angeles, CA; Univ of California, Davis; Northern California Health Care System, Mather)
Clin J Sport Med 22:349-355, 2012

Objective.—Anterior cruciate ligament (ACL) injuries are the most common ligament injury in the United States. These injuries can be career ending for athletes and severely disabling for all individuals. Our objectives are review the epidemiology of these injuries, as well as ACL biomechanics, anatomy, and nonsurgical and surgical management so that generalists as well as sports medicine physicians, orthopedists, and others will have a better understanding of this serious injury as well as choices in its management.

Data Sources.—PubMed was used to identify relevant articles. These articles were then used to identify other sources.

Main Results.—Anterior cruciate ligament injuries occur more commonly in women than in men due to a variety of anatomical factors. The ACL consists of 2 major bundles, the posterolateral and the anteromedial bundles. Forces transmitted through these bundles vary with knee-joint position. Some patients with ACL injuries may not be candidates for surgery because of serious comorbid medical conditions. However, without surgical repair, the knee generally remains unstable and prone to further injury. There are a variety of surgical decisions that can influence outcomes. Single-bundle versus double-bundle repair, whether to leave the ruptured ACL remnant in the knee, the selection of the graft tissue, graft placement, and whether to use the transtibial, far anteromedial portal, or tibial tunnel-independent technique are choices that must be made.

A

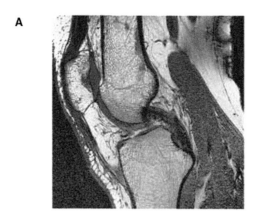

B

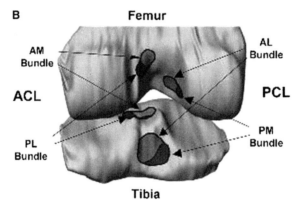

FIGURE 1.—A, MRI of the knee. B, A knee model with ACL and PCL bundle insertion sites for a typical subject. Taken from Li et al[19] with permission. *Editor's Note*: Please refer to original journal article for full references. (Reprinted from Siegel L, Vandenakker-Albanese C, Siegel D. Anterior cruciate ligament injuries: anatomy, physiology, biomechanics, and management. *Clin J Sport Med*. 2012;22:349-355, with permission from Lippincott Williams & Wilkins.)

Conclusions.—With a sound knowledge of the anatomy and kinetics of the knee, newer improved surgical techniques have been developed that can restore proper knee function and have allowed many athletes to resume their careers. These new techniques have also limited the disability in nonathletes (Fig 1).

▶ This is a focused review based on a search of PubMed (and additional sources) regarding issues of interest to clinicians who take care of patients with anterior cruciate ligament (ACL) injuries. The topic headings include the following: factors that contribute to ACL injuries (female sex, neuromuscular and biomechanical risk factors); ACL anatomy (Fig 1) and ACL biomechanics; diagnosis of ACL injuries; nonsurgical (conservative) and surgical management (graft selection, single-bundle vs double-bundle reconstruction, graft placement, femoral tunnel drilling techniques); and postoperative rehabilitation and future directions. The reference list contains some older, classic articles as well as recent more up-to-date research. Although it is not possible in a 7-page journal article to go into great detail on any specific topic, this article provides a convenient and concise overview of the most important and relevant issues in ACL injuries, all in one place.

C. Lebrun, MDCM, MPE, CCFP, Dip Sport Med, FACSM

Application of a Clinic-Based Algorithm as a Tool to Identify Female Athletes at Risk for Anterior Cruciate Ligament Injury: A Prospective Cohort Study With a Nested, Matched Case-Control Analysis

Goetschius J, Smith HC, Vacek PM, et al (Univ of Vermont College of Medicine, Burlington; et al)

Am J Sports Med 40:1978-1984, 2012

Background.—When landing from a jump, the production of increased intersegmental knee abduction moments and coupled valgus motions has been associated with an increased risk of suffering a noncontact anterior cruciate ligament (ACL) injury in one study. This research has led to the development of a clinic-based algorithm that utilizes measures of knee valgus motion, knee flexion range of motion, body mass, tibial length, and quadriceps-to-hamstring strength ratio data to predict the probability of a high knee abduction moment (pKAM) when landing from a jump in female athletes. The ability of this algorithm to identify athletes at increased risk of suffering ACL injury has not been assessed.

Hypothesis.—The pKAM is associated with ACL injury in female athletes.

Study Design.—Case-control study; Level of evidence, 3.

Methods.—This study was based on secondary analysis of data obtained from a previous investigation that focused on the use of the drop vertical jump (DVJ) test to assess the risk of ACL injury in female athletes. The DVJ screenings were performed on 1855 female high school and college athletes over 3 years. Knee valgus motion, knee flexion range of motion, and tibial length were measured from videos of the DVJ obtained during preseason screenings. Mass was measured using a physicians scale, and quadriceps-to-hamstring strength ratio was included using a surrogate value. These data were entered into the clinic-based algorithm that determined the pKAM. The association of pKAM with ACL injury was assessed using conditional logistic regression.

Results.—A total of 20 athletes sustained ACL injury and were matched with 45 uninjured control athletes who were recruited from the same teams. There was no relationship between the risk of suffering ACL injury and pKAM, as determined by the clinic-based algorithm.

Conclusion.—The pKAM was not associated with noncontact ACL injury in our group of injured athletes and matched controls (Figs 1-5).

▶ Anterior cruciate ligament (ACL) injuries in young people are devastating, and not only are they immediately disabling, but they also lead to premature onset of

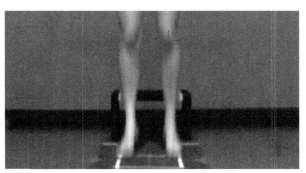

FIGURE 1.—Knee joint center at initial contact with the ground during the landing phase of the drop vertical jump. The + represents the location of the knee joint center at initial contact of the foot with the ground. (Reprinted from Goetschius J, Smith HC, Vacek PM, et al. Application of a clinic-based algorithm as a tool to identify female athletes at risk for anterior cruciate ligament injury: a prospective cohort study with a nested, matched case-control analysis. *Am J Sports Med*. 2012;40:1978-1984, with permission from The Author(s).)

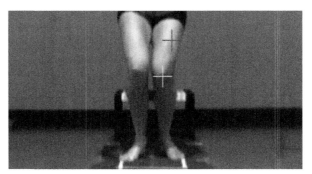

FIGURE 2.—Knee joint center at maximum medial position during the landing phase of the drop vertical jump. The top + represents the location of the knee joint center at initial contact with the ground, and the bottom + is the knee joint center at its maximum medial position during landing. (Reprinted from Goetschius J, Smith HC, Vacek PM, et al. Application of a clinic-based algorithm as a tool to identify female athletes at risk for anterior cruciate ligament injury: a prospective cohort study with a nested, matched case-control analysis. *Am J Sports Med*. 2012;40:1978-1984, with permission from The Author(s).)

osteoarthritis, regardless of operative or conservative management. Female athletes are more prone to ACL injuries than their male colleagues, for a variety of reasons, including biomechanical and neuromuscular factors, some of which are amenable to preventive training programs. Therefore a logical step is to somehow screen large groups of athletes and find those who might benefit from such programs. The risk of suffering a noncontact ACL injury has been associated with increased intersegmental knee abduction moment and valgus angle at the knee, increased foot-floor reaction force, and decreased stance time when landing. These have been measured, using video analyses, in a laboratory setting, during dynamic tests such as the drop vertical jump (DVJ). However, the use of such advanced technology is largely limited to research laboratories able to carry out these complex assessments and are out of reach and impractical for the majority of practicing clinicians. An attempt has been made to develop a clinic-based algorithm to predict the probability of a high knee abduction moment

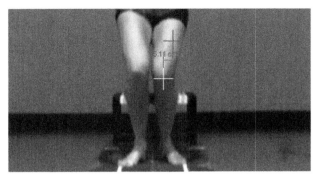

FIGURE 3.—Knee valgus motion during the landing phase of the drop vertical jump (DVJ). The line between the top and bottom + is a measurement of knee motion from initial contact with the ground to the maximum medial position of the knee during the landing portion of the DVJ. (Reprinted from Goetschius J, Smith HC, Vacek PM, et al. Application of a clinic-based algorithm as a tool to identify female athletes at risk for anterior cruciate ligament injury: a prospective cohort study with a nested, matched case-control analysis. *Am J Sports Med.* 2012;40:1978-1984, with permission from The Author(s).)

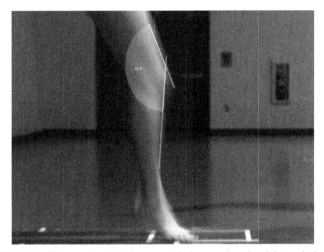

FIGURE 4.—Knee flexion angle at initial contact with the ground produced during the landing phase of the drop vertical jump. (Reprinted from Goetschius J, Smith HC, Vacek PM, et al. Application of a clinic-based algorithm as a tool to identify female athletes at risk for anterior cruciate ligament injury: a prospective cohort study with a nested, matched case-control analysis. *Am J Sports Med.* 2012;40:1978-1984, with permission from The Author(s).)

(pKAM), based on 2-dimensional (2D) video data obtained with standard video cameras (Figs 1-5).[1] These clinic-based surrogate variables have been shown to have a high correlation with the more sophisticated laboratory based 3-dimensional biomechanical measurements obtained by this latter group of researchers. The current study retrospectively analyzes 2D motion analyses of 1855 DVJ screenings on female high school and college athletes over 3 years, as well as a "clinician-friendly" nomogram to allow the evaluation of pKAM.[2] Using a nested case-control analysis (with 1-3 matched control athletes from the same team, and the same age as the 20 athletes who sustained an ACL tear over the 3-year time

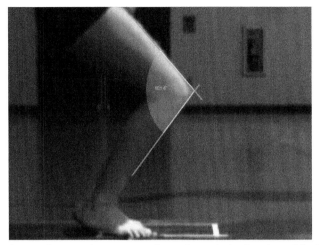

FIGURE 5.—Knee flexion angle at maximum flexion during the landing phase of the drop vertical jump. (Reprinted from Goetschius J, Smith HC, Vacek PM, et al. Application of a clinic-based algorithm as a tool to identify female athletes at risk for anterior cruciate ligament injury: a prospective cohort study with a nested, matched case-control analysis. *Am J Sports Med.* 2012;40:1978-1984, with permission from The Author(s).)

span), and conditional logistic regression, it was determined that the clinic-based algorithm of pKAM was not useful (in this study) for identifying female athletes at increased risk of suffering a noncontact ACL injury. Therefore, additional research is needed to develop such screening tools that can be applied in an efficient manner to large groups of participants. In the meantime, preventive intervention programs will need to be applied to populations as a whole, rather than focusing on just those at increased risk.

C. Lebrun, MDCM, MPE, CCFP, Dip Sport Med, FACSM

References

1. Myer GD, Ford KR, Khoury J, Succop P, Hewett TE. Development and validation of a clinic-based prediction tool to identify female athletes at high risk for anterior cruciate ligament injury. *Am J Sports Med.* 2010;38:2025-2033.
2. Myer DG, Ford KR, Hewett TE. New method to identify athletes at high risk of ACL injury using clinic-based measurements and free-ward computer analysis. *Br J Sports Med.* 2011;45:238-244.

Changes in Self-Reported Knee Function and Health-Related Quality of Life After Knee Injury in Female Athletes
McGuine TA, Winterstein A, Carr K, et al (Univ of Wisconsin-Madison)
Clin J Sport Med 22:334-340, 2012

Objective.—To document the changes in self-reported health-related quality of life and knee function in a cohort of young female athletes who have sustained a knee injury.

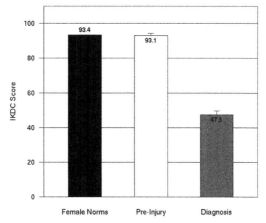

FIGURE 1.—Knee function scores for female normative data as well as all subjects before injury and at diagnosis (mean scores). (Reprinted from Mcguine TA, Winterstein A, Carr K, et al. Changes in self-reported knee function and health-related quality of life after knee injury in female athletes. *Clin J Sport Med*. 2012;22:334-340, with permission from Lippincott Williams & Wilkins.)

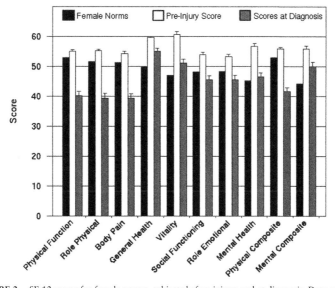

FIGURE 2.—SF-12 scores for female norms, subjects before injury, and at diagnosis. Data reported as the mean (SD) scores. (Reprinted from Mcguine TA, Winterstein A, Carr K, et al. Changes in self-reported knee function and health-related quality of life after knee injury in female athletes. *Clin J Sport Med*. 2012;22:334-340, with permission from Lippincott Williams & Wilkins.)

Design.—Prospective cohort.

Setting.—An outpatient sports medicine clinic and university student health service.

Participants.—A convenience sample of 255 females (age = 17.4 ± 2.4 years) who injured their knee participating in sport or recreational activities. Injuries were categorized as anterior cruciate ligament tears, anterior knee pain, patellar instability, meniscus tear, collateral ligament sprain, and other.

Interventions.—Knee function was assessed with the 2000 International Knee Documentation Committee (IKDC) knee survey. Health-related quality of life was assessed with the SF-12 version 2.0 (acute) survey (SF-12).

Main Outcome Measures.—Dependent variables included the paired differences in the 2000 IKDC and SF-12 subscales, and composite scores from preinjury to diagnosis. Paired differences were assessed with paired t tests ($P < 0.05$) reported as the mean ± SD.

Results.—International Knee Documentation Committee scores at diagnosis were significantly lower than preinjury scores ($P < 0.001$). SF-12 scores were lower ($P < 0.001$) at diagnosis for each subscale (physical functioning, role physical, bodily pain, general health, vitality, social function, role emotional, and mental health) as well as the physical and mental composite scores.

Conclusions.—In addition to negatively affecting knee function, sport medicine providers should be aware that knee injuries can negatively impact the health-related quality of life in these athletes immediately after injury (Figs 1 and 2).

▶ This is a prospective cohort study (convenience sample) of 255 females, presenting to 2 different sport medicine clinics, with specific knee injury diagnoses grouped into 1 of 6 classifications. These were anterior cruciate ligament (ACL) tears: anterior knee pain (AKP), including patellofemoral stress syndrome, patellar tendonitis, fat pad impingement, Osgood-Schlatter disease, medial plica irritation, and iliotibial band syndrome; meniscal tears of the medial or lateral meniscus; collateral ligament sprains (COL) of the medial and lateral collateral ligaments; patellar instability (PAT), including patellar dislocations and subluxations; and other injuries, including contusions, intra-articular loose bodies, osteochondritis dissecans, and fractures. After diagnosis, each subject was asked to complete 2 questionnaires—the 2000 International Knee Documentation Committee Subjective Knee Form—which is a joint-specific, patient-oriented survey that assesses symptoms, as well as function in daily living and sport activities, consisting of 18 multiple choice questions and also a self-reported health-related quality of life (HRQOL) questionnaire, the SF-12 (a shortened version of the widely used SF-36). What is interesting about the design of the study is that the subjects were asked to complete the questionnaire 2 times—the first representing how they considered their knee function (KF) and HRQOL in the week prior to the injury (preinjury), and a second time representing how they were feeling since they sustained their knee injury (diagnosis). Because the subjects were initially examined and enrolled approximately 12 days postinjury (median 12, 25th 7, and 75th

21 days), this approach was justified by the investigators based on the fact that previous researchers have validated the ability of athletes to recall health status up to 4 weeks to 8 weeks before data collection.[1] However, the authors do acknowledge that this is a potential source of bias, where subjects might overestimate their KF and HRQOL before injury. Nevertheless, this study demonstrates that any kind of knee injury, even those considered less serious or not routinely requiring surgical intervention (such as AKP, PAT, and COL) has a significant impact on KF and HRQOL, similar to the more serious ACL injuries (Figs 1 and 2). The authors thus advocate documenting both joint-specific changes and function, as well as HRQOL for athletes who have sustained other common sports injuries. In addition, longitudinal studies to follow the injury rehabilitation process up to and after the return to sport, would be very meaningful, particularly in those subjects who experienced sports-related injuries in adolescence.

C. Lebrun, MDCM, MPE, CCFP, Dip Sport Med, FACSM

Reference

1. Valuri F, Stevenson M, Finch, Hamer P, Elliott B. The validity of a four week self-recall of sports injuries. *Inj Prev.* 2005;11:135-137.

Treatment of Knee Joint Osteoarthritis with Autologous Platelet-Rich Plasma in Comparison with Hyaluronic Acid
Spaková T, Rosocha J, Lacko M, et al (Associated Tissue Bank of Faculty of Medicine UPJS and Univ Hosp of L. Pasteur, Kosice, Slovakia; P. J. Safárik Univ and Univ Hosp of L. Pasteur, Kosice, Slovakia)
Am J Phys Med Rehabil 91:411-417, 2012

Objective.—This study aimed to find a simple, cost-effective, and time-efficient method for the preparation of platelet-rich plasma (PRP), so the acquired benefits will be readily available for multiple procedures in smaller outpatient clinics and to explore the safety and efficacy of the application of PRP in the treatment of degenerative lesions of articular cartilage of the knee.

Design.—The study was designed as a prospective, cohort study with a control group. A total of 120 patients with Grade 1, 2, or 3 osteoarthritis according to the Kellgren and Lawrence grading scale were enrolled in the study. One group of patients was treated using three intra-articular applications of PRP, and the second group of patients was given three injections of hyaluronic acid. Outcome measures included the Western Ontario and McMaster Universities Osteoarthritis Index and the 11-point pain intensity Numeric Rating Scale.

Results.—On average, a 4.5-fold increase in platelet concentration was obtained in the PRP group. No severe adverse events were observed. Statistically significantly better results in the Western Ontario and McMaster Universities Osteoarthritis Index and Numeric Rating Scale scores were recorded in a group of patients who received PRP injections after a 3- and 6-mo follow-up.

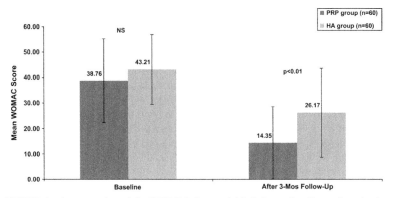

FIGURE 1.—A mean value of the WOMAC Osteoarthritis Index at baseline and at the 3- and 6-mo follow-up in the PRP and HA groups. $P < 0.01$ between groups. WOMAC, Western Ontario and McMaster Universities; NS, nonsignificant; HA, hyaluronic acid; PRP, platelet-rich plasma. (Reprinted from Spaková T, Rosocha J, Lacko M, et al. Treatment of knee joint osteoarthritis with autologous platelet-rich plasma in comparison with hyaluronic acid. *Am J Phys Med Rehabil.* 2012;91:411-417, with permission from Lippincott Williams & Wilkins.)

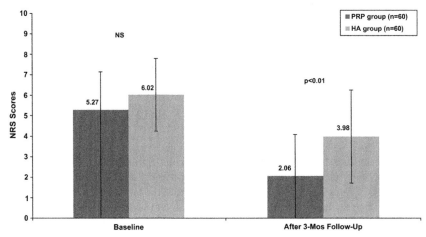

FIGURE 2.—A mean value of NRS at baseline during the 3- and 6-mo follow-up in the PRP and HA groups. $P < 0.01$ between groups. NS, nonsignificant; NRS, 11-point pain intensity Numeric Rating Scale; PRP, plateletrich plasma. (Reprinted from Spaková T, Rosocha J, Lacko M, et al. Treatment of knee joint osteoarthritis with autologous platelet-rich plasma in comparison with hyaluronic acid. *Am J Phys Med Rehabil.* 2012;91:411-417, with permission from Lippincott Williams & Wilkins.)

Conclusions.—Our preliminary findings support the application of autologous PRP as an effective and safe method in the treatment of the initial stages of knee osteoarthritis. Further studies are needed to confirm these results and to investigate the persistence of the beneficial effects observed (Figs 1 and 2).

▶ This was a relatively large prospective study comparing 3 injections of platelet-rich plasma (PRP) with 3 injections of a preparation of hyaluronic acid (HA) in the management of osteoarthritis of the knee. Results at 3 and 6 months demonstrated significantly better outcomes in the PRP group as compared with the HA group, at least in those that were measured (Figs 1 and 2). The Western Ontario and McMaster Universities Osteoarthritis Index assesses quality of life, as well as pain and function, whereas the Numeric Rating Scale primarily documents pain. Theoretically anyway, there appears to be some logic to the use of PRP in osteoarthritis and cartilage repair because of the ability of various growth factors to enhance matrix synthesis. This is related to the recruitment of chondrogenic cells, stimulation of proliferation, and enhancement of cartilage matrix synthesis. There has been quite a bit of basic science research done in this area, but investigations in human subjects are more difficult to carry out. They will require not only accurate grading of osteoarthritis prior to treatment, but characterization of any actual healing that is proposed to take place. In this study, the Kellgren and Lawrence radiographic classification system was used to grade the degree of osteoarthritis in subjects, using non—weight-bearing X-rays and magnetic resonance imaging of the affected knee. The 6-month follow-up period is not long enough to warrant radiological reassessment, but future studies should include much longer follow-ups, more in the range of years, than months. In addition, given the present trend toward a single injection of HA instead of 3 weekly injections, investigations should also be conducted comparing similar single PRP injections. The relative costs of both are similar, but patients may well balk at the thought of having blood drawn on 3 separate occasions as well as having the 3 injections done. Biologically, however, the use of PRP may make better sense because it is thought to actually promote healing, rather than just restore the viscosity and lubrication of the synovial fluid, as HA is purported to do. It will also be necessary to document the platelet concentration, pH of the PRP, and its activation status in all future investigations.

C. Lebrun, MDCM, MPE, CCFP, Dip Sport Med, FACSM

Best tests/clinical findings for screening and diagnosis of patellofemoral pain syndrome: a systematic review

Cook C, Mabry L, Reiman MP, et al (Walsh Univ, North Canton, OH; Kaiser Permanente Med Ctr, Vallejo, CA; Duke Univ School of Medicine, Durham, NC)

Physiotherapy 98:93-100, 2012

Background.—Diagnosis of patellofemoral pain syndrome (PFPS) is commonly performed using a myriad of clinical and imaging-based criteria.

Objectives.—The objective of this systematic literature review was to summarize the research on accuracy of individual clinical tests/findings for PFPS.

Data Sources.—MEDLINE, ProQuest Nursing and Allied Health, Cochrane Trials, PEDro, and CINAHL.

Study Selection or Eligibility Criteria.—PRISMA guidelines were followed for this review. To be considered for review, the study required: (1) a description of a clinical test or tests used for diagnosing PFPS (including a test that was combined with another finding such as patient history), (2) a report of the diagnostic accuracy of the measures (e.g., sensitivity *and* specificity), and (3) an acceptable reference standard for comparison.

Study Appraisal or Synthesis Methods.—Quality Assessment of Studies of Diagnostic Accuracy (QUADAS) scores were completed on each selected article. Sensitivity, specificity, and negative and positive likelihood ratios (LR−/LR+) were calculated for each diagnostic test described.

Results.—The systematic search strategy and hand search revealed 704 potential articles, 9 of which met the criteria for this review; analysing a total of 22 PFPS clinical tests. After assessment using the QUADAS score, 1 of the 9 articles was of high quality. The tests with the highest reported diagnostic value were also associated with studies that had the lowest QUADAS values.

Conclusion.—A majority of the studies that have investigated diagnostic accuracy of clinical tests for PFPS demonstrate notable design or reporting biases, and at this stage, determining the best tests for diagnosis of PFPS is still difficult.

▶ Patellofemoral pain syndrome (PFPS) is a common knee disorder that clinicians encounter frequently in primary care. At the present time, there is no consensus on the specific diagnostic criteria for PFPS, and its diagnosis remains a challenge for clinicians. This systematic review using the Preferred Reporting Items for Systematic Reviews and Meta-Analyses (PRISMA) methodology synthesizes evidence and evaluates the methodological quality of studies regarding the diagnostic validity of clinical physical tests for PFPS that have been published in the literature. However, the methodological quality of included studies was generally, at best, only moderate. This review is interesting for clinicians because it brings much-needed evidence on the best diagnostic validity of clinical physical tests for PFPS. The results should be interpreted with caution, but some tests tended to show better diagnostic validity for PFPS: the Active Instability test, pain during stair climbing, Clarke's test, pain during prolonged sitting, patellar inferior pole tilt, and pain during squatting. It is important to note that for some of these tests the diagnostic accuracy values varied significantly between studies, and many of these studies had notably lower methodological scores, meaning that the results presented may be biased. Generally diagnostic studies with poor methodological quality will tend to overestimate diagnostic accuracy. The findings of this review are nonetheless useful for clinicians and may help design better diagnostic studies in the future. Of note, previously published studies only address the diagnostic validity of specific tests for PFPS when individually performed. This is a limitation because it does not reflect the differential diagnosis process where a clinician uses the patient's history elements and multiple physical tests to make a diagnosis. Future diagnostic studies also need to address this issue to better reflect clinical practice.

F. Desmeules, PT, PhD

The Effects of Group Cycling on Gait and Pain-Related Disability in Individuals With Mild-to-Moderate Knee Osteoarthritis: A Randomized Controlled Trial

Salacinski AJ, Krohn K, Lewis SF, et al (Northern Illinois Univ, DeKalb, IL; Mercy Hosp, Pittsburgh, PA; et al)
J Orthop Sports Phys Ther 42:985-995, 2012

Study Design.—Randomized controlled trial.

Objective.—To determine the effectiveness of a community-based program of stationary group cycling on gait, pain, and physical function in individuals with mild-to-moderate knee osteoarthritis (OA).

Background.—Knee pain and disability are common symptoms in individuals with knee OA. Though exercise for knee OA has acknowledged benefits, it has the potential to aggravate symptoms in some instances.

Methods.—Thirty-seven subjects (27 women, 10 men) with a mean ± SD age of 57.7 ± 9.8 years were randomly assigned to a cycling (n = 19) or control (n = 18) group for a 12-week intervention study. Outcome variables, measured at baseline and 12 weeks, included preferred and maximal gait velocity, a visual analog pain scale at rest and following a 6-minute walk test, muscle strength, and functional-outcome questionnaires. Data were analyzed using mixed-model analyses of variance for group and time differences.

Results.—After 12 weeks, the individuals receiving the cycling intervention showed significantly greater improvements ($P < .05$) for preferred gait velocity (mean difference between groups, 8.7 cm/s; 95% confidence interval [CI]: 2.2, 15.1), visual analog pain scale on the 6-minute walk test (mean difference, 16.5 mm; 95% CI: 2.1, 31.0), the Western Ontario and McMaster Universities Osteoarthritis Index pain subscale (mean difference, 14.9 points; 95% CI: 2.6, 27.0) and stiffness subscale (mean difference, 10.8 points; 95% CI: 0.7, 21.3), the Knee injury and Osteoarthritis Outcome Score pain subscale (mean difference, 13.3 points; 95% CI: 3.4, 23.3), and the Knee Outcome Survey activities of daily living subscale (mean difference, 13.9 points; 95% CI: 2.0, 25.9) compared to controls.

Conclusion.—Stationary group cycling may be an effective exercise option for individuals with mild-to-moderate knee OA and may reduce pain with walking. US trial registration NCT00917618.

Level of Evidence.—Therapy level 1b−.

▶ Knee osteoarthritis (OA) is a common cause of knee pain and may incur significant disability. There has been an important increase in the incidence of knee OA in the past several decades, and predictions suggest this trend will continue for years to come. New simple and accessible cost-efficient nonpharmacological strategies are needed to help these patients. This randomized clinical trial addresses this issue. Although exercise therapy has been found to be effective for knee OA and is now recommended as probably the most important component of a nonpharmacological approach to treat patients with mild to moderate OA, this study chose to use a simpler approach. The intervention under study is the effect on pain and disability in knee OA participants of a cycling exercise class, without any stretching, range of motion, or strengthening exercises. The program consisted of a 12-week adapted spinning class (at least twice a week). Participants showed clinically important and statistically significant improvements compared with a control group in terms of pain and disability measured by 2 validated self-reported questionnaires and during performance tests. This study therefore brings interesting evidence that cardiovascular training through adapted spinning classes may be helpful for this population and could be a viable option to patients who do not have access to physiotherapy treatments. Moreover, because this is a group training intervention, it may increase social support and adherence to treatment.

F. Desmeules, PT, PhD

Musculoskeletal and Estrogen Changes during the Adolescent Growth Spurt in Girls

Wild CY, Steele JR, Munro BJ (Univ of Wollongong, Australia)
Med Sci Sports Exerc 45:138-145, 2013

Introduction.—The adolescent growth spurt is associated with rapid growth and hormonal changes, thought to contribute to the increased anterior cruciate ligament injury risk in girls. However, relatively little is known about these musculoskeletal and estrogen changes during the growth spurt in girls.

Purpose.—To investigate the longitudinal changes in estrogen as well as anterior knee laxity and lower limb strength and flexibility throughout the adolescent growth spurt in girls.

Methods.—Thirty-three healthy girls, age 10–13 yr, in Tanner stage II and 4–6 months from their peak height velocity were recruited. Participants were tested up to four times during the 12 months of their growth spurt, according to the timing of their maturity offset (test 1: maturity offset = −6 to −4 months; test 2: maturity offset = 0 months; test 3: maturity offset = +4 months; test 4: maturity offset = +8 months). During each testing session, anterior knee laxity, lower limb flexibility, and isokinetic strength as well as saliva measures of estradiol concentration were measured.

Results.—A significant ($P = 0.002$) effect of time on anterior knee laxity was found from the time of peak height velocity, although no changes in estradiol concentration were displayed over time ($P = 0.811$). Participants displayed a significant increase ($P < 0.05$) in isokinetic quadriceps strength over time, with no apparent increase in isokinetic hamstring strength.

Conclusions.—We speculate that increased quadriceps strength, combined with increased knee laxity and no accompanying hamstring strength development during the adolescent growth spurt in girls, might contribute to a decrease in their knee joint stability during landing tasks. These musculoskeletal changes could potentially increase anterior cruciate

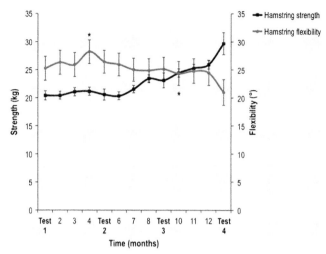

FIGURE 3.—Means ± SE for the month-to-month changes in hamstring flexibility and isometric hamstring strength for 12 months (note that an increase in angle indicates a decrease in hamstring flexibility; *significant main effect of time on the dependent variable, $P < 0.05$). (Reprinted from Wild CY, Steele JR, Munro BJ. Musculoskeletal and estrogen changes during the adolescent growth spurt in girls. *Med Sci Sports Exerc*. 2013;45:138-145, with permission from the American College of Sports Medicine.)

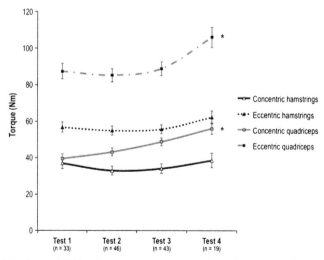

FIGURE 5.—Means ± SE for the concentric and eccentric hamstrings and quadriceps torque (N·m) over the four laboratory test sessions (*significant main effect of time on the strength variable, $P < 0.05$). (Reprinted from Wild CY, Steele JR, Munro BJ. Musculoskeletal and estrogen changes during the adolescent growth spurt in girls. *Med Sci Sports Exerc*. 2013;45:138-145, with permission from the American College of Sports Medicine.)

ligament injury risk at a time of rapid height and lower limb growth (Figs 3 and 5).

▶ Noncontact anterior cruciate ligament (ACL) injuries account for 37% of all knee injuries in pubescent girls. Landing from jumps is an example of an activity that increases ACL injury due to knee laxity. The rapid growth spurt of the lower limb and torso before and after peak height velocity (PHV), respectively, are suspected in the etiology of ACL injury. That is, the rapid change in segmental skeletal length is unmatched by changes in muscular strength and flexibility. They hypothesized that girls would display a consistent increase in hamstring and quadriceps strength without a strength spurt, a decrease in lower limb flexibility around PHV, and a rapid increase in estrogen and anterior knee laxity throughout the growth spurt. Thirty-three girls, ages 10 to 13, began the study in Tanner stage II and were followed up with for up to 4 testing periods over 1 year, with additional home-based testing every month. Girls who reached menarche were excluded from further testing. The offset of PHV was estimated by regression techniques and categorized as 6-to-4 months from PHV, up to +8 months from PHV. In support of the hypothesis, rapid changes in height, flexibility, and knee laxity occurred throughout the growth spurt. The bones grew faster than the musculature. Hamstring flexibility decreased significantly when analyzed monthly. Further, hamstring strength did not increase from month to month, whereas quadriceps strength increased (Figs 3 and 5). Thus, 2 qualities of the hamstrings, flexibility and strength, lagged behind the skeletal growth spurt and may contribute to ACL injury risk. Knee joint laxity increased significantly, but estrogen did not. The clinical recommendation emerging from this study was that girls should be evaluated frequently (monthly) during puberty to evaluate lower limb flexibility. The typical test of touching fingers to the floor is insufficient given that an increase in torso length may mask lower extremity flexibility. Instead, these investigators used goniometry to assess flexibility of the dominant limb, a technique that would likely be in the repertoire of athletic trainers or sports medicine-trained clinicians but not a family practitioner. The longitudinal measures are an asset to the study, but validation of the musculoskeletal changes in a larger study is warranted.

C. M. Jankowski, PhD

A physiotherapy perspective of musculoskeletal imaging in sport
Callaghan MJ (Univ of Manchester, UK)
Br J Radiol 85:1194-1197, 2012

This paper presents a physiotherapy perspective on the role that imaging is now playing in the diagnosis and management of musculoskeletal and sporting injuries. Although the Royal College of Radiologists and the UK Chartered Society of Physiotherapy were founded in the latter part of the nineteenth century, it is 100 years later that developments in the UK NHS have led to increased roles for non-medical healthcare professionals and allied health professionals, such as physiotherapists, in an extended clinical role. Physiotherapists, perhaps because of their knowledge of clinical and applied anatomy, have keenly taken up the opportunities offered to request and interpret imaging in its various forms; the most commonly available are plain radiography, musculoskeletal ultrasound and MRI. This has meant taking formal courses under the auspices of universities with mentorship and tutoring within the clinical setting, which are part of a continuing professional development. The ability to request several forms of imaging has enhanced physiotherapy practice and has increased the appreciation of the responsibilities which accompany this new role.

▶ This is an interesting summary on the use of imaging modalities by physiotherapists, in particular, ultrasound imaging. It is with great interest that we see now emerging new roles for physiotherapists (advanced or extended roles). Although these roles vary from country to country, with these new roles, diagnosis and the use of imaging to aid diagnosis is certainly an exciting development for the physiotherapy profession. It is important to stress how ultrasound imaging is well suited to fall in the hands of physiotherapists. Physiotherapists are experts at diagnosing soft tissue musculoskeletal disorders and have been found to be highly skilled and more competent compared with other health professionals and physicians. Because of its dynamic nature and portability, musculoskeletal ultrasound scan is well suited to aid physiotherapists in the diagnosis of these disorders in the clinic or on the field when following sports events and teams.

Moreover, this article also outlined that once a diagnosis has been established, evidence shows that ultrasound scan may be effectively used for rehabilitation purposes, such as for biofeedback and dynamic assessment of muscles and tendons function. Finally, this review makes the case for the use of ultrasound scan when physiotherapists are able to do injections. Again, it is important to realize that the use of ultrasound scan by physiotherapists has the objective of improving diagnosis, treatment, and access to care for these patients and should be done in the most efficient manner.

F. Desmeules, PT, PhD

The Lichfield bone study: the skeletal response to exercise in healthy young men

Eleftheriou KI, Rawal JS, Kehoe A, et al (Univ College London Hosps, UK; Derriford Hosp, Devon, England; et al)
J Appl Physiol 112:615-626, 2012

The skeletal response to short-term exercise training remains poorly described. We thus studied the lower limb skeletal response of 723 Caucasian male army recruits to a 12-wk training regime. Femoral bone volume was assessed using magnetic resonance imaging, bone ultrastructure by quantitative ultrasound (QUS), and bone mineral density (BMD) using dual-energy X-ray absorptiometry (DXA) of the hip. Left hip BMD increased with training (mean ± SD: $0.85 ± 3.24$, $2.93 ± 4.85$, and $1.89 ± 2.85\%$ for femoral neck, Ward's area, and total hip, respectively;

TABLE 3.—MRI Measurements on Both Left and Right Femurs for Army Recruits Before and After Their 12-wk Training

	Pretraining (All Data)	Pretraining (Paired Data)	Posttraining (Paired Data)	Mean of % Changes	Paired t-test
n	650	399	399		
PV (right)	26,250.3 ± 3,330.6	26,435.7 ± 3,229.5	2,6617.0 ± 3,132.2	0.78 ± 3.14	<0.001
EV (right)	6,149.6 ± 1,927.0	6,136.4 ± 1,876.4	6,121.7 ± 1,801.2	0.44 ± 10.26	0.66
CV (right)	20,100.7 ± 2,622.5	20,299.3 ± 2,505.9	20,495.3 ± 2,449.7	1.09 ± 4.05	<0.001
PV (left)	25,547.7 ± 3,189.0	25,781.0 ± 3,134.9	25,915.7 ± 3,066.4	0.59 ± 2.58	<0.001
EV (left)	6,026.9 ± 1,850.3	6,019.0 ± 1,843.9	6,034.0 ± 1,767.3	1.13 ± 11.75	0.68
CV (left)	19,520.9 ± 2,588.7	19,762.0 ± 2,527.8	19,881.7 ± 2,501.2	0.71 ± 4.05	0.003

Values are means ± SD in mm^3; n, no. of measurements. Similar changes were seen on both legs, with periostial (PV) and cortical volume (CV) increasing significantly after the 12-wk training program ($P \leq 0.003$), with no change seen in the endostial volume (EV) ($P \geq 0.66$).

all $P < 0.001$). Left calcaneal broadband ultrasound attenuation rose $3.57 \pm 0.5\%$ ($P < 0.001$), and left and right femoral cortical volume by 1.09 ± 4.05 and $0.71 \pm 4.05\%$, respectively ($P = 0.0001$ and 0.003), largely through the rise in periosteal volume (0.78 ± 3.14 and $0.59 \pm 2.58\%$ for right and left, respectively, $P < 0.001$) with endosteal volumes unchanged. Before training, DXA and QUS measures were independent of limb dominance. However, the dominant femur had higher periosteal ($25,991.49$ vs. $2,5572$ mm^3, $P < 0.001$), endosteal ($6,063.33$ vs. $5,983.12$ mm^3, $P = 0.001$), and cortical volumes ($19,928$ vs. $19,589.56$ mm^3, $P = 0.001$). Changes in DXA, QUS, and magnetic resonance imaging measures were independent of limb dominance. We show, for the first time, that short-term exercise training in young men is associated not only with a rise in human femoral BMD, but also in femoral bone volume, the latter largely through a periosteal response (Table 3).

▶ It is widely accepted that bone mineral density is increased by physical activity and decreased by immobilization. It is also generally agreed that the bones of the dominant limb are larger than those of the nondominant limb, particularly in athletes. Further, an increase of bone volume has been demonstrated in rodents after 10 weeks of endurance training.[1] However, the direct magnetic resonance imaging demonstration of an increase in human bone dimensions over a short (12-week) basic military training program is a novel finding, and the monitoring of such bone strengthening may have practical relevance to the prevention of fractures among those who have begun training hard.[2-4] The program of strength, endurance, and circuit training and team sports adopted for entry-level military recruits was rigorous, demanding a total energy expenditure of 15 MJ/day (many sedentary people do not spend more than 10 MJ/d), and perhaps because of this rigor it was apparently completed by less than 400 of the 723 recruits. Even with 12 weeks of heavy mechanical loading, the external dimensions of the femur only increased by about 1% (Table 3). Given that the age of the recruits was 20 ½ years, it is possible that some individuals were still growing, and a more precise estimate of exercise-related gains in bone dimensions would require collection of data on a control group. The study would also have been enhanced if it had collected details of diet before recruitment and while undertaking basic training.

R. J. Shephard, MD (Lond), PhD, DPE

References

1. Joo YI, Sone T, Fukunaga M, Lim SG, Onodera S. Effects of endurance exercise on three-dimensional trabecular bone microarchitecture in young growing rats. *Bone.* 2003;33:485-493.
2. Hong SH, Chu IT. Stress fracture of the proximal fibula in military recruits. *Clin Orthop Surg.* 2009;1:161-164.
3. Kiuru MJ, Niva M, Reponen A, Pihlajamäki HK. Bone stress injuries in asymptomatic elite recruits: a clinical and magnetic resonance imagingstudy. *Am J Sports Med.* 2005;33:272-276.
4. Evans RK, Negus C, Antczak AJ, Yanovich R, Israeli E, Moran DS. Sex differences in parameters of bone strength in new recruits: beyond bone density. *Med Sci Sports Exerc.* 2008;40:S645-S653.

Collagen Genes and Exercise-Associated Muscle Cramping

O'Connell K, Posthumus M, Schwellnus MP, et al (Univ of Cape Town, South Africa)

Clin J Sport Med 23:64-69, 2013

Objective.—The authors hypothesized that variants within genes, such as *COL5A1, COL3A1, COL6A1,* and *COL12A1,* that code for connective tissue components of the musculoskeletal system may modulate susceptibility to exercise-associated muscle cramping (EAMC). Specifically, the aim of this study was to investigate if the *COL5A1 rs12722 (C/T), COL3A1* rs1800255 (G/A), *COL6A1* rs35796750 (T/C), and *COL12A1* rs970547 (A/G) polymorphisms are associated with a history of EAMC.

Design.—Retrospective genetic case—control association study.

Setting.—Participants were recruited at triathlon and ultra-marathon events and were asked to report physical activity, medical history, and cramping history.

Participants.—One hundred sixteen participants with self-reported history of EAMC within the past 12 months before an ultra-endurance event were included as cases in this study (EAMC group). One hundred fifty participants with no self-reported history of previous (lifelong) EAMC were included as controls (NON group).

Interventions.—All participants were genotyped for the selected variants.

Main Outcome Measures.—Differences in genotype frequency distributions, for *COL5A1 rs12722, COL3A1* rs1800255, *COL6A1* rs35796750, and *COL12A1* rs970547, among the cases and controls.

Results.—The *COL5A1* CC genotype was significantly overrepresented ($P = 0.031$) among the NON group (21.8%) when compared with the EAMC group (11.1%). No significant genotype differences were found for

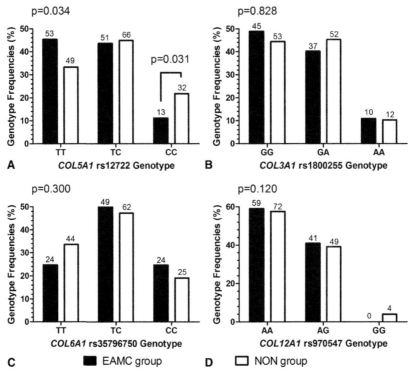

FIGURE 1.—Genotype frequencies for the participants who reported a history of EAMC within 12 months before the event (EAMC group) and those with no self-reported history of previous (lifelong) EAMC (NON group) for (A) *COL5A1* rs12722, (B) *COL3A1* rs1800255, (C) *COL6A1* rs35796750, and (D) *COL12A1* rs970547 polymorphisms. Numbers of participants (n) are indicated above each specific column. Values above the figures refer to the overall *P*-value. *P*-values above a genotype group refer to the pairwise post hoc analysis. (Reprinted from O'Connell K, Posthumus M, Schwellnus MP, et al. Collagen genes and exercise-associated muscle cramping. *Clin J Sport Med*. 2013;23:64-69, with permission from Lippincott Williams & Wilkins.)

the *COL3A1* ($P = 0.828$), *COL6A1* ($P = 0.300$), or *COL12A1* ($P = 0.120$) genotypes between the EAMC and NON groups.

Conclusions.—This study identified, for the first time, the *COL5A1* gene as a potential marker for a history of EAMC (Fig 1).

▶ The origin of exercise-related muscle cramps has long been a puzzling question for sports physicians. Painful, spasmodic, and involuntary contraction of skeletal muscle have followed participation in endurance events, particularly marathons and triathlons, affecting 26% to 67% of contestants in various studies.[1-3] The problem has traditionally been regarded as an expression of heat exposure, dehydration, and resulting disturbances of electrolyte balance,[4-6] although in the case of long-distance athletes, the evidence supporting the role of heat exposure has not been very strong.[7] Cramping usually occurs in localized muscle groups that are actively involved in the event; the duration of the spasm is short (4—5 minutes), and symptoms are commonly relieved by stretching of the affected muscle. These various observations tend to support the alternative, nonthermal hypothesis, that the cramps reflect a change in neuromuscular control, perhaps secondary to muscle fatigue.[7] Some investigators have also pointed to a family history of this problem, thus, opening the way to genetic comparisons between those who are vulnerable to cramping and those who are not. Several genetic variants have recently been linked to a vulnerability to musculoskeletal soft tissue injury.[8-10] O'Connell et al have examined the expression of this group of genes in athletes who are susceptible to cramps. There is a substantial genetic association (Fig 1), which persists after allowing statistically for an effect of these same genes on the individual's competitive performance, although it remains to be seen how far this observation will help in identifying an appropriate remedy. At least it suggests that the cramps are related in some way to the mechanical characteristics of the myofibril rather than to dehydration.

R. J. Shephard, MD (Lond), PhD, DPE

References

1. Norris F, Gasteiger E, Charfield P. An electromyographic study of induced and spontaneous muscle cramps. *Electroencephalogr Clin Neurophysiol.* 1957;9: 139-147.
2. Manjra SI, Schwellnus MP, Noakes TD. Risk factors for exercise associated muscle cramping (EAMC) in marathon runners. *Med Sci Sports Exerc.* 1996; 28:S167.
3. Kantarowski PG, Hiller WD, Garret WE, et al. Cramping studies in 2600 endurance athletes. *Med Sci Sports Exerc.* 1990;22:S104.
4. Bergeron MF. Muscle cramps during exercise—is it fatigue or electrolyte deficit. *Curr Sports Med Rep.* 2008;7:S50-S55.
5. Armstrong LE, Casa DJ, Millard-Stafford M, et al. American College of Sports Medicine position stand. Exertional heat illness during training and competition. *Med Sci Sports Exerc.* 2007;39:556-572.
6. Eichner ER. The role of sodium in heat cramping. *Sports Med.* 2007;37:368-370.
7. Schwellnus MP. Cause of exercise associated muscle cramps (EAMC)— altered neuromuscular control, dehydration or electrolyte depletion? *Br J Sports Med.* 2009;43:401-408.
8. Posthumus M, September AV, O'Cuinneagain D, et al. The COL5A1 gene is associated with increased risk of anterior cruciate ligament ruptures in female participants. *Am J Sports Med.* 2009;37:2234-2240.
9. Mokone GG, Schwellnus MP, Noakes TD, Collins M. The COL5A1 gene and Achilles tendon pathology. *Scand J Med Sci Sports.* 2006;16:19-26.
10. September AV, Cook J, Handley CJ, et al. Variants within the COL5A1 gene are associated with Achilles tendinopathy in two populations. *Br J Sports Med.* 2009; 43:357-365.

Postcontusion Polyphenol Treatment Alters Inflammation and Muscle Regeneration

Kruger MJ, Smith C (Stellenbosch Univ, Matieland, South Africa)
Med Sci Sports Exerc 44:872-880, 2012

Purpose.—Given the major role that oxidants play in cellular damage, and the recent focus on antioxidants as treatment for muscle injuries, the aim of this study was to examine the effect of short-term postinjury

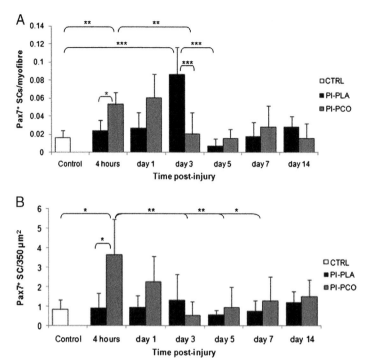

FIGURE 3.—Effect of postcontusion PCO supplementation on Pax-7[+] SC count normalized for the myofiber number (A) and expressed as Pax-7[+] SC count per field of view (B) ($n = 4$ per time point per group). Representative immunofluorescence images are provided as supplementary figures (Supplemental Digital Content 1, http://links.lww.com/MSS/A147). Statistics: *$P < 0.05$, **$P < 0.01$, ***$P < 0.001$. (Reprinted from Kruger MJ, Smith C. Postcontusion polyphenol treatment alters inflammation and muscle regeneration. *Med Sci Sports Exerc.* 2012;44:872-880, with permission from the American College of Sports Medicine.)

grape seed—derived polyphenol supplementation on muscle inflammation and repair processes after contusion injury.

Methods.—Experimental injury of the right gastrocnemius muscle was achieved by drop-mass method (200 g from a height of 50 cm), after which rats were gavaged with either 0.9% saline (placebo—PLA) or 20 mg·kg^{-1}·d^{-1} of proanthocyanidolic oligomer (PCO) from 2 h after contusion injury, for up to 14 d after injury. Blood samples and injured muscle were collected at 4 h and at days 1, 3, 5, 7, and 14 after injury.

Results.—Compared to an uninjured control group, PCO supplementation resulted in an earlier peak in number of activated satellite cells in contusion-injured muscle tissue (4 h for PCO vs day 3 for PLA, $n = 4$ per time point per group) and fetal myosin heavy chain expression (day 5 for PCO, $P < 0.01$ with no change in PLA, $n = 3$ per time point per group), indicative of quicker muscle regeneration. PCO supplementation limited neutrophil infiltration and facilitated earlier macrophage infiltration into the injured area ($n = 4$ per group). PCO also resulted in an earlier return toward control levels of muscle proinflammatory cytokines on day

3 ($P < 0.01$ for interleukin 6 and $P < 0.05$ for tumor necrosis factor α, both $n = 3$ per group).

Conclusions.—Data show that short-term postinjury PCO supplementation was able to quicken muscle regeneration by facilitating earlier recruitment of activated satellite cells and to modulate the immune system in favor of an anti-inflammatory status (Fig 3).

▶ The appropriate treatment of muscle injury following eccentric exercise is one of the more common issues facing the sports physician. Often, therapy is less than optimal, with delayed or incomplete recovery. Anti-inflammatory drugs, either steroid[1] or no-steroid[2] are commonly administered, but their prolonged use and thus the prolonged inhibition of inflammation may encourage the athlete to a premature renewal of exercise (with a risk of repeat injury and permanent scarring) and/or such drugs may inhibit the positive effects of inflammation that appear important for recovery.[3] The long-term prophylactic administration of antioxidants appears to hasten muscle regeneration if injury occurs,[4] and this observation stimulated Kruger and Smith to examine the use of antioxidants in the treatment of standardized muscle contusions in adult rats. The equivalence of injury between animals was established by demonstrating similar increases in creatine kinase levels. The dose of grapeseed-derived polyphenol (20 mg/kg/day) was based on that used in humans, with an adjustment for the higher metabolic rate of rats; dosage began 2 hours after injury, which might also be likely in the case of human injury. Use of the genetic marker Pax-7 allowed the identification of satellite cells when animals were sacrificed at 4 h, 1, 3, 5, 7, and 14 days post-injury. Treatment with the phenol dramatically accelerated the appearance of satellite cells relative to placebo-treated animals (Fig 3), with a greatly blunted pro-inflammatory response, both pointing to the likelihood of faster muscle regeneration. The results should encourage trial of this approach in humans, with assessments of functional recovery in the injured muscle.

R. J. Shephard, MD (Lond), PhD, DPE

References

1. Jarvinen M, Lehto M, Sorvari T, et al. Effect of some antiinflammatory agents on the healing of ruptured muscle. *J Sports Traumatol Rel Res*. 1992;14:19-28.
2. Vignaud A, Cebrian J, Martelly I, et al. Effect of anti-inflammatory and antioxidant drugs on the long-term repair of severely injured mouse skeletal muscle. *Exp Physiol*. 2005;90:487-495.
3. Jarvinen TA, Jarvinen TL, Kaariainen M, et al. Muscle injuries: biology and treatment. *Am J Sports Med*. 2005;33:745-764.
4. Myburgh KH, Kruger MJ, Smith C. Accelerated skeletal muscle recovery after in vivo polyphenol administration. *J Nutr Biochem*. 2011 Nov 11 [Epub ahead of print].

3 Biomechanics, Muscle Strength and Training

Muscle Strength

Muscular strength in male adolescents and premature death: cohort study of one million participants

Ortega FB, Silventoinen K, Tynelius P, et al (Univ of Granada, Spain; Univ of Helsinki, Finland; Karolinska Institutet, Stockholm, Sweden)
BMJ 345:e7279, 2012

Objectives.—To explore the extent to which muscular strength in adolescence is associated with all cause and cause specific premature mortality (<55 years).

Design.—Prospective cohort study.

Setting.—Sweden.

Participants.—1 142 599 Swedish male adolescents aged 16-19 years were followed over a period of 24 years.

Main Outcome Measures.—Baseline examinations included knee extension, handgrip, and elbow flexion strength tests, as well as measures of diastolic and systolic blood pressure and body mass index. Cox regression was used to estimate hazard ratios for mortality according to muscular strength categories (tenths).

Results.—During a median follow-up period of 24 years, 26 145 participants died. Suicide was a more frequent cause of death in young adulthood (22.3%) than was cardiovascular diseases (7.8%) or cancer (14.9%). High muscular strength in adolescence, as assessed by knee extension and handgrip tests, was associated with a 20-35% lower risk of premature mortality due to any cause or cardiovascular disease, independently of body mass index or blood pressure; no association was observed with mortality due to cancer. Stronger adolescents had a 20-30% lower risk of death from suicide and were 15-65% less likely to have any psychiatric diagnosis (such as schizophrenia and mood disorders). Adolescents in the lowest tenth of muscular strength showed by far the highest risk of mortality for different causes. All cause mortality rates (per 100 000 person years) ranged between 122.3 and 86.9 for the weakest and strongest adolescents;

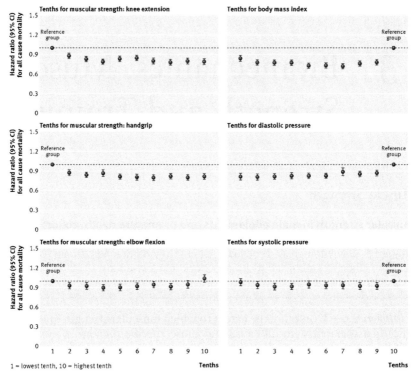

FIGURE 1.—Hazard ratios (95% CI) for relation of muscular strength, body mass index, and blood pressure with all cause premature death. Models were adjusted for birth cohort, conscription age, and conscription office (n = 1 142 599). (Reprinted from Ortega FB, Silventoinen K, Tynelius P, et al. Muscular strength in male adolescents and premature death: cohort study of one million participants. *BMJ.* 2012;345:e7279, with permission from the BMJ Publishing Group Ltd.)

corresponding figures were 9.5 and 5.6 for mortality due to cardiovascular diseases and 24.6 and 16.9 for mortality due to suicide.

Conclusions.—Low muscular strength in adolescents is an emerging risk factor for major causes of death in young adulthood, such as suicide and cardiovascular diseases. The effect size observed for all cause mortality was equivalent to that for well established risk factors such as elevated body mass index or blood pressure (Fig 1).

▶ The finding that low muscular strength is a risk factor for premature death in adolescents was at first inspection quite intriguing, although it has been noted in several earlier reports.[1-4] Strength had a substantial influence on hazard ratios for premature death in a large, 24-year follow-up of young Swedes (Fig 1). It becomes more comprehensible on recalling that the most frequent cause of death (22.3% of incidents in this study) was suicide. Poor cardiorespiratory fitness has previously been associated with psychiatric disturbances,[5-7] but there do not seem any previous investigators who have looked at relationships with muscular strength. There may be some reverse causation, with psychiatric disturbance limiting physical activity. However, there also seems likely to be an influence from adulation of the he-man, muscular individual, leading to a deterioration of self-image in those who are endowed with less brute strength. Such individuals are liable to bullying at school, and their ego is further depressed by the worship of the string "enforcer" rather than the skillful player who is intelligent and considerate of others.[8,9] The time seems ripe for a reconsideration of exactly who deserves recognition on the sports field.

R. J. Shephard, MD (Lond), PhD, DPE

References

1. Fujita Y, Nakamura Y, Hiraoka J, et al. Physical-strength tests and mortality among visitors to health-promotion centers in Japan. *J Clin Epidemiol*. 1995;48:1349-1359.
2. Gale CR, Martyn CN, Cooper C, Sayer AA. Grip strength, body composition, and mortality. *Int J Epidemiol*. 2007;36:228-235.
3. Katzmarzyk PT, Craig CL. Musculoskeletal fitness and risk of mortality. *Med Sci Sports Exerc*. 2002;34:740-744.
4. Ruiz JR, Sui X, Lobelo F, et al. Association between muscular strength and mortality in men: prospective cohort study. *BMJ*. 2008;337:a439.
5. Koivukangas J, Tammelin T, Kaakinen M, et al. Physical activity and fitness in adolescents at risk for psychosis within the Northern Finland 1986 Birth Cohort. *Schizophr Res*. 2010;116:152-158.
6. Wildgust HJ, Beary M. Are there modifiable risk factors which will reduce the excess mortality in schizophrenia? *J Psychopharmacol*. 2010;24:37-50.
7. Beary M, Wildgust HJ. Chronic disease to top agenda. Cardiorespiratory fitness is an important risk factor. *BMJ*. 2011;342:d1152.
8. Greenleaf CA, Petrie TA, Martin SB. Psychosocial variables associated with body composition and cardiorespiratory fitness in middle school students. *Res Q Exerc Sport*. 2010;81:S65-574.
9. Babiss LA, Gangwisch JE. Sports participation as a protective factor against depression and suicidal ideation in adolescents as mediated by self-esteem and social support. *J Dev Behav Pediatr*. 2009;30:376-384.

25(OH) Vitamin D Is Associated with Greater Muscle Strength in Healthy Men and Women

Grimaldi AS, Parker BA, Capizzi JA, et al (Hartford Hosp, CT; et al)
Med Sci Sports Exerc 45:157-162, 2013

Purpose.—The purpose of the study was to examine the relation between serum 25-hydroxy vitamin D (25(OH)D) levels and muscle strength in 419 healthy men and women over a broad age range (20–76 yr).

Methods.—Isometric and isokinetic strength of the arms and legs was measured using computerized dynamometry, and its relation to vitamin D was tested in multivariate models controlling for age, gender, resting HR, systolic blood pressure, diastolic blood pressure, body mass index, maximal oxygen uptake ($\dot{V}O_{2max}$), physical activity counts, and season of vitamin D measurement.

Results.—Vitamin D was significantly associated with arm and leg muscle strength when controlling for age and gender. When controlling for other covariates listed previously, vitamin D remained directly related to both isometric and isokinetic arm strength but only to isometric leg strength.

Conclusion.—These data suggest that there may be a differential effect of vitamin D on upper and lower body strength. The mechanism for this difference remains unclear but could be related to differences in androgenic effects or to differences in vitamin D receptor expression. Our study supports a direct relation between vitamin D and muscle strength and suggests that vitamin D supplementation be evaluated to determine whether it is an effective therapy to preserve muscle strength in adults.

▶ The novel aspect of the study by Grimaldi et al is that the strength measures included upper and lower body muscles tested under isometric and isokinetic conditions. In a cross-sectional analysis of 419 women and men aged 44 ± 16.1 years (mean ± SD), they found that, after controlling for sex and age, higher serum 25-hydroxy vitamin D (25(OH)D) was associated with greater isometric and isokinetic elbow flexion and extension. Interestingly, 25(OH)D was not significantly associated with hand grip strength, a frequently used proxy of total body muscle strength. The lower extremity results were quite similar, with the exception that 25(OH)D was not a significant predictor of isokinetic knee extension (60° and 180° s-1). After adjustment for additional physiologic (eg, $\dot{V}O_{2max}$) and behavioral (eg, physical activity counts) variables and the season of the blood draw, 25(OH)D remained a significant predictor of muscle strength of the elbow but not the knee. The mechanisms underpinning a differential association of 25(OH)D with upper versus lower body muscle strength are unclear. The authors posit that the distribution of type II muscle fibers, concentrations of vitamin D receptors, and androgenic effect of 25(OH)D may explain the inconsistent relations in upper and lower body strength. It is notable that the relation of 25(OH)D to muscle strength was evident in young and middle-aged adults and not isolated to the elderly.

C. M. Jankowski, PhD

Muscle Training and Muscular Injuries

The ACTN3 genotype in soccer players in response to acute eccentric training
Pimenta EM, Coelho DB, Cruz IR, et al (Univ of León, Spain; Federal Univ of Minas Gerais, Brazil; UFMG, Belo Horizonte, Brazil)
Eur J Appl Physiol 112:1495-1503, 2012

Genetic factors can interfere with sporting performance. The identification of genetic predisposition of soccer players brings important information to trainers and coaches for individual training loads adjustment. Different responses to eccentric training could be observed by the genotype referred to as α-actinin-3 (ACTN3) in biomarkers of muscle damage, hormones and inflammatory responses. The aim of this study was to compare acute inflammatory responses, muscle damage and hormonal variations according to the eccentric training in soccer professional athletes with different genetic profiles of ACTN3 (XX, RX and RR). 37 soccer professional athletes (9 XX,

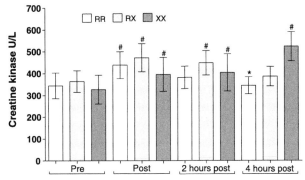

FIGURE 3.—Creatine kinase activity for polymorphism ACTN3. Creatine kinase activity pre, post, 2-h post and 4-h post-eccentric training for the polymorphisms of ACTN3 in professional soccer players. Values are presented as mean ± SEM. *Difference compared to XX in the moment 4-h post ($p < 0.05$). #Difference compared to pre-eccentric training ($p < 0.05$). (Reprinted from Pimenta EM, Coelho DB, Cruz IR, et al. The ACTN3 genotype in soccer players in response to acute eccentric training. *Eur J Appl Physiol.* 2012;112:1495-1503, with permission from Springer-Verlag.)

13 RX, 15 RR) were randomly divided into five stations associated to eccentric muscle contraction and plyometrics. Blood samples were taken from athletes pre-eccentric training, immediately after (post), 2- and 4-h post-eccentric training to determine hormone responses (cortisol and testosterone), muscle damage (CK and α-actin), and inflammatory responses (IL-6). After eccentric training, athletes XX presented higher levels for CK (4-h post), α-actin (post and 2-h post) and cortisol (post) compared to RR and RX athletes. However, RR and RX athletes presented higher levels of testosterone (post) and IL-6 (2 h post and 4 h post) compared to athletes XX. The main conclusion of this study is that professional soccer athletes homozygous to ACTN3XX gene are more susceptible to eccentric damage and present a higher catabolic state, demonstrated by metabolic, hormonal and immune responses post an eccentric training, in comparison to ACTN3RR and ACTN3RX groups (Fig 3).

▶ Soccer is a sport in which sudden changes of speed and direction place heavy eccentric loads on the leg muscles of players, as demonstrated by high levels of serum creatine kinase,[1] inflammatory responses,[2] and increased levels of free radicals and cytokines.[3] Player management would be facilitated if one could identify individuals who were particularly vulnerable to muscle injury, and recent research suggests that a deficiency of α-actinin-3 offers one potential marker.[4] In the study of Pimenta et al, professional soccer players homozygous to the actin3XX gene showed substantially greater eccentric damage and muscle breakdown as shown by creatine kinase readings (Fig 3), α-actinin, and cortisone levels. The authors suggest that players with the XX genotype be allowed longer recovery intervals between training sessions and a differentiated distribution of the training routine.

R. J. Shephard, MD (Lond), PhD, DPE

References

1. Mougios M. Reference intervals for serum creatine kinase in athletes. *Br J Sports Med.* 2007;41:674-678.
2. Ispirlidis I, Fatouros IG, Jamurtas AZ, et al. Time-course of changes in inflammatory and performance responses following a soccer game. *Clin J Sport Med.* 2008; 18:423-431.
3. Ascensão A, Rebelo A, Oliveira E, et al. Biochemical impact of a soccer match - analysis of oxidative stress and muscle damage markers throughout recovery. *Clin Biochem.* 2008;41:841-851.
4. Seto JT, Lek M, Quinlan KG, et al. Deficiency of α-actinin-3 is associated with increased susceptibility to contraction-induced damage and skeletal muscle remodeling. *Hum Mol Genet.* 2011;20:2914-2927.

Contractile function and sarcolemmal permeability after acute low-load resistance exercise with blood flow restriction

Wernbom M, Paulsen G, Nilsen TS, et al (Norwegian School of Sport Sciences, Oslo, Norway)
Eur J Appl Physiol 112:2051-2063, 2012

Conflicting findings have been reported regarding muscle damage with low-intensity resistance exercise with blood flow restriction (BFR) by pressure cuffs. This study investigated muscle function and muscle fibre morphology after a single bout of low-intensity resistance exercise with and without BFR. Twelve physically active subjects performed unilateral knee extensions at 30% of their one repetition maximum (1RM), with partial BFR on one leg and the other leg without occlusion. With the BFR leg, five sets were performed to concentric torque failure, and the free-flow leg repeated the exact same number of repetitions and sets. Biopsies were obtained from vastus lateralis before and 1, 24 and 48 h after exercise. Maximum isometric torque (MVC) and resting tension were measured before and after exercise and at 4, 24, 48, 72, 96 and 168 h post-exercise. The results demonstrated significant decrements in MVC (lasting $\geq$ 48 h) and delayed onset muscle soreness in both legs, and increased resting tension for the occluded leg both acutely and at 24 h post-exercise. The percentage of muscle fibres showing elevated intracellular staining of the plasma protein tetranectin, a marker for sarcolemmal permeability, was significantly increased from 9% before exercise to 27−38% at 1, 24 and 48 h post-exercise for the BFR leg. The changes in the free-flow leg were significant only at 24 h (19%). We conclude that an acute bout of low-load resistance exercise with BFR resulted in changes suggesting muscle damage, which may have implications both for safety aspects and for the training stimulus with BFR exercise.

▶ There has been considerable clinical interest in the possibility of enhancing muscle function by a combination of low-load strength training and vascular occlusion of the active limb; reports have suggested that intensities in the range 20-50% of 1-repetition maximum (RM) can induce hypertrophy comparable with that realized by more conventional strength training.[1,2] However, there have also been reports of moderate to severe delayed-onset muscle soreness following training with vascular occlusion.[3,4] The present study was carried out on relatively fit physical education students at 30% of the 1-RM loading of the quadriceps using the opposite leg for control observations relative to the limb with blood flow occlusion. Muscle biopsies showed that occlusion led to a substantial increase of sarcolemmal permeability, as shown by inward diffusion of the plasma protein tetranectin (Fig 5 in the original article); there were also greater and more long-lasting reductions in maximum voluntary contraction in the occluded limb. The increased membrane permeability may signal a risk of muscular damage with repeated contractions during occlusion; however, there is also some evidence that this increase of permeability plays a useful role in facilitating hypertrophy.[5,6] Further studies of thus type are needed, covering a longer time span.

R. J. Shephard, MD (Lond), PhD, DPE

References

1. Takarada Y, Takazawa H, Sato Y, Takebayashi S, Tanaka Y, Ishii N. Effects of resistance exercise combined with moderate vascular occlusion on muscular function in humans. *J Appl Physiol.* 2000;88:2097-2106.
2. Karabulut M, Abe T, Sato Y, Bemben MG. The effects of low-intensity resistance training with vascular restriction on leg muscle strength in older men. *Eur J Appl Physiol.* 2010;108:147-155.
3. Umbel JD, Hoffman RL, Dearth DJ, Chleboun GS, Manini TM, Clark BC. Delayed-onset muscle soreness induced by low-load blood flow-restricted exercise. *Eur J Appl Physiol.* 2009;107:687-695.
4. Wernbom M, Järrebring R, Andreasson MA, Augustsson J. Acute effects of blood flow restriction on muscle activity and endurance during fatiguing dynamic knee extensions at low load. *J Strength Cond Res.* 2009;23:2389-2395.
5. Miyake K, McNeil PL. Mechanical injury and repair of cells. *Crit Care Med.* 2003; 31:S496-S501.
6. Grembowicz KP, Sprague D, McNeil PL. Temporary disruption of the plasma membrane is required for c-fos expression in response to mechanical stress. *Mol Biol Cell.* 1999;10:1247-1257.

Effect of dehydroepiandrosterone administration on recovery from mix-type exercise training-induced muscle damage

Liao YH, Liao K-F, Kao C-L, et al (Univ of Texas at Austin; Taipei Physical Education College, Taiwan; Taipei Veterans General Hosp and Natl Yang-Ming Univ, Taiwan; et al)
Eur J Appl Physiol 113:99-107, 2013

This study aimed to determine the role of DHEA-S in coping against the exercise training mixing aerobic and resistance components. During 5-day successive exercise training, 16 young male participants (19.2 ± 1.2 years) received either a placebo (flour capsule) or DHEA (100 mg/day) in a double-blinded and placebo-controlled design. Oral DHEA supplementation significantly increased circulating DHEA-S by 2.5-fold, but a protracted drop (~35%) was observed from Day 3 during training. In the Placebo

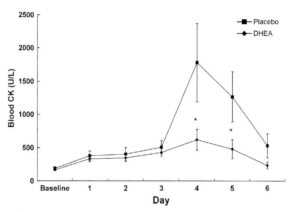

FIGURE 4.—Blood creatine kinase (CK) level changes during exercise training. Blood creatine kinase (CK) level changes by treatment measured pre-training (Day 0, baseline), during training (Day 1–Day 5), and post-training (Day 6) with DHEA ($n = 8$) or placebo ($n = 8$) administration. *Significant difference between Placebo and DHEA groups ($p < 0.05$). (With kind permission from Springer Science+Business Media: Liao YH, Liao K-F, Kao C-L, et al. Effect of dehydroepiandrosterone administration on recovery from mix-type exercise training-induced muscle damage. *Eur J Appl Physiol.* 2013;113:99-107, with permission from Springer-Verlag.)

group, only a minimal DHEA-S reduction ($\sim 17\%$) was observed. Changes in testosterone followed a similar pattern as DHEA-S. Muscle soreness was elevated significantly on Day 2 for both groups to a similar extent. Lower muscle soreness was observed in the DHEA-supplemented group on Day 3 and Day 6. In the Placebo group, training increased circulating creatine kinase (CK) levels by approximately ninefold, while only a threefold increase was observed in the DHEA-supplemented group. This mix-type exercise training improved glucose tolerance in both groups, while lowering the insulin response to the glucose challenge, but no difference between treatments was observed. Our results suggest that DHEA-S may play a role in protecting skeletal muscle from exercise training-induced muscle damage (Fig 4).

▶ A variety of treatments has recently been proposed to reduce training-induced muscular injuries. The report of Liao and associates shows a dramatic response to oral dehydroepiandrosterone (DHEA) given orally (100 mg/d) over 5 days of training that included a pattern of resistance training designed to maximize muscle damage (Fig 4). DHEA is the main precursor of testosterone, and concentrations often seem to be reduced by heavy exercise or stress.[1] Moreover, although aerobic and resistance exercise both normally improve insulin sensitivity and increase glycemic control,[2,3] eccentric exercise reduces insulin sensitivity in association with a prolonged decrease in DHEA.[1] The importance of decreasing the creatine kinase response to eccentric exercise by DHEA therapy may be questioned; should one treat changes in laboratory data rather than the patient's symptoms? Certainly, the changes in delayed-onset muscle soreness induced by DHEA were relatively small, and there was no change in glucose tolerance relative to control subjects. Moreover, creatine kinase release may reflect a change in permeability of the muscle sarcolemma that is important to muscle hypertrophy. Possibly, the processes of muscle repair or hypertrophy after eccentric exercise consume increased amounts of DHEA, and, if plasma levels are increased, repair and hypertrophy are hastened, thus allowing creatine kinase levels to return to normal. Some investigators have also suggested an anti-inflammatory effect of DHEA, with reduced levels of tumor necrosis factor—α and interleukin-6.[4,5] Further research should examine changes in muscle strength between treated and placebo groups to be sure that it is really a good idea to reduce the leakage of creatine kinase!

R. J. Shephard, MD (Lond), PhD, DPE

References

1. Tsai Y, Chou S, Lin Y, et al. Effect of resistance exercise on dehydroepiandrosterone sulfate concentrations during a 72-h recovery: relation to glucose tolerance and insulin response. *Life Sci.* 2006;79:1281-1286.
2. Holloszy JO. Exercise-induced increase in muscle insulin sensitivity. *J Appl Physiol.* 2005;99:338-343.
3. Lai Y, Chen C, Kuo C. Exercise and type 2 diabetes. *Adaptive Med.* 2009;1:1-16.
4. Brignardello E, Runzo C, Aragno M, et al. Dehydroepiandrosterone administration counteracts oxidative imbalance and advanced glycation end product formation in type 2 diabetic patients. *Diabetes Care.* 2007;30:2922-2927.
5. Straub RH, Konecna L, Hrach S, et al. Serum dehydroepiandrosterone (DHEA) and DHEA sulfate are negatively correlated with serum interleukin-6 (IL-6), and DHEA inhibits IL-6 secretion from mononuclear cells in man in vitro: possible link between endocrinosenescence and immunosenescence. *J Clin Endocrinol Metab.* 1998;83:2012-2017.

Predictors of low back pain in physically active conscripts with special emphasis on muscular fitness

Taanila HP, Suni JH, Pihlajamäki HK, et al (The UKK Inst, Tampere, Finland; Centre for Military Medicine, Lahti, Finland; et al)
Spine J 12:737-748, 2012

Background Context.—Association between low physical fitness and low back pain (LBP) is contradictory in previous studies.

Purpose.—The objective of the present prospective cohort study was to investigate the predictive associations of various intrinsic risk factors in young conscripts for LBP, with special attention to physical fitness.

Study Design.—A prospective cohort study.

Patient Sample.—A representative sample of Finnish male conscripts. In Finland, military service is compulsory for male citizens and 90% of young men enter into the service.

Outcome Measures.—Incidence of LBP and recurrent LBP prompting a visit at the garrison health clinic during 6-month military training.

Methods.—Four successive cohorts of 18- to 28-year-old male conscripts (N = 982) were followed for 6 months. Conscripts with incidence of LBP were identified and treated at the garrison clinic. Predictive associations between intrinsic risk factors and LBP were examined using multivariate Cox proportional hazard models.

Results.—The cumulative incidence of LBP was 16%, the incidence rate being 1.2 (95% confidence interval [CI], 1.0–1.4) per 1,000 person-days. Conscripts with low educational level had increased risk for incidence of LBP (hazard ratio [HR], 1.6; 95% CI, 1.1–2.3). Conscripts with low dynamic trunk muscle endurance and low aerobic endurance simultaneously (ie, having coimpairment) at baseline also had an increased risk for incidence of LBP. The strongest risk factor was coimpairment of trunk muscular endurance in tests of back lift and push-up (HR, 2.8; 95% CI, 1.4–5.9).

Conclusions.—The increased risk for LBP was observed among young men who had a low educational level and poor fitness level in both muscular and aerobic performance.

▶ The link between physical activity, fitness, and low back pain risk is commonly accepted, but the data are far from consistent.[1,2] In this study, the strongest risk factors for low back pain (and recurrent) were low education level and low aerobic capacity (12-minute running test) and trunk muscular endurance (situp, pushup, and back lift tests). Basic military training and similar occupations are physically demanding for the back and require adequate physical fitness, supporting efforts to establish minimum physical fitness standards for recruits.

D. C. Nieman, DrPH

References

1. Wedderkopp N, Kjaer P, Hestbaek L, Korsholm L, Leboeuf-Yde C. High-level physical activity in childhood seems to protect against low back pain in early adolescence. *Spine J.* 2009;9:134-141.
2. Hamberg-van Reenen HH, Ariëns GA, Blatter BM, van Mechelen W, Bongers PM. A systematic review of the relation between physical capacity and future low back and neck/shoulder pain. *Pain.* 2007;130:93-107.

Kinesio Taping in Treatment and Prevention of Sports Injuries: A Meta-Analysis of the Evidence for its Effectiveness
Williams S, Whatman C, Hume PA, et al (Auckland Univ of Technology, New Zealand)
Sports Med 42:153-164, 2012

Kinesio tape (KT) is an elastic therapeutic tape used for treating sports injuries and a variety of other disorders. Chiropractor, Dr Kenso Kase, developed KT taping techniques in the 1970s. It is claimed that KT supports injured muscles and joints and helps relieve pain by lifting the skin and allowing improved blood and lymph flow. The profile of KT rose after the tape was donated to 58 countries for use during the 2008 Olympic Games, and was seen on high-profile athletes. Practitioners are asking whether they should use KT over other elastic adhesive tapes. The aim of this review was to evaluate, using meta-analysis, the effectiveness of KT in the treatment and prevention of sports injuries. Electronic databases including SPORTDiscus™, Scopus, MEDLINE, ScienceDirect and sports medicine websites were searched using keywords 'kinesio taping/tape'. From 97 articles, ten met the inclusion criteria (article reported data for effect of KT on amusculoskeletal outcome and had a control group) and were retained for meta-analyses. Magnitude-based inferences were used to assess clinical worth of positive outcomes reported in studies. Only two studies investigated sports-related injuries (shoulder impingement), and just one of these involved injured athletes. Studies attending to musculoskeletal outcomes in healthy participants were included on the basis that these outcomes may have implications for the prevention of sporting injuries. The efficacy of KT in pain relief was trivial given there were no clinically important results. There were inconsistent range-of-motion outcome results, with at least small beneficial results seen in two studies, but trivial results in two other studies across numerous joint measurements. There was a likely beneficial effect for proprioception regarding grip force sense error, but no positive outcome for ankle proprioception. Seven outcomes relating to strength were beneficial, although there were numerous trivial findings for quadriceps and hamstrings peak torque, and grip strength measures. KT had some substantial effects on muscle activity, but it was unclear whether these changes were beneficial or harmful. In conclusion, there was little quality evidence to support the use of KT over other types of elastic taping in themanagement or prevention of sports injuries. KT may have a small beneficial role in improving strength, range of motion in certain injured cohorts and force sense error compared with other tapes, but further studies are needed to confirm these findings. The amount of case study and anecdotal support for KT warrants well designed experimental research, particularly pertaining to sporting injuries, so that practitioners can be confident that KT is beneficial for their athletes.

▶ Taping has long been used for the prevention and treatment of different kinds of injuries, and there are numerous potential mechanisms that help explain its proposed benefits: increased proprioception and muscle activation, passive joint stabilization, and it has also been shown to reduce pain. More recently Kinesio taping (KT) has emerged as a new type of taping that may increase proprioceptive feedback to joints and muscles as it is placed in a stretch position on the skin, and then exerts a pulling force across the skin and surrounding structures. KT has been used mostly in athletes, and interest in the colorful taping bands has been generated as many world-class athletes participating in recent Olympics were using them. This systematic review is interesting as it tries to draw conclusions on the effectiveness of KT. This systematic review included 10 studies with limited methodological quality, and no firm conclusions could be drawn from the available data, but for injured subjects KT may have a small beneficial effect on strength, on muscle force sense, and active range of motion. At this time, the authors concluded that there is no evidence to support the use of KT for reduction of pain, ankle proprioception, and increase in muscle activity. Of note, the authors could not make any recommendation regarding the efficacy of KT for the prevention of injuries.

F. Desmeules, PT, PhD

Operative Versus Nonoperative Management of Acute Achilles Tendon Ruptures: A Quantitative Systematic Review of Randomized Controlled Trials

Wilkins R, Bisson LJ (The State Univ of New York at Buffalo)
Am J Sports Med 40:2154-2160, 2012

Background.—Despite several randomized controlled trials comparing operative to nonoperative management of Achilles tendon ruptures, the optimal management of this condition remains the subject of significant debate. Rerupture is a known complication, but most level I studies have not shown a significant difference in the incidence of reruptures when comparing operative to nonoperative management.

Purpose.—The goal of this systematic review was to identify all randomized controlled trials comparing operative and nonoperative management of Achilles tendon ruptures and to meta-analyze the data with reruptures being the primary outcome. Secondary outcomes including strength, time to return to work, and other complications were analyzed as well.

Study Design.—Meta-analysis.

Methods.—We searched multiple online databases to identify English-language, prospective randomized controlled trials comparing open surgical repair of acute Achilles tendon ruptures to nonoperative management. Rerupture was our primary outcome. Secondary outcomes included strength, time to return to work, deep infections, sural nerve sensory disturbances, noncosmetic scar complaints, and deep venous thrombosis. Coleman methodology scores were calculated for each included study.

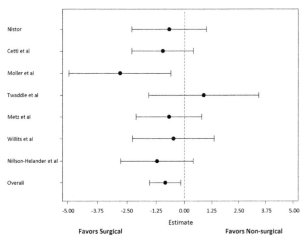

FIGURE 1.—Analysis of reruptures expressed as log odds ratios. (Reprinted from Wilkins R, Bisson LJ. Operative versus nonoperative management of acute Achilles tendon ruptures: a quantitative systematic review of randomized controlled trials. *Am J Sports Med.* 2012;40:2154-2160, with permission from The Author(s).)

Data were extracted from all qualifying articles and, when appropriate, pooled and meta-analyzed.

Results.—Seven level I trials involving 677 patients met inclusion criteria. Coleman scores were 95, 95, 95, 89, 78, 97, and 92. Open repair was associated with a significantly lower rerupture rate compared with nonoperative treatment (3.6% vs 8.8%; odds ratio, 0.425; 95% confidence interval, 0.222-0.815). The incidence of deep infections was significantly higher for patients treated with surgery ($P = .0113$). The incidences of noncosmetic scar complaints and sural nerve sensory disturbances were also significantly higher in patients treated with surgery ($P < .001$ for each). Strength measurements were not standardized and therefore could not be meta-analyzed.

Conclusion.—Open surgical repair of acute Achilles tendon ruptures significantly reduces the risk of reruptures when compared with nonoperative management. Several other complications, which are clearly avoided with nonoperative treatment, occur with a significantly higher incidence when surgical repair is performed. The available literature makes it difficult to compare the return of strength in the involved lower extremity after operative or nonoperative management. Future studies may focus on testing strength in a more functional and reproducible manner than isokinetic testing (Fig 1).

▶ Achilles tendon rupture occurs mainly in active people and athletes who take part in sports, especially stop-and-go sports. The incidence of Achilles tendon ruptures makes it a relatively frequent pathology seen in sports medicine or physiotherapy clinics, and the incidence has been reported to be increasing. Despite being a fairly common pathology, controversies exist regarding the best treatment options to effectively treat this injury. Historically, surgery was advocated, but, more recently, studies evaluating a conservative approach including casting the ankle with a non—weight-bearing period and then mobilization to allow tendon healing have shown no differences in rates of reruptures and with fewer surgical complications. Previous meta-analyses could not formally conclude in favor of one option over the other, most possibly because of low statistical power. This meta-analysis includes new recent randomized, controlled trials and concluded that surgery (open repair) was associated with a significantly lower rerupture rate compared with conservative treatment (3.6% vs 8.8%; odds ratio, 0.425; 95% confidence interval, 0.222—0.815) (Fig 1). However, the complication rate, most importantly, deep infections, was higher for surgery, but was, however, low (2.36% of all cases). For athletes who put more biomechanical demand on the Achilles tendon, the surgical option may be the most appropriate option, but all options should be discussed with the patient, and common decision making should be achieved with knowledge of the current evidence.

F. Desmeules, PT, PhD

Effectiveness of PhysioDirect telephone assessment and advice services for patients with musculoskeletal problems: pragmatic randomised controlled trial

Salisbury C, Montgomery AA, Hollinghurst S, et al (Univ of Bristol, UK; et al)
BMJ 346:f43, 2013

Objectives.—To assess the clinical effectiveness, effect on waiting times, and patient acceptability of PhysioDirect services in patients with musculoskeletal problems, compared with usual care.

Design.—Pragmatic randomised controlled trial to assess equivalence in clinical effectiveness. Patients were individually randomised in a 2:1 ratio to PhysioDirect or usual care.

Setting.—Four physiotherapy services in England.

Participants.—Adults (aged ≥18 years) referred by general practitioners or self referred for musculoskeletal physiotherapy.

Interventions.—PhysioDirect services invited patients to telephone a physiotherapist for initial assessment and advice, followed by face-to-face physiotherapy if necessary. Usual care involved patients joining a waiting list for face-to-face treatment.

Main Outcome Measures.—Numbers of appointments, waiting time for treatment, and non-attendance rates. Primary outcome was physical health (SF-36v2 physical component score) at six months. Secondary outcomes included four other measures of health outcome, mental component score and scales from the SF-36v2, time lost from work, and patient satisfaction and preference. Participants were not blind to allocation, but outcome data were collected blind to allocation.

Results.—Of 1506 patients allocated to PhysioDirect and 743 to usual care, 85% provided primary outcome data at six months (1283 and 629 patients, respectively). PhysioDirect patients had fewer face-to-face appointments than usual care patients (mean 1.91 v 3.11; incidence rate ratio 0.59 (95% confidence interval 0.53 to 0.65)), a shorter waiting time (median 7 days v 34 days; arm time ratio 0.32 (0.29 to 0.35)), and lower rates of non-attendance (incidence rate ratio 0.55 (0.41 to 0.73)). After six months' follow-up, the SF-36v2 physical component score was equivalent between groups (adjusted difference in means −0.01 (−0.80 to 0.79)). Health outcome measures suggested a trend towards slightly greater improvement in the PhysioDirect arm at six week follow-up and no difference at six months. There was no difference in time lost from work. PhysioDirect patients were no more satisfied with access to physiotherapy than usual care patients, but had slightly lower satisfaction overall at six months (difference in satisfaction −3.8% (−7.3% to −0.3%); $P = 0.031$). PhysioDirect patients were more likely than usual care patients to prefer PhysioDirect in future. No adverse events were detected.

Conclusions.—PhysioDirect is equally clinically effective compared with usual care, provides faster access to physiotherapy, and seems to be safe. However, it could be associated with slightly lower patient satisfaction.

▶ Timely access to appropriate primary care is an important problem in many health care systems. Telephone triage, assessment, and advice have been implemented in many countries with long wait times to see primary care practitioners. The PhysioDirect project is innovative because it uses physiotherapists as telephone consultants for patients suffering from musculoskeletal (MSK) disorders. MSK disorders are 1 of the leading reasons for consultation in primary care, and with the aging of the population in many countries, access to appropriate primary care for patients suffering from MSK disorders will likely worsen. In many countries, direct access to physiotherapy treatment is not possible, and patients need to see a physician to get a referral. Evidence shows that the diagnosis of MSK disorders by physicians is often not optimal and they tend to refer less to physiotherapy.[1] Also, physiotherapy is often part of the private sector and many patients do not have insurance or the financial means to pay for initial assessment and treatment. The PhysioDirect model may therefore help patients to get an initial quick assessment and advice to manage their condition. This randomized controlled trial, conducted in the United Kingdom, therefore compared usual care (physicians visit and referral to physiotherapy) to direct telephone access to physiotherapy (PhysioDirect). Using various validated outcome measures, the authors did not find any differences in clinical outcomes between the two types of care. Only in terms of satisfaction, patients in the PhysioDirect program showed a slightly lower satisfaction level. Although the authors did not specifically measure economic costs, patients in the PhysioDirect program had a shorter wait for physiotherapy treatments, fewer face-to-face appointments, and fewer physiotherapy consultations, which provides indirect support for the economic efficiency of this model.

F. Desmeules, PT, PhD

Reference

1. Desmeules F, Roy JS, Macdermid JC, Champagne F, Hinse O, Woodhouse LJ. Advanced practice physiotherapy in patients with musculoskeletal disorders: a systematic review. *BMC Musculoskelet Disord.* 2012;13:107.

4 Physical Activity, Cardiorespiratory Physiology and Immune Function

Physical Activity

Physical activity education in the undergraduate curricula of all UK medical schools. Are tomorrow's doctors equipped to follow clinical guidelines?
Weiler R, Chew S, Coombs N, et al (Univ College London Hosp NHS Foundation Trust, UK; UCL-PARG (Univ College London Population Health Domain Physical Activity Res Group), UK)
Br J Sports Med 46:1024-1026, 2012

Physical activity (PA) is a cornerstone of disease prevention and treatment. There is, however, a considerable disparity between public health policy, clinical guidelines and the delivery of physical activity promotion within the National Health Service in the UK. If this is to be addressed in the battle against non-communicable diseases, it is vital that tomorrow's doctors understand the basic science and health benefits of physical activity. The aim of this study was to assess the provision of physical activity teaching content in the curricula of all medical schools in the UK. Our results, with responses from all UK medical schools, uncovered some alarming findings, showing that there is widespread omission of basic teaching elements, such as the Chief Medical Officer recommendations and guidance on physical activity. There is an urgent need for physical activity teaching to have dedicated time at medical schools, to equip tomorrow's doctors with the basic knowledge, confidence and skills to promote physical activity and follow numerous clinical guidelines that support physical activity promotion.

▶ Although this study was conducted in UK medical schools, I suspect that findings from a survey of North American teaching departments would be very similar. On average, the UK schools were allocating a total of only 4.2 hours of instruction

91

to exercise medicine, compared with an average of 109 hours for pharmacology. Moreover, only half of the medical schools were teaching the Chief Medical Officer's guidelines for physical activity (the British equivalent of the Surgeon General's report). Many physicians currently give very limited exercise advice to their patients because they feel poorly qualified to do so, yet doctors remain one of the key groups who can influence patient behavior. If national goals of greater physical activity are to be achieved, the curricula of medical schools need to be reviewed and changed. One hopeful feature of this British survey is an indication that the presentation of these data may have begun such a process in Great Britain.

R. J. Shephard, MD (Lond), PhD, DPE

Can a single question provide an accurate measure of physical activity?
Milton K, Clemes S, Bull F (Loughborough Univ, Leicestershire, UK; Univ of Western Australia, Perth, Australia)
Br J Sports Med 47:44-48, 2013

Objective.—The 'single-item measure' was developed as a short self-report tool for assessing physical activity. The aim of this study was to test the criterion validity of the single-item measure against accelerometry.

Design.—Participants (n = 66, 65% female, age: 39 ± 11 years) wore an accelerometer (ActiGraph GT3X) over a 7-day period and on day 8, completed the single-item measure. The number of days of ≥30 min of accelerometer-determined moderate to vigorous intensity physical activity (MVPA) were calculated using two approaches; first by including all minutes of MVPA and second by including only MVPA accumulated in bouts of ≥10 min (counts/min ≥1952). Associations between the single-item measure and accelerometer were examined using Spearman correlations and 95% limits of agreement. Percent agreement and κ statistic were used to assess agreement between the tools in classifying participants as sufficiently/insufficiently active.

Results.—Correlations between the number of days of ≥30 min MVPA recorded by the single-item and accelerometer ranged from 0.46 to 0.57. Participants underreported their activity on the single-item measure (−1.59 days) when compared with all objectively measured MVPA, but stronger congruence was observed when compared with MVPA accumulated in bouts of ≥10 min (0.38 days). Overall agreement between the single-item and accelerometry in classifying participants as sufficiently/insufficiently active was 58% (k = 0.23, 95% CI 0.05 to 0.41) when including all MVPA and 76% (k = 0.39, 95% CI 0.14 to 0.64) when including activity undertaken in bouts of ≥10 min.

Conclusions.—The single-item measure is a valid screening tool to determine whether respondents are sufficiently active to benefit their health.

▶ I have long argued that a brief physical activity questionnaire gives as much (and sometimes more!) useful information as the very long instruments that some laboratories have devised.[1] Certainly, the average doctor does not have time to oversee the accurate completion or to analyze a lengthy questionnaire. There are a number of brief questionnaires already available,[2] but the attraction of the instrument proposed by Milton et al is that it is phrased in such a way as to examine whether the patient is meeting the currently recommended minimum standards of weekly physical activity. The question asked is rather long, but it is quite specific to this objective: "In the past week, on how many days have you done a total of 30 min or more of physical activity, which was enough to raise your breathing rate? This may include sport, exercise and brisk walking, cycling for recreation, or to get to and from places, but it should not include housework or physical activity that may be part of your job." The agreement of yes/no responses with accelerometer data was about as good as previously reported for the best of questionnaires, either short or long (correlations of 0.46 to 0.57). Although this is relatively low and implies a substantial proportion of discrepancies, part of the error variance arises from the accelerometer, which is good at recording walking but does not measure all types of activity. Further evaluation is needed on a substantially larger sample, but this new instrument may prove a helpful tool in office consultations.

R. J. Shephard, MD (Lond), PhD, DPE

References

1. Godin G, Shephard RJ. A simple method to assess exercise behavior in the community. *Can J Appl Sport Sci.* 1985;10:141-146.
2. Milton K, Bull FC, Bauman A. Reliability and validity testing of a single-item physical activity measure. *Br J Sports Med.* 2011;45:203-208.

Evidence-based intervention in physical activity: lessons from around the world

Heath GW, for the Lancet Physical Activity Series Working Group (Univ of Tennessee at Chattanooga and Univ of Tennessee College of Medicine; et al)

Lancet 380:272-281, 2012

Promotion of physical activity is a priority for health agencies. We searched for reviews of physical activity interventions, published between 2000 and 2011, and identified effective, promising, or emerging interventions from around the world. The informational approaches of community-wide and mass media campaigns, and short physical activity messages targeting key community sites are recommended. Behavioural and social approaches are effective, introducing social support for physical activity within communities and worksites, and school-based strategies that encompass physical education, classroom activities, after-school sports, and active transport. Recommended environmental and policy approaches include creation and improvement of access to places for physical activity with informational outreach activities, community-scale and street-scale urban design and land use, active transport policy and practices, and community-wide policies and planning. Thus, many approaches lead to acceptable increases in physical activity among people of various ages, and from different social groups, countries, and communities.

▶ Although most healthy practitioners now recognize the health value of regular physical activity, many are much less certain of their ability to persuade the public to adopt such behavior. The review of Heath and associates offers some modest encouragement, based on the effect sizes reported in previous reviews; the most effective approaches apparently are after-school programs for children and adolescents and web-based or pedometer-based programs for adults (Fig 1 in the original article).

R. J. Shephard, MD (Lond), PhD, DPE

Effectiveness of intervention on physical activity of children: systematic review and meta-analysis of controlled trials with objectively measured outcomes (EarlyBird 54)
Metcalf B, Henley W, Wilkin T (Plymouth Univ Campus, UK; Univ of Exeter Campus, UK)
BMJ 345:e5888, 2012

Objective.—To determine whether, and to what extent, physical activity interventions affect the overall activity levels of children.

Design.—Systematic review and meta-analysis.

Data Sources.—Electronic databases (Embase, Medline, PsycINFO, SPORTDiscus) and reference lists of included studies and of relevant review articles.

Study Selection.—*Design*: Randomised controlled trials or controlled clinical trials (cluster and individual) published in peer reviewed journals.

Intervention: Incorporated a component designed to increase the physical activity of children/adolescents and was at least four weeks in duration.

Outcomes: measured whole day physical activity objectively with accelerometers either before or immediately after the end of the intervention period.

Data Analysis.—Intervention effects (standardised mean differences) were calculated for total physical activity, time spent in moderate or vigorous physical activity, or both for each study and pooled using a weighted random effects model. Meta-regression explored the heterogeneity of intervention effects in relation to study participants, design, intervention type, and methodological quality.

Results.—Thirty studies (involving 14 326 participants; 6153 with accelerometer measured physical activity) met the inclusion criteria and all were eligible for meta-analysis/meta-regression. The pooled intervention effect across all studies was small to negligible for total physical activity (standardised mean difference 0.12, 95% confidence interval 0.04 to 0.20; $P < 0.01$) and small for moderate or vigorous activity (0.16, 0.08 to 0.24; $P < 0.001$). Meta-regression indicated that the pooled intervention effect

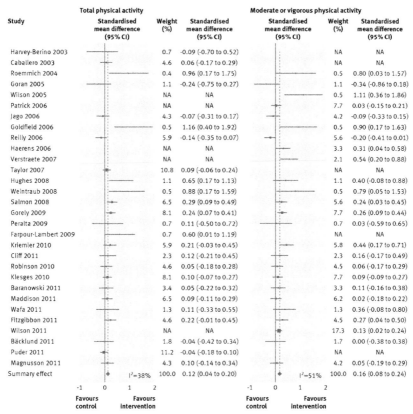

FIGURE 2.—Forest plot showing standardised mean difference in change in physical activity between intervention and control groups for each included study. NA=not available. (Reprinted from Metcalf B, Henley W, Wilkin T. Effectiveness of intervention on physical activity of children: Systematic review and meta-analysis of controlled trials with objectively measured outcomes (EarlyBird 54). *BMJ*. 2012;345:e5888, with permission from the BMJ Publishing Group Ltd.)

did not differ significantly between any of the subgroups (for example, for total physical activity, standardised mean differences were 0.07 for age <10 years and 0.16 for ≥10 years, P = 0.19; 0.07 for body mass index across the entire range and 0.22 for exclusively overweight/obese children, P = 0.07; 0.12 for study duration ≤6 months and 0.09 for >6 months, P = 0.71; 0.15 for home/family based intervention and 0.10 for school based intervention, P = 0.53; and 0.09 for higher quality studies and 0.14 for lower quality studies, P = 0.52).

Conclusions.—This review provides strong evidence that physical activity interventions have had only a small effect (approximately 4 minutes more walking or running per day) on children's overall activity levels. This finding may explain, in part, why such interventions have had limited success in reducing the body mass index or body fat of children (Fig 2).

▶ This is at first inspection a disappointing article for those who are engaged in health promotion. Despite a possible bias to the publication of research yielding positive results, as shown by a funnel plot of the data, a careful meta-analysis of 30 large and seemingly well-performed studies on children and adolescents under the age of 16 years, conducted between 2003 and 2011, suggests that, at best, efforts to encourage greater physical activity induced the equivalent of an additional 4 minutes of walking or running per day (Fig 2). The studies that were reviewed provided a sample of 6153 children whose activity had been examined by various types of accelerometer. One explanatory hypothesis suggested by the authors is that the exercise interventions simply replaced some other facet of a child's active leisure.[1] Certainly this is an important point to check following any physical activity intervention. A further question may be the period for which activity was measured: the accelerometers were worn for periods varying from 1 to 21 days; short periods of wear do not yield representative data, and in some of the children studied, the baseline activity would likely have been increased by a reactive response to the wearing of the accelerometer. However, most of the studies included a control group, so a reactive response should not have been a serious issue that would have compromised the results.

A possible message for sports physicians is that health promotional efforts should be directed toward required physical education sessions. All of the minimum physical activity that a child requires for good health could be provided by an hour of well-structured physical education per day. A study of primary school students was able to integrate an hour of quality physical education into the students' day without prejudice to their academic learning or reducing their leisure activities.[2] However, if such an approach is to be advocated, it is important that the physical education teachers concerned are closely monitored to ensure that the curricular time allocated to them is devoted to vigorous physical activity rather than waiting to use specialized equipment or time spent explaining tactics to be used in the sport.[3]

R. J. Shephard, MD (Lond), PhD, DPE

References

1. Frémeaux AE, Mallam KM, Metcalf BS, et al. The impact of school-time activity on total physical activity: the activitystat hypothesis (EarlyBird 46). *Int J Obes (Lond)*. 2011;35:1277-1283.
2. Shephard RJ, Lavallée H. Impact of enhanced physical education in the prepubescent child: Trois Riviéres revisited. *Pediatr Ex Sci*. 1993;5:177-189.
3. Goode RC, Virgin A, Romet T, et al. Effects of a short period of physical activity in adolescent boys and girls. *Can J Appl Sport Sci*. 1976;1:241-250.

Young Children and Parental Physical Activity Levels: Findings from the Canadian Health Measures Survey

Adamo KB, Langlois KA, Brett KE, et al (Children's Hosp of Eastern Ontario Res Inst, Ottawa, Canada; Statistics Canada, Ottawa, Ontario)
Am J Prev Med 43:168-175, 2012

Background.—Physical inactivity is a global public health concern. The relationship between dependent children in the home and parental physical activity has not been quantified using objective measures, nor has the relative association of the physical activity levels of mothers and fathers been examined.

Purpose.—To investigate the association of children of different ages in the home on two measures of parental physical activity: daily moderate-to-vigorous physical activity (MVPA) and likelihood of meeting the guideline of 150 minutes of MVPA per week accumulated in 10-minute bouts.

Methods.—Data were from the 2007–2009 Canadian Health Measures Survey ($n = 2315$), and analyses were conducted between February and December 2011. MVPA was measured directly using accelerometry. Linear (minutes of MVPA) and logistic (meeting physical activity guidelines) regression models were performed to determine if the presence, number of children, or the age of the youngest child at home was associated with parental physical activity. All models were adjusted for parental age, marital status, household income, employment, and BMI.

Results.—Mothers whose youngest child was aged <6 years and fathers whose youngest was aged 6–11 years engaged in fewer minutes of daily MVPA than those without dependent children. Linear regression results identified that in comparison to those without children, women whose youngest child in the home was aged <6 years participated in 7.7 minutes less activity per day ($p = 0.007$) whereas men engaged in 5.7 fewer minutes

TABLE 2.—Average Minutes of Daily MVPA, By Gender

	Women (n=1237)		Men (n=1078)	
	n	Average (95% CI)	n	Average (95% CI)
Has a dependent child in the home				
No	656	22.9 (19.2, 26.6*)	623	30.8 (25.4, 36.3)
Yes	581	21.1 (18.1, 24.0)	455	25.4 (20.7, 30.0)
Number of dependent children in the home				
0	656	22.9 (19.2, 26.6*)	623	30.8 (25.4, 36.3)
1	230	21.3 (17.7, 24.9)	197	25.7 (21.4, 30.0)
≥2	351	20.9 (17.3, 24.5)	258	25.0 (19.3, 30.7)
Age of youngest dependent child in the home (years)				
0 (no dependent children)	656	22.9 (19.2, 26.6*)	623	30.8 (25.4, 36.3)
<6	231	17.7** (13.8, 21.6*)	210	25.6 (23.9, 27.2)
6–11	221	23.8 (20.3, 27.3)	139	23.7** (16.6, 30.9)
12–17	129	22.9 (18.5, 27.2)	106	26.3[a] (15.8, 36.8)

MVPA, moderate-to-vigorous physical activity.
[a]Data should be interpreted with caution because of high sampling variability (coefficient of variation ≥16.6 and <33.3).
*Significantly different from men in the same category/column ($p<0.05$).
**Significantly different from those of the same gender with no dependent children in the home ($p<0.05$).

per day, or 54 and 40 minutes per week less, respectively. Similarly, logistic regression analyses indicated that both women and men were less likely to meet guidelines if their youngest child in the home was aged <6 years (OR = 0.31, 95% CI = 0.11, 0.87; OR = 0.34, 95% CI = 0.13, 0.93).

Conclusions.—The physical activity level of parents with young children present in the home was lower than that of those without children. Given the many physiologic, psychological, and social benefits of healthy active living, research efforts should continue to focus on strategies to encourage parents with young children to establish or re-engage in a physically active lifestyle, not only for their own health but to model healthy behavior for the next generation (Table 2).

▶ This article suggests that the addition of young children to a household decreases daily physical activity (Table 2). It is a viewpoint that would surprise many mothers of small children, although several other authors have made similar suggestions based on self-reported activity levels.[1-3] The present dataset was collected by accelerometer and on this basis may be considered as "objective." The findings formed a part of the 2007-2009 Canadian Health Measures Survey. There is little question that an accelerometer is more accurate than questionnaire data, particularly when quantitating daily levels of physical activity. However, it does not record all forms of activity, and (with a few of the more modern types of equipment) it does not measure the intensity of exercise. An accelerometer responds mostly to deliberate walking, and it is possible that those with young families replaced walking by some other type of activity, particularly lifting and carrying of the child in the case of the very young. The methodology of the present study was less than ideal. The actometer was worn for 7 consecutive days, and this is not a sufficient period either to overcome any reactive response to wearing of the instrument or to provide representative data on the activity of an individual across seasons.[4] Moreover, the authors' conclusion is based on a small apparent decrease in the minutes of moderate-to-vigorous activity per day (without any consideration of whether the intensity of activity was increased). Finally, in order to be counted, each burst of activity had to last for at least 10 minutes, and it is likely that activities with young children require repeated but much shorter bursts of movement, mirroring the activity patterns of the children. The authors may be correct, but I would side with those mothers who find they are working much harder when they are caring for a young child.

R. J. Shephard, MD (Lond), PhD, DPE

References

1. Bellows-Riecken KH, Rhodes RE. A birth of inactivity? A review of physical activity and parenthood. *Prev Med.* 2008;46:99-110.
2. Pereira MA, Rifas-Shiman SL, Kleinman KP, et al. Predictors of change in physical activity during and after pregnancy: project viva. *Am J Prev Med.* 2007;32: 312-319.
3. Gennaro S, Fehder W. Health behaviors in postpartum women. *Fam Community Health.* 2000;22:16-26.
4. Shephard RJ, Aoyagi Y. Objective monitoring of physical activity in older adults: clinical and practical implications. Phys Therap Rev 15: 170–182.

Daily Step Target to Measure Adherence to Physical Activity Guidelines in Children

Colley RC, Janssen I, Tremblay MS (Children's Hosp of Eastern Ontario Res Inst, Ottawa, Ontario, Canada; Queen's Univ, Kingston, Ontario, Canada)
Med Sci Sports Exerc 44:977-982, 2012

Purpose.—There is a lack of robust evidence to support a daily step count target that equates to current physical activity guidelines in children and youth. This information would be useful to researchers and practitioners who are using pedometers to monitor physical activity.

Methods.—Accelerometer and pedometer data collected on children and youth age 6−19 yr in the Canadian Health Measures Survey were used in this analysis ($n = 1613$). Correlation analyses of daily step counts and minutes of moderate-to-vigorous physical activity (MVPA) by age and sex were completed. The daily step count equivalent to 60 min of MVPA was derived using linear regression by age and sex. Cross-validation, including receiver operating curve analysis, was completed to compare the new cut points to one currently used as a proxy estimate of 60 min of daily MVPA (13,500 steps per day) as well as a range of possible step count targets between 8000 and 15,000 steps per day.

Results.—Daily step counts were correlated with daily minutes of MVPA ($r = 0.81$, $P < 0.0001$). The step count equivalents to 60 min of MVPA ranged between 11,290 and 12,512 steps per day (R^2 range = 0.59−0.74). A step count target of 12,000 steps per day resulted in closer population estimates of meeting the physical activity guideline (as measured as minutes of MVPA by accelerometer) as well as improved balance between sensitivity and specificity when compared with any cut point between 8000 and 15,000 steps per day, including the currently used daily step count target of 13,500 steps per day.

Conclusions.—We propose that 12,000 steps per day be used as a target to determine whether children and youth age 6−19 yr are meeting the current physical activity guideline of 60 min of daily MVPA (Table 1).

▶ Recent physical activity guidelines for children have recommended that children should accumulate at least 60 minutes of moderate to vigorous physical activity per day.[1-3] However, the monitoring of success in achieving this goal has been hampered by difficulty in ascertaining how much activity was actually being performed, with "social desirability" and other factors leading to large errors in the usual questionnaire estimates of physical activity patterns.[4] The development of inexpensive pedometers and pedometer/accelerometers has now provided a potential alternative and somewhat more objective source of such information (although with a single pedometer, much childhood activity such as cycling remains unrecorded). There remains some disagreement on the daily pedometer step count corresponding to the desired volume of physical activity.[4,5] Previous approaches to setting a target count have included correlating findings with a desirable body mass index[6] and observing the step count recorded when performing an appropriate intensity of activity on a treadmill. These authors use an

TABLE 1.—Sample Size (Individuals and Days), Mean MVPA, and Mean Steps Per Day
Presented by Age and Sex

	Sample Size	No. of Valid Days	MVPA (min·d^{-1})	Steps Per Day
6—10 yr	719	4493	63.7 ± 39.3	12,530 ± 5188
Boys	373	2335	69.3 ± 41.9	13,274 ± 5384
Girls	346	2158	57.6 ± 35.3	11,728 ± 4843
11—14 yr	500	3082	53.5 ± 39.6	11,185 ± 5240
Boys	254	1560	58.9 ± 43.3	11,835 ± 5560
Girls	246	1522	48.1 ± 34.6	10,518 ± 4802
15—19 yr	394	2304	45.3 ± 39.3	10,098 ± 5229
Boys	185	1075	50.8 ± 40.2	10,992 ± 5518
Girls	209	1229	40.5 ± 37.9	9316 ± 4830
All boys	812	4970	62.0 ± 42.6	12,328 ± 5548
All girls	801	4909	50.4 ± 36.4	10,749 ± 4924
Total sample	1613	9879	56.2 ± 40.1	11,543 ± 5306

accelerometer both to accumulate daily step count and to detect the number of minutes of vigorous activity performed during the day. Using this approach, the average count corresponding to the arbitrary 60 minute requirement is around 12 000 steps per day at most ages (Table 1). However, there is much to be said for basing the desired step count on the body's response as in the earlier BMI standards,[6] rather than seeking a somewhat arbitrary duration of activity. The BMI data point to a target of 12 000 steps per day in girls, but to the higher figure of 15 000 steps per day in boys.

R. J. Shephard, MD (Lond), PhD, DPE

References

1. Tremblay MS, Warburton DE, Janssen I, et al. New Canadian physical activity guidelines. *Appl Physiol Nutr Metab.* 2011;36:36-46.
2. *US Department of Health and Human Services.* 2008 *Physical Activity Guidelines for Americans.* Washington, DC: ODPHP; 2008. http://www.health.gov/paguidelines.
3. *World Health Organization. Global Recommendations on Physical Activity for Health.* Geneva, Switzerland: WHO; 2010. http://www.who.int/dietphysicalactivity/factsheet_recommendations/en/index.html.
4. Adamo KB, Prince SA, Tricco AC, Connor-Gorber S, Tremblay M. A comparison of indirect versus direct measures for assessing physical activity in the pediatric population: a systematic review. *Int J Pediatr Obes.* 2009;4:2-27.
5. Laurson KR, Eisenmann JC, Welk GJ, Wickel EE, Gentile DA, Walsh DA. Evaluation of youth pedometer-determined physical activity guidelines using receiver operator characteristic curves. *Prev Med.* 2008;46:419-424.
6. Tudor-Locke C, Pangrazi RP, Corbin CB, et al. BMI-referenced standards for recommended pedometer-determined steps/day in children. *Prev Med.* 2004;38:857-864.

Advantage of Distance- versus Time-Based Estimates of Walking in Predicting Adiposity

Williams PT (Lawrence Berkeley Natl Laboratory, CA)
Med Sci Sports Exerc 44:1728-1737, 2012

Purpose.—Physical activity recommendations are defined in terms of time spent being physically active (e.g., 30 min of brisk walking, $5 \, d \cdot wk^{-1}$). However, walking volume may be more naturally assessed by distance than by time. Analyses were therefore performed to test whether time or distance provides the best metric for relating walking volume to estimated total and regional adiposity.

Methods.—Linear and logistic regression analyses were used to relate exercise dose to body mass index (BMI), body circumferences, and obesity in a cross-sectional sample of 12,384 female and 3434 male walkers who reported both usual distance walked and time spent walking per week on survey questionnaires. Metabolic equivalent hours per day ($MET \cdot h \cdot d^{-1}$, $1 \, MET = 3.5 \, mL \, O2 \cdot kg^{-1} \cdot min^{-1}$) were calculated from the time and pace, or distance and pace, using published compendium values.

Results.—Average MET-hours per day walked was 37% greater when calculated from time spent walking versus usual distance in women and was 32% greater in men. Per MET-hours per day, declines in BMI and circumferences (slope $\pm$ SE) were nearly twice as great, or greater, for distance- versus time-derived estimates for kilograms per squared meter of BMI (females $= -0.58 \pm 0.03$ vs -0.31 ± 0.02, males $= -0.35 \pm 0.04$ vs -0.15 ± 0.02), centimeter of waist circumference (females $= -1.42 \pm 0.07$ vs -0.72 ± 0.04, males $= -0.96 \pm 0.10$ vs -0.45 ± 0.07), and reductions in the odds for total obesity (odds ratio: females $= 0.72$ vs 0.84, males $= 0.84$ vs 0.92) and abdominal obesity (females $= 0.74$ vs 0.85, males $= 0.79$ vs 0.91, all comparisons significant).

Conclusions.—Distance walked may provide a better metric of walking volume for epidemiologic obesity research, and better public health targets for weight control, than walking duration. Additional research is required to determine whether these results, derived in a sample that regularly walks for exercise, apply more generally (Table 2).

▶ Rather than telling a patient to walk for 30 minutes per day, we have always specified a distance to be covered, using the time element simply to set the pace of walking or jogging.[1] Much of 30 minutes of walking may be spent getting ready for exercise or talking with friends met along the way; comparisons with accelerometer data have shown that self-reports of exercise times greatly exaggerate the amount of physical activity that has been performed and the proportion of people who are engaging in recommended daily levels of physical activity.[2,3] However, within limits the energy expenditure needed to walk a given distance is independent of the time spent in covering this distance. Thus, if the main element of a daily physical activity program is walking (as is commonly the case in studies of obesity), it makes more sense to base estimates on the distance that is covered rather than on the time that is spent. Williams demonstrates here

TABLE 2.—Cross-Sectional Regression Slopes (TSE) of BMI and Body Circumference Measurements Versus MET-Hours Per Day of Walking and Other Physical Activities to the Test of the Exchangeability Premise

Estimation Method	BMI (kgm^{-2}) Distance	Time	Waist Circumference (cm) Distance	Time	Hip Circumference (cm) Distance	Time
Females						
Walking coefficient	−0.58 ± 0.03*	−0.31 ± 0.02*	−1.42 ± 0.07*	−0.72 ± 0.04*	−1.19 ± 0.06*	−0.62 ± 0.04*
Nonwalking exercise coefficient	−0.11 ± 0.01*	−0.13 ± 0.01*	−0.25 ± 0.03**	−0.30 ± 0.03*	−0.26 ± 0.03*	−0.30 ± 0.03*
Walking − nonwalking difference (95% confidence interval)	−0.47* (−0.53 to −0.41)	−0.19* (−0.23 to −0.14)	−1.16* (−1.31 to −1.02)	−0.42* (−0.52 to −0.31)	−0.93* (−1.07 to −0.79)	−0.32 (−0.42 to −0.23)
Walking coefficient	−0.58 ± 0.03*	−0.32 ± 0.02*	−1.42 ± 0.07*	−0.72 ± 0.04*	−1.19 ± 0.06*	−0.63 ± 0.04*
Vigorous exercise coefficient	−0.12 ± 0.01**	−0.14 ± 0.02*	−0.26 ± 0.04**	−0.32 ± 0.04*	−0.29 ± 0.03*	−0.33 ± 0.03*
Nonwalking moderate exercise coefficient	−0.07 ± 0.03***	−0.07 ± 0.03***	−0.18 ± 0.07***	−0.19 ± 0.07***	−0.14 ± 0.06****	−0.14 ± 0.07****
Light exercise coefficient	−0.46 ± 0.11**	−0.49 ± 0.11**	−0.75 ± 0.26***	−0.80 ± 0.26***	−0.64 ± 0.24***	−0.68 ± 0.24***
Walking − nonwalking moderate exercise difference (95% confidence interval)	−0.51* (−0.58 to −0.43)	−0.24** (−0.31 to −0.18)	−1.24* (−1.43 to −1.05)	−0.53** (−0.69 to −0.37)	−1.05* (−1.23 to −0.87)	−0.49* (−0.64 to −0.34)
Males						
Walking coefficient	−0.35 ± 0.04*	−0.15 ± 0.03**	−0.96 ± 0.10*	−0.45 ± 0.07**		
Nonwalking exercise coefficient	−0.09 ± 0.02**	−0.09 ± 0.02**	−0.25 ± 0.05**	−0.27 ± 0.05**		
Walking − nonwalking difference (95% confidence interval)	−0.27** (−0.36 to −0.18)	−0.05 (−0.12 to 0.01)	−0.71** (−0.94 to −0.49)	−0.18*** (−0.34 to −0.02)		
Walking coefficient	−0.35 ± 0.04*	−0.14 ± 0.03**	−0.96 ± 0.10*	−0.46 ± 0.07**		
Vigorous exercise coefficient	−0.10 ± 0.02**	−0.11 ± 0.02**	−0.27 ± 0.06**	−0.30 ± 0.06**		
Nonwalking moderate exercise coefficient	−0.07 ± 0.04***	−0.07 ± 0.04***	−0.21 ± 0.09****	−0.21 ± 0.09****		
Light exercise coefficient	0.03 ± 0.11	0.05 ± 0.11	−0.21 ± 0.28	−0.17 ± 0.28		
Walking − nonwalking moderate exercise difference (95% confidence interval)	−0.28** (−0.38 to −0.17)	−0.07 (−0.16 to 0.01)	−0.75** (−1.02 to −0.48)	−0.244 (−0.46 to −0.02)		

Values were adjusted for age, education, current smoking status, and intakes of meat, fruit, and alcohol.
In the model:
Dependent variable = intercept + α × Walking$_{Distance}$ + β × Nonwalking exercise + covariates
Dependent variable = intercept + α × Walking$_{Time}$ + β × Nonwalking exercise + covariates
Significance of the regression coefficients coded: *$P < 10^{-15}$, **$P < 0.0001$, ***$P < 0.01$, ****$P < 0.05$, ‡$P < 0.001$.

that the use of self-reported walking time led to a 30% to 40% overestimate of physical activity relative to distance in a group of adults who on average reported walking 2.7-2.9 km per day. Errors probably become greater if the individual is not taking a deliberate daily walk. The use of time as a measure may be particularly fallacious if interest is focused on all "walks" > 10 minutes in duration, as is the case in many current epidemiological studies. In Williams' study, using distance rather than time as the appropriate index also increased the cross-sectional association with measures such as body mass index and waist circumference (Table 2). These findings suggest that the usual time-based exercise recommendations for the general public may need to be reconsidered in favor of distance-based prescriptions. But if this is done, it is important that distance also does not become exaggerated. In our cardiac studies,[1] patients have always measured the distance with a car odometer before beginning their rehabilitation program.

R. J. Shephard, MD (Lond), PhD, DPE

References

1. Shephard RJ. *Ischemic heart disease and exercise*. London (UK): Croom Helm; 1981.
2. Luke A, Dugas LR, Durazo-Arvizu RA, Cao G, Cooper RS. Assessing physical activity and its relationship to cardiovascular risk factors: NHANES 2003-2006. *BMC Public Health*. 2011;11:387.
3. Colley RC, Garriguet D, Janssen I, Craig CL, Clarke J, Tremblay MS. Physical activity of Canadian adults: accelerometer results from the 2007 to 2009 Canadian Health Measures Survey. *Health Rep*. 2011;22:7-14.

Initial Validation of an Exercise "Vital Sign" in Electronic Medical Records
Coleman KJ, Ngor E, Reynolds K, et al (Kaiser Permanente Southern California, Pasadena, CA; et al)
Med Sci Sports Exerc 44:2071-2076, 2012

Purpose.—The objective of this study is to describe the face and discriminant validity of an exercise vital sign (EVS) for use in an outpatient electronic medical record.

Methods.—Eligible patients were 1,793,385 adults 18 yr and older who were members of a large health care system in Southern California. To determine face validity, median total self-reported minutes per week of exercise as measured by the EVS were compared with findings from national population-based surveys. To determine discriminant validity, multivariate Poisson regression models with robust variance estimation were used to examine the ability of the EVS to discriminate between groups of patients with differing physical activity (PA) levels on the basis of demographics and health status.

Results.—After 1.5 yr of implementation, 86% (1,537,798) of all eligible patients had an EVS in their electronic medical record. Overall, 36.3% of patients were completely inactive (0 min of exercise per week), 33.3% were insufficiently active (more than 0 but less than 150 min·wk^{-1}), and 30.4% were sufficiently active (150 min or more per week). As compared with national population-based surveys, patient reports of PA were lower but followed similar patterns. As hypothesized, patients who were older, obese, of a racial/ethnic minority, and had higher disease burdens were more likely to be inactive, suggesting that the EVS has discriminant validity.

Conclusions.—We found that the EVS has good face and discriminant validity and may provide more conservative estimates of PA behavior when compared with national surveys. The EVS has the potential to provide information about the relationship between exercise and health care use, cost, and chronic disease that has not been previously available at the population level.

▶ This practice-based research supports the implementation of physical activity as a vital sign in the outpatient health care setting. The health care system Kaiser Permanente incorporated questions about exercise into the measurement of vital signs for every outpatient visit in the Southern California region. This exercise vital sign (EVS) was used to identify adult patients who were not meeting the 2008 Physical Activity Guidelines for Americans[1] to engage in at least 150 minutes per week of moderate-to-vigorous intensity physical activity. The electronic health system was modified to include 2 exercise questions that were posed to patients by a medical assistant: 1) "On average, how many days per week do you engage in moderate-to-strenuous exercise (like a brisk walk)" and 2) "On average, how many minutes do you engage in exercise at this level?" It took less than 1 minute to administer the EVS questions. Over 1 year of implementation, the EVS was obtained in 86% (1.5 million) of eligible patients. Face and discriminant validity were good as compared with 2 national surveys (Behavior Risk Factor Surveillance System [BRFSS] and National Health and Nutrition Examination Survey [NHANES]), and the expected trends in physical activity across age, gender, and ethnic/racial strata were found. Only 30.4% of patients self-reported that they were sufficiently active ($\geq$150 min/week) as compared with about 50% in the BRFSS and NHANES. Demographic differences and the terms used to describe exercise and exercise intensity could account for some of the differences in physical activity in the EVS compared with the reference databases. Whether the EVS is used to initiate counseling to increase physical activity and what that method of counseling will comprise are areas for future research.

C. M. Jankowski, PhD

Reference

1. Physical Activity Guidelines for Americans Web site [Internet]. Washington DC: Department of Health and Human Services. http://www.health.gov/paguidelines/guidelines/default.aspx. Accessed November 16, 2012.

Advantage of Distance- versus Time-Based Estimates of Walking in Predicting Adiposity

Williams PT (Lawrence Berkeley Natl Laboratory, CA)
Med Sci Sports Exerc 44:1728-1737, 2012

Purpose.—Physical activity recommendations are defined in terms of time spent being physically active (e.g., 30 min of brisk walking, $5 \, d \cdot wk^{-1}$). However, walking volume may be more naturally assessed by distance than by time. Analyses were therefore performed to test whether time or distance provides the best metric for relating walking volume to estimated total and regional adiposity.

Methods.—Linear and logistic regression analyses were used to relate exercise dose to body mass index (BMI), body circumferences, and obesity in a cross-sectional sample of 12,384 female and 3434 male walkers who reported both usual distance walked and time spent walking per week on survey questionnaires. Metabolic equivalent hours per day ($MET \cdot h \cdot d^{-1}$, $1 \, MET = 3.5 \, mL \, O2 \cdot kg^{-1} \cdot min^{-1}$) were calculated from the time and pace, or distance and pace, using published compendium values.

Results.—Average MET-hours per day walked was 37% greater when calculated from time spent walking versus usual distance in women and was 32% greater in men. Per MET-hours per day, declines in BMI and circumferences (slope $\pm$ SE) were nearly twice as great, or greater, for distance- versus time-derived estimates for kilograms per squared meter of BMI (females $= -0.58 \pm 0.03$ vs -0.31 ± 0.02, males $= -0.35 \pm 0.04$ vs -0.15 ± 0.02), centimeter of waist circumference (females $= -1.42 \pm 0.07$ vs -0.72 ± 0.04, males $= -0.96 \pm 0.10$ vs -0.45 ± 0.07), and reductions in the odds for total obesity (odds ratio: females $= 0.72$ vs 0.84, males $= 0.84$ vs 0.92) and abdominal obesity (females $= 0.74$ vs 0.85, males $= 0.79$ vs 0.91, all comparisons significant).

Conclusions.—Distance walked may provide a better metric of walking volume for epidemiologic obesity research, and better public health targets for weight control, than walking duration. Additional research is required to determine whether these results, derived in a sample that regularly walks for exercise, apply more generally.

▶ This study challenges the use of time versus distance metrics for physical activity guidelines. The data indicate that distance walked is a better self-assessment of activity volume than time spent walking and is more strongly related to excess body weight. In agreement with other research, time-based estimates overestimated a person's exercise dose by 32%—37% for walking when compared with distance-based estimates.[1] The goal is to decrease the influence of bias in self-reported physical activity. Most studies show that people overestimate their physical activity by substantial amounts. For example, the National Health and Nutrition Examination Survey showed that only less than 1% of adults met current physical activity guidelines as measured by accelerometry (16) compared with 42% as assessed by time-by-intensity—based calculations from self-reported questionnaire data.[2,3] In Canada, only 15% of adults engaged in 150 min/wk or more of physical activity when objectively measured compared with 65% when using self-reported time and intensity.[4,5] Taken together, the data from this study and others call into doubt the utility of time-based activity guidelines for the general population.

D. C. Nieman, DrPH

References

1. Prince SA, Adamo KB, Hamel ME, Hardt J, Gorber SC, Tremblay M. A comparison of direct versus self-report measures for assessing physical activity in adults: a systematic review. *Int J Behav Nutr Phys Act.* 2008;5:56.
2. Luke A, Dugas LR, Durazo-Arvizu RA, Cao G, Cooper RS. Assessing physical activity and its relationship to cardiovascular risk factors: NHANES 2003-2006. *BMC Public Health.* 2011;11:387.
3. Sisson SB, Camhi SM, Church TS, et al. Leisure time sedentary behavior, occupational/domestic physical activity, and metabolic syndrome in U.S. men and women. *Metab Syndr Relat Disord.* 2009;7:529-536.
4. Bryan SN, Katzmarzyk PT. Are Canadians meeting the guidelines for moderate and vigorous leisure-time physical activity? *Appl Physiol Nutr Metab.* 2009;34:707-715.
5. Colley RC, Garriguet D, Janssen I, Craig CL, Clarke J, Tremblay MS. Physical activity of Canadian adults: accelerometer results from the 2007 to 2009 Canadian Health Measures Survey. *Health Rep.* 2011;22:7-14.

Estimated Time Limit: A Brief Review of a Perceptually Based Scale
Coquart JB, Eston RG, Noakes TD, et al (Université de Rouen, Mont Saint Aignan, France; Univ of South Australia, Adelaide, Australia; Univ of Cape Town, South Africa; et al)
Sports Med 42:845-855, 2012

The ability to predict performance is of great interest for athletes and coaches. It is helpful for the selection of athletes to a team, the prescription of individualized training and the determination of the optimal pacing strategy. However, it is often difficult to judge the time to exhaustion without maximal exercise testing, which is often difficult to schedule during a competitive season. Consequently, the purpose of this review is to presen a recent tool based on subjective prediction of time to exhaustion than can be achieved without requiring a maximal effort. This tool is the estimated time limit (ETL) scale. This review summarizes all experimentations that have studied the ETL scale. These studies suggest that the ETL scale may be used to predict time to exhaustion (Fig 1).

▶ It is a common experience to see an athlete who misjudges his or her speed and who becomes exhausted before reaching the finish line. But at the same time, most people—whether athletes or not—have some ability to predict how much longer they can continue at a given rate of exercising. In the days when the Douglas bag was used to measure maximal oxygen intake, it was common for the investigator to obtain the critical gas sample by asking test candidates to signal when they could continue running for just 30 seconds longer. The development of a formal scale to predict time to exhaustion (Fig 1) is analogous to the Rating of Perceived

How long would you be able to perform an exercise
at this intensity to exhaustion?

20	
19	2 minutes
18	
17	4 minutes
16	
15	8 minutes
14	
13	15 minutes
12	
11	30 minutes
10	
9	1 hour
8	
7	2 hours
6	
5	4 hours
4	
3	8 hours
2	
1	more than 16 hours

FIGURE 1.—Estimated time limit scale (reproduced from Garcin et al.,[10] with permission). *Editor's Note*: Please refer to original journal article for full references. (Reprinted from Coquart JB, Eston RG, Noakes TD, et al. Estimated time limit: a brief review of a perceptually based scale. *Sports Med*. 2012;42:845-855, with permission from Springer International Publishing AG.)

Exertion (RPE)[1] and is an interesting idea. Marcora has suggested that the score reported on a scale of this type depends on a person's ability to combine the immediate RPE with an accumulated memory of how rapidly RPE increases at any given perception of effort.[2] It will be interesting to see whether this tool proves of practical value to athletes as they learn to refine their pacing ability, and whether it can also be of help in developing more effective regimens for the training of endurance performance in the general public.

R. J. Shephard, MD (Lond), PhD, DPE

References

1. Borg G. *Borg's Exertion and Pain Scales*. Champaign, IL: Human Kinetics; 1998.
2. Marcora S. Counterpoint: afferent feedback from fatigued locomotor muscles is not an important determinant of endurance exercise performance. *J Appl Physiol*. 2010;108:454-457.

Aerobic Fitness Affects Cortisol Responses to Concurrent Challenges
Webb HE, Rosalky DS, Tangsilsat SE, et al (Mississippi State Univ, Starkville; The Univ of New South Wales, Sydney, Australia; et al)
Med Sci Sports Exerc 45:379-386, 2013

Purpose.—Studies have demonstrated that a combination of mental and physical challenge can elicit exacerbated state anxiety, effort sense, and cortisol responses above that of a single stimulus. However, an analysis of the effects of aerobic fitness on the responses of cortisol to concurrent mental

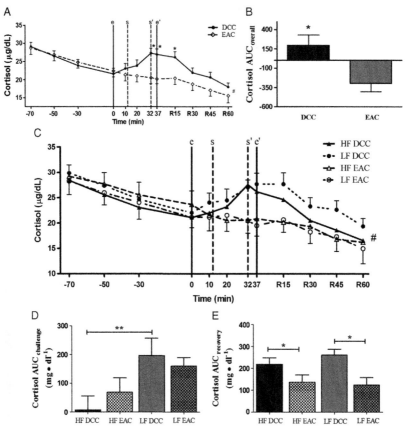

FIGURE 3.—Cortisol responses of participants across time in the EAC and DCC between conditions (A) and between fitness levels and condition across time (B). Significant differences were seen between the DCC and EAC (*$P < 0.05$) and across time (#$P < 0.05$). Cortisol AUC responses are presented as (C) AUC$_{overall}$ (0−R60 min), (D) AUC$_{challenge}$ (0−37 min), and (E) AUC$_{recovery}$ (37−R60 min) between fitness levels, with differences between the conditions found for AUC$_{overall}$ and AUC$_{recovery}$ (*$P < 0.05$) and between fitness levels and condition for AUC$_{challenge}$(**$P < 0.05$). *Points* represent the cortisol values at specific time points during the protocol; *vertical lines* depict SE of the means. The *solid vertical lines* extending from the ordinate represent the conclusion of the exercise (é) component, whereas *vertical dotted lines* extending from the ordinate represent the start of the mental challenge (s) and the end of the mental challenge (ś). (Reprinted from Webb HE, Rosalky DS, Tangsilsat SE, et al. Aerobic fitness affects cortisol responses to concurrent challenges. *Med Sci Sports Exerc.* 2013;45:379-386, with permission from the American College of Sports Medicine.)

and physical stress between below average and above average fitness individuals has not been conducted. This study examined the effects of a combination of acute mental challenges and physical stress on psychological and cortisol responses between eight individuals of below average fitness (low fit (LF), $\dot{V}O_{2max} = 36.58 \pm 3.36$ mL·kg^{-1}·min^{-1}) and eight individuals of above average fitness (high fit (HF), $\dot{V}O_{2max} = 51.18 \pm 2.09$ mL·kg^{-1}·min^{-1}).

Methods.—All participants completed two experimental conditions. An exercise-alone condition (EAC) consisted of cycling at 60% $\dot{V}O_{2max}$ for

37 min, and a dual-challenge condition (DCC) included concurrent participation in a mental challenge for 20 min while cycling.

Results.—The DCC resulted in increases in state anxiety ($P = 0.018$), perceived overall workload ($P = 0.001$), and exacerbated cortisol responses ($P = 0.04$). Furthermore, LF participants had a greater overall cortisol response in the DCC compared with the EAC (DCC = 346.83 ± 226.92; EAC = −267.46 ± 132.32; $t_7 = 2.49$, $P = 0.04$), whereas HF participants demonstrated no difference between conditions (DCC = 38.91 ± 147.01; EAC = −324.60 ± 182.78; $t_7 = 1.68$, $P = 0.14$).

Discussion.—LF individuals seem to demonstrate unnecessary and unfavorable responses to the DCC compared with HF individuals, particularly concerning cortisol. The exacerbated cortisol responses in LF individuals have implications for harmful consequences such as increased risk of cardiovascular disease (Fig 3).

▶ Previous authors have shown that fitness attenuates the cortisol response to either physical or mental stress. This article makes the point that fit individuals are also better able to handle a combination of vigorous physical activity and mental stress, with a smaller cumulative release of cortisol (Fig 3). They thus avoid such possible adverse consequences of excessive cortisol release as lean tissue breakdown, insulin resistance, and cardiovascular disease.[1-3] The issue seems important for occupations such as the military, fire-fighting, and emergency medical technicians, where heavy physical work is sometimes combined with severe psychological stress. Differences between the fit and unfit subjects are statistically convincing. However, the sample size is quite small, and confidence in the data is further attenuated by presentation of an excessive array of digits for each variable. Moreover, the challenges imposed (37 minutes of cycle ergometry at 60% of maximal oxygen intake, together with performance of the Stroop test and some mental arithmetic) are much less than those likely in "real life," and certainly do not present any danger to life or limb. Although it would be more difficult to quantitate the corresponding variables on the job, there remains scope to document the magnitude of this benefit on larger samples of fit and unfit individuals as they undertake the challenging phases of their normal work.

R. J. Shephard, MD (Lond), PhD, DPE

References

1. Christiansen JJ, Djurhuus CB, Gravholt CH, et al. Effects of cortisol on carbohydrate, lipid, and protein metabolism: studies of acute cortisol withdrawal in adrenocortical failure. *J Clin Endocrinol Metab.* 2007;92:3553-3559.
2. Dickerson SS, Kemeny ME. Acute stressors and cortisol responses: a theoretical integration and synthesis of laboratory research. *Psychol Bull.* 2004;130:355-391.
3. Ho RC, Neo LF, Chua AN, Cheak AA, Mak A. Research on psychoneuroimmunology: does stress influence immunity and cause coronary artery disease? *Ann Acad Med Singapore.* 2010;39:191-196.

Leisure Time Physical Activity of Moderate to Vigorous Intensity and Mortality: A Large Pooled Cohort Analysis

Moore SC, Patel AV, Matthews CE, et al (Natl Cancer Inst, Bethesda, MD; American Cancer Society, Atlanta, GA; et al)
PLoS Med 9:e1001335, 2012

Background.—Leisure time physical activity reduces the risk of premature mortality, but the years of life expectancy gained at different levels remains unclear. Our objective was to determine the years of life gained after age 40 associated with various levels of physical activity, both overall and according to body mass index (BMI) groups, in a large pooled analysis.

Methods and Findings.—We examined the association of leisure time physical activity with mortality during follow-up in pooled data from six prospective cohort studies in the National Cancer Institute Cohort Consortium, comprising 654,827 individuals, 21—90 y of age. Physical activity was categorized by metabolic equivalent hours per week (MET-h/wk). Life expectancies and years of life gained/lost were calculated using direct adjusted survival curves (for participants 40+ years of age), with 95% confidence intervals (CIs) derived by bootstrap. The study includes a median 10 y of follow-up and 82,465 deaths. A physical activity level of 0.1—3.74 MET-h/wk, equivalent to brisk walking for up to 75 min/wk, was associated with a gain of 1.8 (95% CI: 1.6—2.0) y in life expectancy relative to no leisure time activity (0 MET-h/wk). Higher levels of physical activity were associated with greater gains in life expectancy, with a gain of 4.5 (95% CI: 4.3—4.7) y at the highest level (22.5+ MET-h/wk, equivalent to brisk walking for 450+ min/wk). Substantial gains were also observed in each BMI group. In joint analyses, being active (7.5+ MET-h/wk) and normal weight (BMI 18.5—24.9) was associated with a gain of 7.2 (95% CI: 6.5—7.9) y of life compared to being inactive (0 MET-h/wk) and obese (BMI 35.0+). A limitation was that physical activity and BMI were ascertained by self report.

Conclusions.—More leisure time physical activity was associated with longer life expectancy across a range of activity levels and BMI groups (Fig 1).

▶ Over the past 30 years, Paffenbarger et al have argued, first from occupational comparisons and subsequently from a study of the leisure activities reported by a group of Harvard alumni, that the choice of an active lifestyle can add as much as 2 years to the average lifespan.[1] However, their conclusion was based on an association rather than a controlled experiment, and although various attempts were made to control statistically for associated variables, fears have remained that those who engage in regular vigorous activity are not typical of the general population; rather, they include a high proportion of former smokers and those motivated to exercise by a history of cancer or heart disease.[2] The new meta-analysis by Moore et al examines the issue of exercise and life expectancy prospectively in 6 studies, covering an impressive sample of 654 827 adults who were followed for an average of 10 years. Careful statistical adjustments of the data

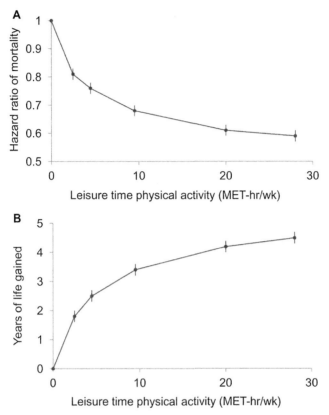

FIGURE 1.—Leisure time physical activity level and hazard ratios for mortality and gains in life expectancy after age 40. The points shown represent the HR (A) or years of life gained (B) for each of the physical activity categories examined, and the vertical lines represent the 95% CIs for that physical activity category. The reference category for both (A) and (B) is 0.0 MET-h/wk of leisure time physical activity. The lines connecting the points help to illustrate the dose—response relationship between physical activity and risk of mortality; the shape of the association shown here is similar to that obtained using spline modeling (Figure S1 in the original article). HRs were calculated in models stratified by study that used age as the underlying time scale. Multivariable models were adjusted for gender, alcohol consumption (0, 0.1—14.9, 15.0—29.9, 30.0+ g/d), education (did not complete high school, completed high school, post-high-school training, some college, completed college), marital status (married, divorced, widowed, unmarried), history of heart disease, history of cancer, BMI (<18.5, 18.5—19.9, 20—22.4, 22.5—24.9, 25—27.4, 27.5—29.9, 30+ kg/m^2), and smoking status (never, former, current). Years of life expectancy gained after age 40 were derived using direct adjusted survival curves [31,32] for participants who were 40+ y of age at baseline (97.5% of participants). *Editor's Note*: Please refer to original journal article for full references. (Reprinted from Moore SC, Patel AV, Matthews CE, et al. Leisure time physical activity of moderate to vigorous intensity and mortality: a large pooled cohort analysis. *PLoS Med.* 2012;9:e1001335, © 2012 National Center for Biotechnology Information.)

were made for age, sex, educational attainment, some chronic diseases, and unhealthy lifestyles, including smoking and drinking, and a clear benefit of regular physical activity was still seen. Relative to those who were sedentary, those individuals who reported energy expenditures up to 3.74 metabolic equivalent hours per week (equal to 75 minutes of brisk walking per week) had a lifespan advantage of 1.8 years. A doubling of weekly energy expenditure, to the widely recommended

150 minutes of brisk walking per week, was associated with an advantage of 3.4 to 4.5 years (Fig 1). The comparison of obesity plus inactivity with a normal body mass and >150 minutes of exercise per week was particularly striking (a life expectancy advantage of 7.2 years to the more active and thinner subjects). Although these data are still "associations" and do not address the equally important issue of quality-adjusted life expectancy, they are enough to convince me of the importance of regular exercise.

R. J. Shephard, MD (Lond), PhD, DPE

References

1. Paffenbarger RS Jr, Hyde RT, Wing AL, Hsieh CC. Physical activity, all-cause mortality, and longevity of college alumni. *N Engl J Med.* 1986;314:605-613.
2. Active adults live longer. *BMJ.* 2012;345:e7641.

Biomechanical, cardiorespiratory, metabolic and perceived responses to electrically assisted cycling
Sperlich B, Zinner C, Hébert-Losier K, et al (Univ of Wuppertal, Germany; German Sport Univ Cologne, Germany; Mid Sweden Univ, Östersund)
Eur J Appl Physiol 112:4015-4025, 2012

The aims of the present study were to characterize the effects of cycling in varying terrain with the assistance of an electric motor with respect to (1) power output, velocity, and electromyography (EMG) signals; (2) cardiorespiratory parameters; (3) energy expenditure (EE); (4) rate of perceived exertion (RPE) and enjoyment and to compare these effects with those of non-assisted cycling. Eight sedentary women (age: 38 ± 15 years, BMI: 25.3 ± 2.1 kg m^{-2}) cycled 9.5 km on varying terrain (change in elevation: 102 m, maximum incline: 5.8 %) at their own pace, once with and once without motorized assistance, in randomized order. With electrical assistance, the mean power output (−29%); EMG patterns of the m. biceps femoris (−49%), m. vastus lateralis (−33%), m. vastus medialis (−37%), and m. gastrocnemius medialis (−29%); heart rate (−29.1%); oxygen uptake (−33.0%); respiratory exchange ratio (−9.0%); and EE (−36.5%) were all lower, whereas the mean cycling speed was higher ($P < 0.05$) than that without such assistance. In addition, following assisted exercise the mean blood lactate concentration and RPE were lower ($P < 0.05$) and ratings of enjoyment higher ($P < 0.05$). Moreover, motorized cycling was associated with (1) lower EMG with higher power output and speed; (2) less cardiorespiratory and metabolic effort; (3) lower respiratory exchange ratio; (4) lower RPE with more enjoyment; and (5) sufficient EE, according to present standards, to provide health benefits. Thus, electrically assisted cycling may represent an innovative approach to persuading reluctant sedentary women to exercise (Table 3).

▶ There is substantial evidence linking active commuting by bicycle with enhanced cardiovascular health.[1,2] Although the practice of cycling to and from

TABLE 3.—Mean (±SD) Data of Power Outputs, Velocity of Cycling, Breathing Frequency, Ventilation, Heart Rate, Oxygen Uptake, RER, Energy Expenditure, and the Amplitudes of EMG Signals During Five Laps of Cycling in Varying Terrain with (the e-Bike) or Without (the Conventional Bike) Electrical Assistance

Parameter	Terrain (Lap 1–5)								All Terrain combined		
	Uphill 1		Downhill 1		Uphill 2		Flat				
	e-Bike	Conventional	e-Bike	Conventional	e-Bike	Conventional	e-Bike	Conventional	e-Bike	Conventional	Cohen's d
Mean power output (W)	89 ± 35	105 ± 49*	73 ± 37	116 ± 32*	84 ± 27	122 ± 39*	76 ± 33	120 ± 33*	80 ± 33	113 ± 33	1.00
Velocity of cycling (km h^{-1})	13.9 ± 4.9	9.9 ± 2.3*	18.5 ± 5.4	17.2 ± 2.9	15.4 ± 5.2	12.6 ± 3.2*	15.5 ± 3.9	14.1 ± 5.0	15.8 ± 5.6	13.7 ± 4.1	0.40
Breathing frequency (L min^{-1})	31 ± 4	32 ± 5	30 ± 4	33 ± 5	31 ± 4	33 ± 6	30 ± 5	32 ± 5	31 ± 4	33 ± 5	0.44
Ventilation (L min^{-1})	36.9 ± 6.8	50.3 ± 13.2*	37.9 ± 7.2	54.2 ± 12.0*	37.9 ± 6.3	54.4 ± 12.3*	37.6 ± 10.2	54.9 ± 9.2*	37.6 ± 6.7	52.6 ± 12.0*	1.54
Heart rate (bpm)	108 ± 18	136 ± 17*	104 ± 20	133 ± 21*	105 ± 17	137 ± 16*	100 ± 20	140 ± 19*	105 ± 20	133 ± 19*	1.53
Oxygen uptake (mL min^{-1})	1,340 ± 373	1,824 ± 450*	1,271 ± 356	1,656 ± 418*	1,390 ± 358	1,942 ± 439*	1,330 ± 380	1,839 ± 356*	1,333 ± 351	1,774 ± 430*	1.12
Oxygen uptake (mL min^{-1} kg^{-1})	18.3 ± 4.6	25.7 ± 4.8*	16.9 ± 3.2	23.2 ± 4.6*	18.9 ± 4.3	27.4 ± 5.3*	18.0 ± 3.3	25.7 ± 5.3*	18.0 ± 3.8	25.5 ± 4.8*	1.73
O$_2$-cost of exercise (mL min^{-1} W^{-1})	15.1 ± 5.5	17.3 ± 7.2	17.4 ± 4.7	14.3 ± 8.0	16.5 ± 5.3	15.9 ± 6.4	17.5 ± 3.6	15.3 ± 5.6	16.6 ± 4.8	15.7 ± 6.8	0.15
RER	0.85 ± 0.07	0.91 ± 0.06	0.91 ± 0.07	1.07 ± 0.08*	0.84 ± 0.05	0.91 ± 0.07*	0.86 ± 0.06	0.96 ± 0.06*	0.86 ± 0.06	0.94 ± 0.10*	0.97
METs	5.2 ± 1.2	7.2 ± 1.5*	4.8 ± 0.9	6.5 ± 1.3*	5.8 ± 2.8	7.7 ± 1.6*	5.1 ± 1.2	7.3 ± 1.2*	5.2 ± 1.7	7.1 ± 1.4*	1.22
EMG amplitude (μV)											
Biceps femoris	17.9 ± 4.5	57.6 ± 39.1	19.0 ± 5.6	29.1 ± 17.8	14.6 ± 2.8	22.6 ± 2.8	13.6 ± 1.9	18.0 ± 6.7	16.3 ± 15.7	31.8 ± 23.2*	0.78
Vastus lateralis	35.3 ± 20.4	52.5 ± 30.5	20.6 ± 11.5	30.0 ± 16.5	39.0 ± 22.0	57.9 ± 32.4	21.8 ± 15.1	32.1 ± 18.4	28.9 ± 26.8	43.1 ± 40.0*	0.41
Vastus medialis	43.3 ± 11.2	68.6 ± 26.1	24.3 ± 6.6	36.0 ± 6.1	46.6 ± 13.0	75.4 ± 23.4	25.7 ± 10.6	39.2 ± 9.2	35.0 ± 32.2	54.8 ± 50.2*	0.46
Gastrocnemius medialis	30.4 ± 13.7	52.7 ± 11.7	23.2 ± 10.0	28.7 ± 16.2	34.0 ± 16.3	41.9 ± 25.8	19.7 ± 7.0	27.3 ± 15.4	26.8 ± 25.6	37.6 ± 32.6*	0.36

bpm beats per minute; RER respiratory exchange ratio; MET metabolic equivalent of task.
*Indicates statistical differences at P < 0.05 between the e-bike and the conventional bike cycling mode.

work may identify individuals with a healthy overall lifestyle, the energy expenditures involved in cycling at a moderate speed seem enough to enhance the cardiorespiratory fitness of the average person. However, 1 negative motivational factor for the older person who initially is not in very good physical condition is the final hill on the return journey. It is thus interesting to evaluate how far a small auxiliary electric motor overcomes this deterrent. Some recent studies suggest that cycling a distance of around 5 km does provide a useful cardiovascular stimulus, even if the bicycle is equipped with a small electric motor.[3,4] The study by Sperlich et al demonstrates that effort dropped by about 30% when there was assistance from the motor, but in previously sedentary middle-aged women, enjoyment of the experience was increased and the rating of perceived exertion dropped from 14.3 to 8.3 units; the speed of cycling also increased, allowing commutes to be completed in a more reasonable time. The oxygen consumption, both on the flat and uphill tended to drop to around 5 METs, with a heart rate around 55% of maximum (as opposed to 69% of maximum on a conventional bicycle) (Table 3). Thus, to develop the same total energy expenditure (if desiring to lose weight), a person would need to increase his or her weekly cycling distance by some 30%. The currently recommended health objective for aerobic activity was met by using an electrically assisted bicycle over a distance of 10 km 3 or 4 times per week, corresponding with the likely daily commuting distance for many North Americans.

R. J. Shephard, MD (Lond), PhD, DPE

References

1. Shephard RJ. Is active commuting the answer to population health? *Sports Med.* 2008;38:751-758.
2. Shephard RJ. The exercising commuter: is commuting a healthy way to be active? *Curr Cardiovasc Risk Rep.* 2012;6:299-306.
3. Gojanovic B, Welker J, Iglesias K, Daucourt C, Gremion G. Electric bikes as a new active transportation modality to promote health. *Med Sci Sports Exerc.* 2011;43: 2204-2210.
4. Simons M, Van Es E, Hendriksen I. Electrically assisted cycling: a new mode for meeting physical activity guidelines? *Med Sci Sports Exerc.* 2009;41:2097-2102.

Active Transportation and Cardiovascular Disease Risk Factors in U.S. Adults

Furie GL, Desai MM (Yale School of Medicine, New Haven, CT)
Am J Prev Med 43:621-628, 2012

Background.—Evidence of associations between active transportation (walking and bicycling for transportation) and health outcomes is limited. Better understanding of this relationship would inform efforts to increase physical activity by promoting active transportation.

Purpose.—This study examined associations between active transportation and cardiovascular disease risk factors in U.S. adults.

Methods.—Using the 2007–2008 and 2009–2010 cycles of the National Health and Nutrition Examination Survey (NHANES), adults (N = 9933) were classified by level of active transportation. Multivariable linear and logistic regression analyses controlled for sociodemographic characteristics, smoking status, and minutes/week of non-active transportation physical activity. Analyses were conducted in 2011.

Results.—Overall, 76% reported no active transportation. Compared with no active transportation, mean BMI was lower among individuals with low (−0.9, 95% CI = −1.4, −0.5) and high (−1.2, 95% CI = −1.7, −0.8) levels of active transportation. Mean waist circumference was lower in the low (−2.2 cm, 95% CI = −3.2, −1.2) and high (−3.1 cm, 95% CI = −4.3, −1.9) active transportation groups. The odds of hypertension were 24% lower (AOR = 0.76, 95% CI = 0.61, 0.94) and 31% lower (AOR = 0.69, 95% CI = 0.58, 0.83) among individuals with low and high levels of active transportation, respectively, compared with no active transportation. High active transportation was associated with 31% lower odds of diabetes (AOR = 0.69, 95% CI = 0.54, 0.88). Active transportation was not associated with high-density lipoprotein level.

Conclusions.—Active transportation was associated with more-favorable cardiovascular risk factor profiles, providing additional justification for infrastructure and policies that permit and encourage active transportation.

▶ About 4 in 10 US adults do not engage in the minimum 150 minutes/week of moderate physical activity recommended by the Department of Health and Human Services.[1] There are many barriers to regular physical activity, and chief among them is lack of time. Walking and bicycling to work, school, or other scheduled duties is attractive to many people because it is more purposeful than swimming laps, running 400-m repeats on a track, or cycling on an indoor ergometer. Active transportation is popular in Europe.[2] For example, in Germany, the proportion of individuals reporting walking or cycling for transportation is 2 and 7 times greater, respectively, than in the United States.[3] This difference is facilitated by a vast network of trails in Germany that make active transportation easy, appealing, and time effective. This study shows that another benefit of active transportation is lowered cardiovascular disease risk factors, and this finding is consistent with other similar studies of US adults.[4]

D. C. Nieman, DrPH

References

1. Tucker JM, Welk GJ, Beyler NK. Physical activity in U.S.: adults compliance with the Physical Activity Guidelines for Americans. *Am J Prev Med.* 2011;40:454-461.
2. Pucher J, Buehler R, Bassett DR, Dannenberg AL. Walking and cycling to health: a comparative analysis of city, state, and international data. *Am J Public Health.* 2010;100:1986-1992.
3. Buehler R, Pucher J, Merom D, Bauman A. Active travel in Germany and the U.S. Contributions of daily walking and cycling to physical activity. *Am J Prev Med.* 2011;41:241-250.
4. Gordon-Larsen P, Boone-Heinonen J, Sidney S, Sternfeld B, Jacobs DR Jr, Lewis CE. Active commuting and cardiovascular disease risk: the CARDIA study. *Arch Intern Med.* 2009;169:1216-1223.

Sustained and Shorter Bouts of Physical Activity Are Related to Cardiovascular Health

Glazer NL, Lyass A, Esliger DW, et al (Boston Univ School of Medicine, MA; Natl Heart, Lung and Blood Inst's Framingham Heart Study, MA; Loughborough Univ, UK; et al)

Med Sci Sports Exerc 45:109-115, 2013

Purpose.—Whereas greater physical activity (PA) is known to prevent cardiovascular disease (CVD), the relative importance of performing PA in sustained bouts of activity versus shorter bouts of activity on CVD risk is not known. The objective of this study was to investigate the relationship between moderate-to-vigorous PA (MVPA), measured in bouts ≥ 10 and <10 min, and CVD risk factors in a well-characterized community-based sample of white adults.

Methods.—We conducted a cross-sectional analysis of 2109 participants in the Third Generation Cohort of the Framingham Heart Study (mean age - $= 47$ yr, 55% women) who underwent objective assessment of PA by accelerometry over 5–7 d. Total MVPA, MVPA done in bouts ≥ 10 min ($MVPA_{10+}$), and MVPA done in bouts < 10 min ($MVPA_{<10}$) were calculated. MVPA exposures were related to individual CVD risk factors, including measures of adiposity and blood lipid and glucose levels, using linear and logistic regression.

Results.—Total MVPA was significantly associated with higher HDL levels and with lower triglycerides, BMI, waist circumference, and Framingham risk score ($P < 0.0001$). $MVPA_{<10}$ showed similar statistically significant associations with these CVD risk factors ($P < 0.001$). Compliance with national guidelines (150 min of total MVPA) was significantly related to lower BMI, triglycerides, Framingham risk score, waist circumference, higher HDL, and a lower prevalence of obesity and impaired fasting glucose ($P < 0.001$ for all).

Conclusions.—Our cross-sectional observations on a large middle-age community-based sample confirm a positive association of MVPA with a healthier CVD risk factor profile and indicate that accruing PA in bouts < 10 min may favorably influence cardiometabolic risk. Additional investigations are warranted to confirm our findings (Table 3).

▶ The idea that the accumulation of short bursts of activity might be beneficial to health was first advanced by Murphy and Hardman.[1] Such a suggestion is popular with health promotion gurus who have difficulty in persuading people to exercise for 30 minutes at a stretch, and it has some logic at least as far the metabolism of excess energy is concerned, although for the enhancement of physical fitness, a certain duration of "strain" may be required. A more recent review of this issue concluded that there was insufficient evidence on the value of short periods of activity in studies where the intensity and total volume of physical activity had been controlled adequately relative to longer periods of exercise.[2] Evidence is particularly limited concerning the health significance of exercise bouts shorter than 10 minutes. The 7-day Actical accelerometer data of Glazer and associates

TABLE 3.—Relations of MVPA Measures to CVD Risk Factors

	Total MVPA[a]		MVPA10+[b]		MVPA<10[c]		
	β Coefficient	P	β Coefficient	P	β Coefficient	P	P for Comparison*
Triglycerides (mg·dL^{-1})	−3.8 (0.58)	<0.0001	−3.17 (0.81)	<0.0001	−4.42 (0.99)	<0.0001	0.48
HDL (mg·dL^{-1})	1.14 (0.18)	<0.0001	1.45 (0.34)	<0.0001	0.87 (0.26)	0.001	0.17
SBP (mm Hg)	−0.33 (0.15)	0.03	−0.19 (0.24)	0.44	−0.46 (0.23)	0.05	0.47
DBP (mm Hg)	−0.08 (0.10)	0.42	−0.16 (0.17)	0.35	0.01 (0.15)	0.96	0.55
Framingham risk score (%)	−0.19 (0.04)	<0.0001	−0.10 (0.07)	0.16	−0.28 (0.06)	<0.0001	0.08
Waist circumference (cm)	−1.01 (0.14)	<0.0001	−1.17 (0.20)	<0.0001	−0.86 (0.22)	<0.0001	0.36
BMI (kg·m^{-2})	−0.38 (0.05)	<0.0001	−0.46 (0.08)	<0.0001	−0.30 (0.09)	0.0007	0.27
Glucose (mg·dL^{-1})	−0.30 (0.16)	0.05	−0.29 (0.19)	0.12	−0.29 (0.28)	0.29	0.99
	Odds Ratio (95% CI)	P	Odds Ratio (95% CI)	P	Odds Ratio (95% CI)	P	
Hypertension	0.97 (0.91–1.023)	0.37	0.93 (0.84–1.04)	0.23	0.98 (0.89–1.08)	0.70	0.55
Obesity	0.85 (0.80–0.90)	<0.0001	0.83 (0.74–0.93)	0.0001	0.86 (0.78–0.94)	0.002	0.67
IGT	0.97 (0.92–1.03)	0.37	0.96 (0.87–1.07)	0.50	0.97 (0.90–1.06)	0.59	0.86
DM	0.93 (0.80–1.08)	0.36	0.86 (0.66–1.13)	0.28	0.97 (0.79–1.20)	0.81	0.48

β's and odds ratios are presented per 10 min·d−1 of MVPA. Statistical significance was set at $P < 0.001$ (Bonferroni correction for 12 CVD risk factors and 3 exposure variables.
[a]Adjusted for age, sex, average accelerometer wear time (total wear time/number of days worn), education level, and self-reported general health.
[b]Adjusted for age, sex, average accelerometer wear time, education level, self-reported general health, and MVPA<10.
[c]Adjusted for age, sex, average accelerometer wear time, education level, self-reported general health, and MVPA10+.
*P comparing β coefficient from MVPA10+ model versus MVPA<10 model.

were obtained on a large population sample spread over each of the 4 seasons of the year, and their data confirm that short periods of physical activity show a favorable association with metabolic risk (body mass index, waist circumference, cholesterol, and triglycerides; Table 3). One limitation of the data, as in many studies of this type, is that there was no control for a possible association between a higher level of physical activity and other aspects of a healthy lifestyle, including a more prudent diet. Also, the hip-mounted accelerometer did not capture such forms of exercise as cycling and resistance training. Although there is growing evidence that short bouts of activity can contribute to some aspects of metabolic health, in my view it would be a mistake to allow those counseling patients to avoid recommending longer regular bouts of activity that can also improve cardiovascular fitness.

R. J. Shephard, MD (Lond), PhD, DPE

References

1. Murphy MH, Hardman AE. Training effects of short and long bouts of brisk walking in sedentary women. *Med Sci Sports Exerc.* 1998;30:152-157.
2. Murphy MH, Blair SN, Murtagh EM. Accumulated versus continuous exercise for health benefit: a review of empirical studies. *Sports Med.* 2009;39:29-43.

Sustained and Shorter Bouts of Physical Activity Are Related to Cardiovascular Health

Glazer NL, Lyass A, Esliger DW, et al (Boston Univ School of Medicine, MA; Natl Heart, Lung and Blood Insts Framingham Heart Study, MA; Loughborough Univ, UK; et al)

Med Sci Sports Exerc 45:109-115, 2013

Purpose.—Whereas greater physical activity (PA) is known to prevent cardiovascular disease (CVD), the relative importance of performing PA in sustained bouts of activity versus shorter bouts of activity on CVD risk is not known. The objective of this study was to investigate the relationship between moderate-to-vigorous PA (MVPA), measured in bouts ≥ 10 and <10 min, and CVD risk factors in a well-characterized community-based sample of white adults.

Methods.—We conducted a cross-sectional analysis of 2109 participants in the Third Generation Cohort of the Framingham Heart Study (mean age = 47 yr, 55% women) who underwent objective assessment of PA by accelerometry over 5–7 d. Total MVPA, MVPA done in bouts ≥ 10 min ($MVPA_{10+}$), and MVPA done in bouts <10 min ($MVPA_{<10}$) were calculated. MVPA exposures were related to individual CVD risk factors, including measures of adiposity and blood lipid and glucose levels, using linear and logistic regression.

Results.—Total MVPA was significantly associated with higher HDL levels and with lower triglycerides, BMI, waist circumference, and Framingham risk score ($P < 0.0001$). $MVPA_{<10}$ showed similar statistically significant associations with these CVD risk factors ($P < 0.001$). Compliance with national guidelines (≥150 min of total MVPA) was significantly related to lower BMI, triglycerides, Framingham risk score, waist circumference, higher HDL, and a lower prevalence of obesity and impaired fasting glucose ($P < 0.001$ for all).

Conclusions.—Our cross-sectional observations on a large middle-age community-based sample confirm a positive association of MVPA with a healthier CVD risk factor profile and indicate that accruing PA in bouts <10 min may favorably influence cardiometabolic risk. Additional investigations are warranted to confirm our findings.

▶ National guidelines recommend accumulating 150 min/wk or more of physical activity in bouts of 10 minutes or longer.[1] This recommendation, however, is not based on definitive research data and imposes a potential barrier to individuals who prefer accumulating 150 min/wk in shorter duration bouts. Of interest, approximately half of the middle-age adult population in this study met the recommendation of at least 150 min/wk of total physical activity, but only 12% engaged in this level of activity in bouts of 10 minutes or longer. Compliance with national physical activity guidelines was associated with a statistically significant lower cardiovascular disease risk factor burden and lower prevalence of obesity and impaired glucose tolerance, regardless of how physical activity was accrued. The important message is that individuals can forget the 10-minute rule and concentrate on accumulating 150 min/wk any way they can (eg, climbing the stairs, carrying groceries from the store to the car, taking 5-minute walks during breaks at work).

D. C. Nieman, DrPH

Reference

1. Physical Activity Guidelines Advisory Committee. *Physical Activity Guidelines Advisory Committee Report.* Washington, DC: Department of Health and Human Services; 2008.

Years of Life Gained Due to Leisure-Time Physical Activity in the U.S.
Janssen I, Carson V, Lee I-M, et al (Queen's Univ, Kingston, Ontario, Canada; Brigham and Women's Hosp, Boston, MA; et al)
Am J Prev Med 44:23-29, 2013

Background.—Physical inactivity is an important modifiable risk factor for noncommunicable disease. The degree to which physical activity affects the life expectancy of Americans is unknown.

Purpose.—This study estimated the potential years of life gained due to leisure-time physical activity in the U.S.

Methods.—Data from the National Health and Nutrition Examination Survey (2007–2010); National Health Interview Study mortality linkage (1990–2006); and U.S. Life Tables (2006) were used to estimate and compare life expectancy at each age of adult life for inactive (no moderate

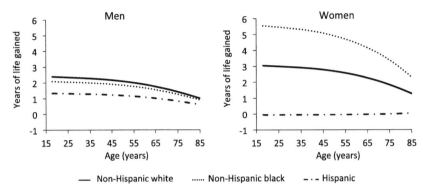

FIGURE.—Potential years of life gained in the active category across the adult lifespan. (Reprinted from American Journal of Preventive Medicine. Janssen I, Carson V, Lee I-M, et al. Years of life gained due to leisure-time physical activity in the U.S. *Am J Prev Med.* 2013;44:23-29, Copyright 2013, with permission from Elsevier.)

to vigorous physical activity); somewhat-active (some moderate to vigorous activity but <500 MET minutes/week); and active (≥500 MET minutes/week of moderate to vigorous activity) adults. Analyses were conducted in 2012.

Results.—Somewhat-active and active non-Hispanic white men had a life expectancy at age 20 years that was ~2.4 years longer than that for the inactive men; this life expectancy advantage was 1.2 years at age 80 years. Similar observations were made in non-Hispanic white women, with a higher life expectancy within the active category of 3.0 years at age 20 years and 1.6 years at age 80 years. In non-Hispanic black women, as many as 5.5 potential years of life were gained due to physical activity. Significant increases in longevity were also observed within somewhat-active and active non-Hispanic black men; however, among Hispanics the years-of-life-gained estimates were not significantly different from 0 years gained.

Conclusions.—Leisure-time physical activity is associated with increases in longevity (Fig).

▶ This study is consistent with others showing that physical activity has a strong effect on increasing life expectancy (Fig).[1] Lack of time is the number 1 reason people give for not engaging in a regular physical activity program, but this study showed that non-Hispanics can expect to gain 2.3–5.6 hours of life for every hour of moderate physical activity, and 5.2–11.3 hours of life for every hour of vigorous physical activity they accumulate during adulthood. This is an amazing return for the time investment and is important information to share with busy individuals.

D. C. Nieman, DrPH

Reference

1. Wen CP, Wai JP, Tsai MK, et al. Minimum amount of physical activity for reduced mortality and extended life expectancy: a prospective cohort study. *Lancet.* 2011; 378:1244-1253.

Exercise Frequency Is Related to Psychopathology but Not Neurocognitive Function

Knab AM, Nieman DC, Sha W, et al (Appalachian State Univ, Kannapolis, NC; Appalachian State Univ, Boone, NC; et al)
Med Sci Sports Exerc 44:1395-1400, 2012

Introduction.—In this study, we measured neurocognitive function, perceived stress, quality of life (QOL), and psychopathology in community-dwelling adults, with data contrasted across tertiles of exercise frequency.

Methods.—A group of 998 adults (age 18−85 yr) was measured for neurocognitive function using a computerized neuropsychological test from CNS Vital Signs (Morrisville, NC). They also completed the Brief Symptom Inventory (BSI), which measures psychopathology, as well as the World Health Organization QOL questionnaire and the Perceived Stress Scale. General linear modeling was used to examine relationships between exercise frequency and neurocognitive function, BSI, QOL, and the Perceived Stress Scale. Backward selection in the GLMSELECT procedure in SAS (version 9.1.3; SAS Institute, Inc., Cary, NC) was used to identify confounding variables including age, gender, body mass index, marital status, education level, stress level, alcohol, smoking, and chronic disease. A contrast to test linear trend was performed after adjusting for confounders. Pairwise comparisons were performed across exercise frequency tertiles using the Tukey−Kramer method.

Results.—*P* values for trend tests and pairwise comparisons were nonsignificant for all five cognition function domains across exercise frequency tertiles after adjustment for confounders. Age and education level emerged as the best correlates of neurocognitive function. *P* values for trend were significant for all BSI domains and indices, QOL, and perceived stress, across exercise frequency tertiles.

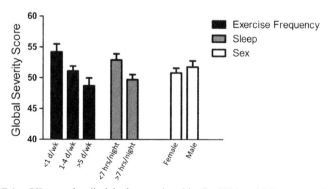

FIGURE 1.—GSI scores for all of the factors selected by the GLM model. Data are antilogs of least squares means after model adjustment (±95% confidence intervals). Factors selected are plotted in rank order of importance with the *P* for trend value reported for each factor (*P* for trend < 0.001). (Reprinted from Knab AM, Nieman DC, Sha W, et al. Exercise frequency is related to psychopathology but not neurocognitive function. *Med Sci Sports Exerc.* 2012;44:1395-1400, with permission from the American College of Sports Medicine.)

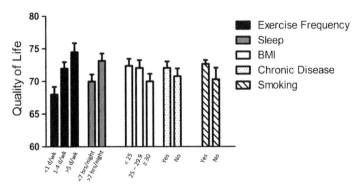

FIGURE 2.—QOL scores for all of the factors selected by the GLM model. Data are antilogs of least squares means after model adjustment (± 95% confidence intervals). Factors selected are plotted in rank order of importance with the P for trend value reported for each factor (P for trend < 0.001). (Reprinted from Knab AM, Nieman DC, Sha W, et al. Exercise frequency is related to psychopathology but not neurocognitive function. *Med Sci Sports Exerc.* 2012;44:1395-1400, with permission from the American College of Sports Medicine.)

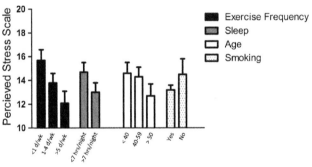

FIGURE 3.—PSS scores for all of the factors selected by the GLM model. Data are antilogs of least squares means after model adjustment (± 95% confidence intervals). Factors selected are plotted in rank order of importance with the P for trend value reported for each factor (P for trend < 0.001). (Reprinted from Knab AM, Nieman DC, Sha W, et al. Exercise frequency is related to psychopathology but not neurocognitive function. *Med Sci Sports Exerc.* 2012;44:1395-1400, with permission from the American College of Sports Medicine.)

Conclusions.—In conclusion, nine BSI psychopathology domains, perceived stress, and QOL but not five neurocognitive function domains were modestly but significantly associated with aerobic exercise frequency in a heterogeneous group of community-dwelling adults after adjustment for demographic and lifestyle factors (Figs 1-3).

▶ In this heterogeneous group of adults, higher exercise frequency was associated, after adjustment for demographic and lifestyle factors, to several measures of psychopathology including decreased overall psychological distress (Fig 1), higher quality of life (Fig 2), and decreased perceived stress (Fig 3). However, exercise frequency was not related to neurocognitive function. Mental cognition may be enhanced transiently after acute exercise,[1] but evidence showing chronic improvements with long-term exercise training is inconsistent. The link between exercise training and improved mental cognition is better established in elderly populations, especially those with impaired cognitive skills.[2] In general, regular physical activity can be counted on to lower feelings of distress and improve overall psychological well-being, but not to improve cognitive function.

D. C. Nieman, DrPH

References

1. Lucas SJ, Ainslie PN, Murrell CJ, Thomas KN, Franz EA, Cotter JD. Effect of age on exercise-induced alterations in cognitive executive function: relationship to cerebral perfusion. *Exp Gerontol.* 2012;47:541-551.
2. Langlois F, Vu TT, Chassé K, Dupuis G, Kergoat MJ, Bherer L. Benefits of physical exercise training on cognition and quality of life in Frail Older adults. *J Gerontol B Psychol Sci Soc Sci.* 2012 Aug 28 [Epub ahead of print].

Serum Creatine Kinase Activity and Its Relationship With Renal Function Indices in Professional Cyclists During the Giro d'Italia 3-Week Stage Race
Colombini A, Corsetti R, Marco M, et al (Istituto Ortopedico Galeazzi, Milano, Italy; Pro Cycling Team Liquigas Cannondale Med Board, Sesto al Reghena, Italy; Universitary Foundation of Itaperuna, Brazil; et al)
Clin J Sport Med 22:408-413, 2012

Objective.—To analyze the behavior of total creatine kinase (CK) and other muscular damage markers and to compare CK activity and renal function indices in professional cyclists during a 3-week stage race.

Design.—Prospective, noncomparative, interventional.

Setting.—The athletes were recruited during the 2011 Giro d'Italia.

Participants.—Nine professional road cyclists from the Liquigas-Cannondale team and competing in the race.

Assessment of Risk Factors.—Blood samples were collected on the day before the start of the race, on day 12, and on the final day (day 22) of the race.

Main Outcome Measures.—Creatinine and cystatin C concentrations, CK, lactate dehydrogenase (LDH), and aspartate aminotransferase (AST) activities were measured. The estimated glomerular filtration rate was calculated according to equations based on creatinine, cystatin C, or both.

Results.—Creatine kinase and AST activity increased during the second part of the race, and LDH activity progressively increased during the entire course of the race. There was a negative correlation between CK activity and the delta prerace-day 12 of glomerular filtration rate, as obtained with simple cystatin C or with Chronic Kidney Disease Epidemiology Collaboration (CKD-EPI) creatinine and cystatin C equations.

Conclusions.—The effect of prolonged strenuous muscular effort on biochemical laboratory parameters in professional road cyclists was confirmed. The correlation observed between renal function and CK activity underscores that measurement of cystatin C is more accurate than creatinine

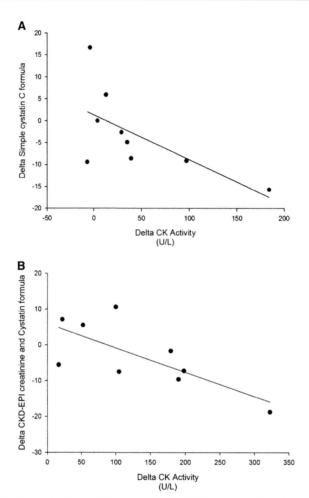

FIGURE 3.—Correlation between delta prerace-day 12 of GFR, as obtained with the simple cystatin C equation (A) or the CKD-EPI creatinine and cystatin C equation (B), and delta prerace-day 12 of CK activity. (Reprinted from Colombini A, Corsetti R, Marco M, et al. Serum creatine kinase activity and its relationship with renal function indices in professional cyclists during the Giro d'Italia 3-week stage race. *Clin J Sport Med.* 2012;22:408-413, with permission Lippincott Williams & Wilkins.)

alone in the evaluation of renal function and that it is unaffected by response to physical stress—induced muscular damage (Fig 3).

▶ Exertional rhabdomyolysis is a potential complication of participation in various types of ultraendurance sport. It is caused by excessive muscle microtrauma,[1,2] including the direct effects of increased concentrations of oxidant species on the muscle membranes. A high serum creatine kinase (CK) offers one of the best measures of the severity of such muscle damage.[3,4] The article by Colombini et al demonstrates a progressive rise of serum CK over the course of the Giro d'Italia, and a correlation between the increase of CK on day 12 of the event and the corresponding deterioration in glomerular flow rate (Fig 3). One problem when estimating the glomerular filtration rate of athletes is that the standard equation (which is based on creatinine excretion) is influenced by the individual's muscle mass. Colombini et al show a closer correlation between deterioration of renal function and CK release when glomerular filtration rates are estimated from an equation based on both creatinine excretion and cystatin C,[5] the latter measure being independent of muscle mass. One puzzling feature of their data is that although CK was negatively related to renal function at day 12, this was not the case at day 29 of the race, when the increase of CK was even larger than on day 12. It remains to be explored whether this is simply a problem of a small sample size or whether the subjects were making some sort of adaptation by the end of the event.

R. J. Shephard, MD (Lond), PhD, DPE

References

1. Clarkson PM, Hubal MJ. Exercise-induced muscle damage in humans. *Am J Phys Med Rehabil*. 2002;81:S52-S69.
2. Skenderi KP, Kavouras SA, Anastasiou CA, Yiannakouris N, Matalas AL. Exertional rhabdomyolysis during a 246-km continuous running race. *Med Sci Sports Exerc*. 2006;38:1054-1057.
3. Banfi G, Colombini A, Lombardi G, Lubkowska A. Metabolic markers in sports medicine. *Adv Clin Chem*. 2012;56:1-54.
4. Vincent HK, Vincent KR. The effect of training status on the serum creatine kinase response, soreness and muscle function following resistance exercise. *Int J Sports Med*. 1997;18:431-437.
5. Colombini A, Corsetti R, Graziani R, Lombardi G, Lanteri P, Banfi G. Evaluation of creatinine, cystatin C and eGFR by different equations in professional cyclists during the Giro d'Italia 3-weeks stage race. *Scand J Clin Lab Invest*. 2012;72:114-120.

Performance Trends and Cardiac Biomarkers in a 30-km Cross-Country Race, 1993–2007

Aagaard P, Sahlén A, Braunschweig F, et al (Karolinska Univ Hosp, Stockholm, Sweden)
Med Sci Sports Exerc 44:894-899, 2012

Purpose.—Long-distance running events enjoy increasing popularity in all ages. Whereas the health benefits of regular moderate exercise are undisputed, the net health effects of single or repeated participation in endurance events of marathon type remain to be determined. We wanted to investigate performance trends over time and the relationship between race performance and cardiac biomarker levels among participants in a large annual 30-km cross-country race.

Methods.—We analyzed a database containing age, gender, run times, and previous race participation of 124,608 runners finishing the Lidingöloppet (30 km) between 1993 and 2007. In 249 male runners age ≥45 yr, we also performed a thorough cardiovascular examination, including measuring

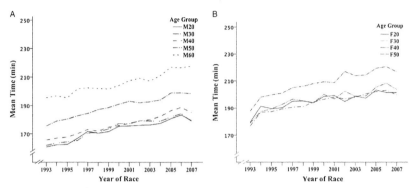

FIGURE 1.—Performance as measured by mean run time in different male (A) and female (B) age groups in the Lidingöloppet 30-km cross-country race, 1993–2007. For definition of age groups, see "Methods" section. (Reprinted from Aagaard P, Sahlén A, Braunschweig F, et al. Performance trends and cardiac biomarkers in a 30-km cross-country race, 1993–2007. *Med Sci Sports Exerc.* 2012;44:894-899, with permission from the American College of Sports Medicine.)

the cardiac biomarkers N-terminal pro—brain natriuretic peptide (NT-proBNP) and troponin.

Results.—Total participation increased 56% with the largest gains in younger female and older male runners. Mean run times rose from 164 ± 27 min in 1993 to 184 ± 33 min in 2007 ($P < 0.001$) in men and from 179 ± 26 to 203 ± 32 in women ($P < 0.001$) after a strong linear relationship (men, $r = 0.98$; women, $r = 0.93$). Increased run times were seen in the mean, top, and bottom quartiles as well as in the top and bottom 5% of all age and gender groups. In the substudy among 249 older male runners, not only higher body mass index, older age, and fewer previous race participations but also higher baseline NT-proBNP was independently associated with increased run time.

Conclusions.—Whereas participation in the Lidingöloppet increased, fitness deteriorated over time in both genders and in all ages. In a subset of older male athletes, longer run times were associated with higher levels of NT-proBNP. The present findings may support the usefulness of preparticipation evaluation to ensure appropriate fitness and cardiovascular health in long-distance race participants (Fig 1).

▶ The great preponderance of studies in the literature have pointed to a progressive improvement in athletic records,[1] and it is good to be reminded that such gains in performance apply only to a small handful of the top participants in a mass endurance event such as a marathon run. Although the total number of contestants is often greater than there would have been 20 years ago, the analysis of these authors shows that for the average person, the times that are achieved have become substantially poorer (Fig 1), reflecting either involvement of a broader cross-section of the population or a deterioration in fitness standards. The association of slower race times with higher baseline levels of the heart failure biomarker *N*-terminal pro—brain natriuretic peptide (NT-proBNP) and postrace increases in both cardiac and inflammatory markers suggest that there may be an increase in the small cardiac risk of an endurance run associated with the participation of more poorly prepared or unfit contestants in such events.[2] From the clinical viewpoint, NT-proBNP is a strong marker of cardiac risk.[3] Although marathon participation may stimulate some people to engage in prolonged training, for those who are not prepared to accept such discipline, it may be prudent to consider less-demanding forms of physical activity.

R. J. Shephard, MD (Lond), PhD, DPE

References

1. Jokl P, Sethi PM, Cooper AJ. Master's performance in the New York City Marathon 1983–1999. *Br J Sports Med.* 2004;38:408-412.
2. Thompson PD, Franklin BA, Balady GJ, et al. Exercise and acute cardiovascular events placing the risks into perspective: a scientific statement from the American heart association Council on Nutrition, physical activity, and Metabolism and the Council on Clinical Cardiology. *Circulation.* 2007;115:2358-2368.
3. Wang TJ, Larson MG, Levy D, et al. Plasma natriuretic peptide levels and the risk of cardiovascular events and death. *N Engl J Med.* 2004;350:655-663.

Aggravation of Exercise-Induced Intestinal Injury by Ibuprofen in Athletes
Van Wijck K, Lenaerts K, Van Bijnen AA, et al (Top Inst Food and Nutrition, Wageningen, The Netherlands; Maastricht Univ Med+, The Netherlands)
Med Sci Sports Exerc 44:2257-2262, 2012

Introduction.—Nonsteroidal anti-inflammatory drugs are commonly used by athletes to prevent anticipated exercise-induced pain, thereby putatively improving physical performance. However, these drugs may have potentially hazardous effects on the gastrointestinal (GI) mucosa during strenuous physical exercise. The aim of the current study was to determine the effect of oral ibuprofen administration before exercise on GI integrity and barrier function in healthy individuals.

Methods.—Nine healthy, trained men were studied on four different occasions: 1) 400 mg ibuprofen twice before cycling, 2) cycling without ibuprofen, 3) 400 mg ibuprofen twice at rest, and 4) rest without ibuprofen intake. To assess small intestinal injury, plasma intestinal fatty acid binding protein (I-FABP) levels were determined, whereas urinary excretion of orally ingested multisugar test probes was measured using liquid chromatography and mass spectrometry to assess GI permeability.

Results.—Both ibuprofen consumption and cycling resulted in increased I-FABP levels, reflecting small intestinal injury. Levels were higher after cycling with ibuprofen than after cycling without ibuprofen, rest with ibuprofen, or rest without ibuprofen (peak I-FABP, 875 ± 137, 474 ± 74, 507 ± 103, and 352 ± 44 pg·mL^{-1}, respectively, $P < 0.002$). In line, small intestinal permeability increased, especially after cycling with ibuprofen (0–2 h urinary lactulose/rhamnose ratio, 0.08 (0.04–0.56) compared with 0.04 (0.00–0.20), 0.05 (0.01–0.07), and 0.01 (0.01–0.03), respectively), reflecting loss of gut barrier integrity. Interestingly, the extent of intestinal injury and barrier dysfunction correlated significantly ($R_S = 0.56$, $P < 0.001$).

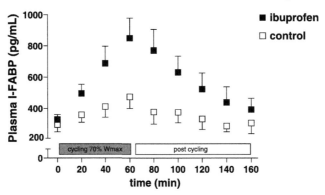

FIGURE 1.—Ibuprofen significantly increases plasma I-FABP levels in rest and during cycling. A. Plasma I-FABP levels in athletes during and after cycling with prior intake of ibuprofen compared with cycling without ibuprofen ($P < 0.0001$). *Squares* represent mean data, with the SEM as *black lines*. (Reprinted from Van Wijck K, Lenaerts K, Van Bijnen AA, et al, Aggravation of exercise-induced intestinal injury by ibuprofen in athletes. *Med Sci Sports Exerc.* 2012;44:2257-2262, with permission from the American College of Sports Medicine.)

Conclusion.—This is the first study to reveal that ibuprofen aggravates exercise-induced small intestinal injury and induces gut barrier dysfunction in healthy individuals. We conclude that nonsteroidal anti-inflammatory drugs consumption by athletes is not harmless and should be discouraged (Fig 1A).

▶ At the arduous 160-km Western States Endurance Run (WSER), we showed that runners developed significant muscle damage and soreness leading to unusually high inflammation.[1-3] To cope with the pain and inflammation, 70% of WSER athletes used ibuprofen. An unexpected finding from our research was that ibuprofen use was ineffective and potentially harmful. We showed that ibuprofen users (600 mg and 1200 mg ibuprofen the day before and during the race, respectively) compared with nonusers experienced the same degree of muscle damage and soreness. Moreover, ibuprofen use caused a small leakage of colon bacteria into the circulation that promoted even more inflammation (25% to 88%, depending on the biomarker) and oxidative stress, with a side effect of mild kidney dysfunction. We were unable to measure any benefit of using ibuprofen by WSER athletes, only harm. Every indication from our research was that ibuprofen amplified inflammation and oxidative stress while providing no relief from exercise effort or muscle damage and soreness. The data from this study showed that even moderate ibuprofen use amplified exercise-induced cell damage in the small intestine (Fig 1A) and adds to previous research that athletes would do well to not mix ibuprofen use with exertion.

D. C. Nieman, DrPH

References

1. Nieman DC, Henson DA, Dumke CL, et al. Ibuprofen use, endotoxemia, inflammation, and plasma cytokines during ultramarathon competition. *Brain Behav Immun.* 2006;20:578-584.

2. McAnulty SR, Owens JT, McAnulty LS, et al. Ibuprofen use during extreme exercise: effects on oxidative stress and PGE2. *Med Sci Sports Exerc.* 2007;39: 1075-1079.
3. Nieman DC, Dumke CL, Henson DA, McAnulty SR, Gross SJ, Lind RL. Muscle damage is linked to cytokine changes following a 160-km race. *Brain Behav Immun.* 2005;19:398-403.

Cardiorespiratory Physiology

The current standard measure of cardiorespiratory fitness introduces confounding by body mass: the DR's EXTRA study

Savonen K, Krachler B, Hassinen M, et al (Kuopio Res Inst of Exercise Medicine, Finland; et al)

Int J Obes 36:1135-1140, 2012

Objective.—Cardiorespiratory fitness is currently estimated by dividing maximal oxygen consumption (VO_{2max}) by body weight (per-weight standard). However, the statistically correct way to neutralize the effect of weight on VO_{2max} in a given population is adjustment for body weight by regression techniques (adjusted standard). Our objective is to quantify the bias introduced by the per-weight standard in a population distributed across different categories of body mass.

Design.—This is a cross-sectional study.

Subjects and Methods.—Baseline measures from participants of the Dose-Responses to Exercise Training Study (DR's EXTRA), 635 men (body mass index (BMI): $19-47 \, kg \, m^{-2}$) and 638 women (BMI: $16-49 \, kg \, m^{-2}$) aged 57—78 years who performed oral glucose tolerance tests and maximal exercise stress tests with direct measurement of VO_{2max}. We compare the increase in VO_{2max} implied by the per-weight standard with the real increase of VO_{2max} per kg body weight. A linear logistic regression model estimates odds for abnormal glucose metabolism (either impaired fasting glycemia or impaired glucose tolerance or Type 2 diabetes) of the least-fit versus most-fit quartile according to both per-weight standard and adjusted standard.

Results.—The per-weight standard implies an increase of VO_{2max} with $20.9 \, ml \, min^{-1}$ in women and $26.4 \, ml \, min^{-1}$ in men per additional kg body weight. The true increase per kg is only $7.0 \, ml \, min^{-1}$ (95% confidence interval: 5.3—8.8) and $8.0 \, ml \, min^{-1}$ (95% confidence interval: 5.3—10.7), respectively. Risk for abnormal glucose metabolism in the least-fit quartile of the population is overestimated by 52% if the per-weight standard is used.

Conclusions.—In comparisons across different categories of body mass, the per-weight standard systematically underestimates cardiorespiratory fitness in obese subjects. Use of the per-weight standard markedly inflates associations between poor fitness and co-morbidities of obesity (Fig 1).

▶ Maximal oxygen intake is used sufficiently often as a measure in sports medicine that the appropriate handling of the data becomes an important issue. The most common method is simply to divide the peak oxygen intake by the individual's body mass, or (less appropriately) to make this same calculation for grouped

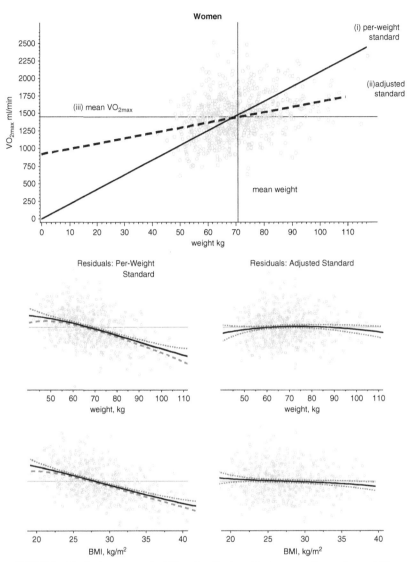

FIGURE 1.—Maximal oxygen uptake (VO_{2max}) and body weight in women: Expected normal VO_{2max} according to per-weight standard (i), adjusted standard (ii) and mean standard (iii). Residual distribution for per-weight standard and adjusted standard by body weight and body mass. Per-weight equation: $VO_{2max} = 20.91 \times weight$; regression equation: $VO_{2max} = 951 + 7.03 \times weight$. (Reprinted from Savonen K, Krachler B, Hassinen M, et al. The current standard measure of cardiorespiratory fitness introduces confounding by body mass: the DR's EXTRA study. *Int J Obes.* 2012;36:1135-1140, with permission from Macmillan Publishers Limited.)

data. The theoretical problem with this approach is that the relationship between maximal oxygen intake and body mass is not a straight line passing through zero on both axes (Fig 1). Pediatric work physiologists have argued that when comparing individuals of widely differing size, it is more appropriate to make an allometric comparison—that is, by calculating the regression of maximal oxygen intake on body mass. Often, when dealing with adults, interindividual differences in body masses are fairly small, and in practice there is then not much to choose between ratio and allometric treatment of the data. However, as Savonen et al point out, differences can become important in those who are grossly obese, and the use of ratios can inflate estimates of the side effects of poor fitness in those who are morbidly obese. A further issue is whether data should indeed be related to body mass. This approach penalizes the cardiorespiratory performance of those who are obese, because their cardiorespiratory attainment is diminished by a substantial additional mass of biologically largely inert fat. In some respects, this is a fair penalty to apply to their fitness assessment, because the physical work involved in most forms of physical activity increases with the individual's body mass. The performance of the heart itself is best indicated by oxygen transport expressed in L/min, but when comparing individuals, this gives an advantage to a tall person. Probably the fairest way to examine the condition of the heart alone is to express oxygen transport as a function of standing height. And if the range of heights is substantial, this comparison should again be made by regression rather than by calculating a simple ratio.

R. J. Shephard, MD (Lond), PhD, DPE

Effect of Respiratory Muscle Training on Exercise Performance in Healthy Individuals: A Systematic Review and Meta-Analysis
Illi SK, Held U, Frank I, et al (Inst of Human Movement Sciences, Zurich, Switzerland; Univ of Zurich, Switzerland)
Sports Med 42:707-724, 2012

Objectives.—Two distinct types of specific respiratory muscle training (RMT), i.e. respiratory muscle strength (resistive/threshold) and endurance (hyperpnoea) training, have been established to improve the endurance performance of healthy individuals. We performed a systematic review and meta-analysis in order to determine the factors that affect the change in endurance performance after RMT in healthy subjects.

Data Sources.—A computerized search was performed without language restriction in MEDLINE, EMBASE and CINAHL and references of original studies and reviews were searched for further relevant studies.

Review Methods.—RMT studies with healthy individuals assessing changes in endurance exercise performance by maximal tests (constant load, time trial, intermittent incremental, conventional [non-intermittent] incremental) were screened and abstracted by two independent investigators. A multiple linear regression model was used to identify effects of subjects' fitness, type of RMT (inspiratory or combined inspiratory/expiratory muscle strength training, respiratory muscle endurance training), type of exercise test, test duration and type of sport (rowing, running, swimming, cycling) on changes in performance after RMT. In addition, a meta-analysis was performed to determine the effect of RMT on endurance performance in those studies providing the necessary data.

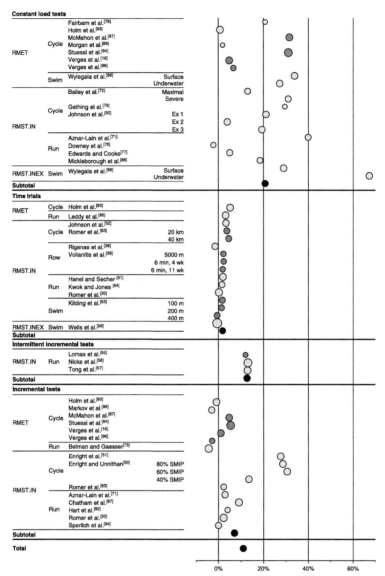

FIGURE 4.—Mean difference in the effect of respiratory muscle training on exercise performance between intervention and sham-training/no-training control groups. Dark grey circles: average mean difference of each type of exercise test. Medium grey circles: tests also included in the forest plot of figure 2. Light grey circles: tests not included in the meta-analysis because data to calculate the confidence interval was not provided. The size of the circles represents the number of subjects included in the study. **RMET** = respiratory muscle endurance training; **RMST.IN** = inspiratory muscle strength training; **RMST.INEX** = inspiratory and expiratory muscle strength training; **SMIP** = sustained maximal inspiratory pressure (i.e. maximal pressure generation capacity from residual volume to total lung capacity). (Reprinted from Illi SK, Held U, Frank I, et al. Effect of respiratory muscle training on exercise performance in healthy individuals: a systematic review and meta-analysis. *Sports Med.* 2012;42:707-724, with permission from Springer International Publishing AG.)

Results.—The multiple linear regression analysis including 46 original studies revealed that less fit subjects benefit more from RMT than highly trained athletes (6.0% per $10 \, mL \cdot kg^{-1} \cdot min^{-1}$ decrease in maximal oxygen uptake, 95% confidence interval [CI] 1.8, 10.2%; $p = 0.005$) and that improvements do not differ significantly between inspiratory muscle strength and respiratory muscle endurance training ($p = 0.208$), while combined inspiratory and expiratory muscle strength training seems to be superior in improving performance, although based on only 6 studies (+12.8% compared with inspiratory muscle strength training, 95% CI 3.6, 22.0%; $p = 0.006$). Furthermore, constant load tests (+16%, 95% CI 10.2, 22.9%) and intermittent incremental tests (+18.5%, 95% CI 10.8, 26.3%) detect changes in endurance performance better than conventional incremental tests (both $p < 0.001$) with no difference between time trials and conventional incremental tests ($p = 0.286$). With increasing test duration, improvements in performance are greater (+0.4% per minute test duration, 95% CI 0.1, 0.6%; $p = 0.011$) and the type of sport does not influence the magnitude of improvements (all $p < 0.05$). The meta-analysis, performed on eight controlled trials revealed a significant improvement in performance after RMT, which was detected by constant load tests, time trials and intermittent incremental tests, but not by conventional incremental tests.

Conclusion.—RMT improves endurance exercise performance in healthy individuals with greater improvements in less fit individuals and in sports of longer durations. The two most common types of RMT (inspiratory muscle strength and respiratory muscle endurance training) do not differ significantly in their effect, while combined inspiratory/expiratory strength training might be superior. Improvements are similar between different types of sports. Changes in performance can be detected by constant load tests, time trials and intermittent incremental tests only. Thus, all types of RMT can be used to improve exercise performance in healthy subjects but care must be taken regarding the test used to investigate the improvements (Fig 4).

▶ Respiratory muscle training seems likely to have a beneficial effect on physical performance, mainly in those individuals whose effort is limited by the sensation of dyspnea. This depends in part on the fraction of the vital capacity that is used at each breath (the threshold in a sedentary person is about 50% of vital capacity) and in part on fatigue of the chest muscles (most likely in prolonged bouts of exercise).[1,2] Both are probably more likely to occur in a sedentary person, and, despite some possible issues with publication bias, this seems to be borne out by the careful meta-analysis of the authors of this article. They distinguish 2 potential types of respiratory muscle training—endurance and strength training—but find benefit from both tactics (Fig 4). One might have expected maximal benefit in activities where the respiratory muscles also contributed to exercise, as in rowing and kayaking, but this was not demonstrated in the available studies. Although benefit was larger in sedentary as opposed to athletic individuals, some benefit was seen in athletes, and potential respiratory limitations might be worth considering by the serious competitor.

R. J. Shephard, MD (Lond), PhD, DPE

References

1. Mador MJ, Acevedo FA. Effect of respiratory muscle fatigue on subsequent exercise performance. *J Appl Physiol.* 1991;70:2059-2065.
2. Verges S, Sager Y, Erni C, Spengler CM. Expiratory muscle fatigue impairs exercise performance. *Eur J Appl Physiol.* 2007;101:225-232.

Physical Fitness

Systemic Acid Load from the Diet Affects Maximal-Exercise RER

Niekamp K, Zavorsky GS, Fontana L, et al (Saint Louis Univ, MO; Marywood Univ, Scranton, PA; Washington Univ School of Medicine, St Louis, MO)
Med Sci Sports Exerc 44:709-715, 2012

A maximal-exercise RER (RER_{max}) ≥ 1.10 is commonly used as a criterion to determine whether a "true" maximal oxygen uptake ($\dot{V}O_{2max}$) has been attained during maximal-effort exercise testing. Because RER_{max} is heavily influenced by CO_2 production from acid buffering during maximal exercise, we postulated that dietary acid load, which affects acid–base regulation, might contribute to variability in RER_{max}.

Purpose.—The study's purpose was to determine whether a habitual dietary intake that promotes systemic alkalinity results in higher RER_{max} during $\dot{V}O_{2max}$ testing.

Methods.—Sedentary men and women (47–63 yr, $n = 57$) with no evidence of cardiovascular disease underwent maximal graded treadmill exercise tests. $\dot{V}O_{2max}$ and RER_{max} were measured with indirect calorimetry. Habitual diet was assessed for its long-term effect on systemic acid–base status by performing nutrient analysis of food diaries and using this information to calculate the potential renal acid load (PRAL). Participants were grouped into tertiles on the basis of PRAL.

Results.—The lowest PRAL tertile (alkaline PRAL) had higher RER_{max} values (1.21 ± 0.01, $P \leq 0.05$) than the middle PRAL tertile (1.17 ± 0.01) and highest PRAL tertile (1.15 ± 0.01). There were no significant differences (all $P \geq 0.30$) among PRAL tertiles for RER at submaximal exercise intensities of 70%, 80%, or 90% $\dot{V}O_{2max}$. After controlling for age, sex, $\dot{V}O_{2max}$, and HR_{max}, regression analysis demonstrated that 19% of the variability in RER_{max} was attributed to PRAL ($r = -0.43$, $P = 0.001$). Unexpectedly, HR_{max} was lower ($P \leq 0.05$) in the low PRAL tertile (164 ± 3 beats·min^{-1}) versus the highest PRAL tertile (173 ± 3 beats·min^{-1}).

Conclusions.—These results suggest that individuals on a diet that promotes systemic alkalinity may more easily achieve the RER_{max} criterion of ≥ 1.10, which might lead to false-positive conclusions about achieving maximal effort and $\dot{V}O_{2max}$ during graded exercise testing (Fig 1).

▶ Conventional wisdom has argued that if an oxygen consumption plateau is not attained during a measurement of maximal oxygen intake, the quality of the patient's effort can be judged by reference to the arterialized blood lactate, the heart rate, and the respiratory gas exchange ratio (RER). Commonly, a good effort

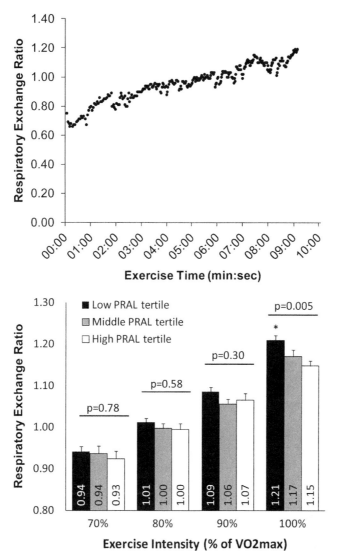

FIGURE 1.—RER during submaximal- and maximal-intensity exercise. The *top panel* depicts the breath-by-breath changes in RER during progressive-intensity exercise to exhaustion from a representative exercise test. The *bottom panel* depicts the mean (± SEM) RER values for subjects in each PRAL tertile during submaximal- and maximal-intensity exercise. *P* values are from ANOVA tests comparing means among PRAL (mEq·d^{-1}) tertiles. *$P \leq 0.05$ versus the middle and high PRAL tertiles. (Reprinted from Niekamp K, Zavorsky GS, Fontana L, et al. Systemic acid load from the diet affects maximal-exercise RER. *Med Sci Sports Exerc.* 2012;44:709-715, with permission from the American College of Sports Medicine.)

is associated with an RER value of greater than 1.10,[1-3] although plainly both heart rate and RER are also influenced by the anxiety level of the individual who is being tested, and the RER is also likely to be affected by the sensitivity of central and peripheral chemoreceptors. These authors make the interesting suggestion that interindividual differences in diet can be sufficient to influence systemic alkalinity and thus become a further factor modifying the RER response to maximal aerobic exercise; depending on food choices, an individual's blood pH can vary by 0.03 pH units[3,4] and the urinary pH by 1.0 units.[5] Fruits and vegetables promote alkalinity, and meat and cheese promote acidity. The effect on RER at maximal effort seems of practical importance (Fig 1), although there is a slight possibility of subject selection, since a low RER was associated with a low heart rate, and the authors plan further trials where diet is altered experimentally. The effects of alkalinity might be even greater given an extreme diet, medication, or use of the alkalis by a sprinter, and this variable should certainly be kept in mind when evaluating stress tests.

R. J. Shephard, MD (Lond), PhD, DPE

References

1. Shephard RJ. *Endurance Fitness.* 2nd ed. Toronto, Ontario: University of Toronto Press; 1977.
2. Midgley AW, McNaughton LR, Polman R, Marchant D. Criteria for determination of maximal oxygen uptake: a brief critique and recommendations for future research. *Sports Med.* 2007;37:1019-1028.
3. Robergs RA, Ghiasvand F, Parker D. Biochemistry of exercise-induced metabolic acidosis. *Am J Physiol Regul Integr Comp Physiol.* 2004;287:R502-R516.
4. Giannini S, Nobile M, Sartori L, et al. Acute effects of moderate dietary protein restriction in patients with idiopathic hypercalciuria and calcium nephrolithiasis. *Am J Clin Nutr.* 1999;69:267-271.
5. Buclin T, Cosma M, Appenzeller M, et al. Diet acids and alkalis influence calcium retention in bone. *Osteoporos Int.* 2001;12:493-499.

Blood and Immune Function

Negative Interaction between Indomethacin and Exercise in Mice

Enos RT, Davis JM, McClellan JL, et al (Univ of South Carolina, Columbia)
Int J Sports Med 34:191-195, 2013

We examined the possible negative interaction of the combined use of the NSAID indomethacin (IND) and exercise in mice. Mice were assigned to one of 4 groups: Exercise 2.5 mg/kg IND (Ex-2.5), Sedentary 2.5 mg/kg IND (Sed-2.5), Exercise 5.0 mg/kg IND (Ex-5.0) and Sedentary 5.0 mg/kg IND (Sed-5.0). Mice were given IND (gavage) 1 h prior to exercise (treadmill run at 30 m/min, 8% grade for 90 min) or rest for 14 consecutive days. Run times, body weight and mortality were recorded daily. Sed-5.0 was highly toxic and caused 70% mortality compared to Sed-2.5, which was well tolerated (0% mortality) ($P < 0.05$). While the addition of exercise had no greater effect on mortality in Ex-5.0, it increased it in the 2.5 group (52% vs. 0%; $P < 0.05$). Run time was reduced from baseline beginning on day 2 (Ex-5.0), or day 3 (Ex-2.5) ($P < 0.05$). Body weight (recorded in the 2.5 mg/kg groups only) was decreased from baseline in Ex-2.5 and Sed-2.5 ($P < 0.05$), but this effect occurred earlier and was of greater magnitude in Ex-2.5. Exercise combined with IND use can lead to serious side effects in mice. Future research is needed to test the hypothesis that this

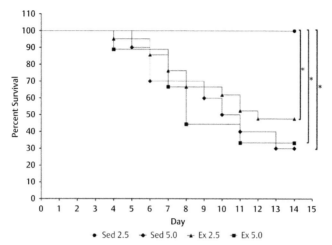

FIGURE 1.—Effect of IND and exercise on mortality in mice. Mice were given either 2.5 mg/kg or 5.0 mg/kg IND daily and 1 h prior to exercise for 14 consecutive days. Mortality was recorded daily (n = 9—21/group). *$P < 0.05$. (Reprinted from Enos RT, Davis JM, McClellan JL, et al. Negative interaction between indomethacin and exercise in mice. *Int J Sports Med.* 2013;34:191-195, © 2013, Thieme Medical Publishers, Inc.)

effect is due to increased GI permeability and whether humans are also at risk (Fig 1).

▶ It has long been recognized that prolonged endurance exercise can reduce intestinal blood flow to the point that the gut wall becomes more permeable to endotoxins, with potential for the development of a life-threatening endotoxemia.[1] Nonsteroidal anti-inflammatory drugs (NSAIDS) are gastrointestinal irritants, and they can cause a similar effect to heavy exercise.[2] Given the frequent heavy use of NSAIDS by endurance competitors, there is a danger that the combined effects on the gut wall could have serious consequences for an athlete.[3,4] The combined risk was evaluated in mice running up an 8% grade at 30 m/min for 90 minutes per day. Some animals were given the normal clinical indomethacin dosage of 2.5 mg/kg, and some who received a dose of 5 mg/kg simulated the athlete who personally elects to overdose with NSAIDS. The latter dose was highly toxic for the mice; even without exercise, 70% of the sedentary animals died. However, when they were given the normal therapeutic dose, the sedentary animals had zero mortality, whereas 52% of those who took 2.5 mg/kg and exercised died (Fig 1). Associated signs of poor health in the NSAIDS + exercise group were a decrease of body mass (probably from gastrointestinal inflammation, with a decreased intake of food and water) and a decrease of total run time. Although this study does warn of a possible danger in humans, the mice are evidently more sensitive to NSAIDS because it seems unlikely that an indomethacin dose of 5 mg/kg would ever be lethal in humans. There is a need for further studies looking at athletes who are using various doses of NSAIDS, measuring blood levels of endotoxins before and after prolonged endurance effort.

R. J. Shephard, MD (Lond), PhD, DPE

References

1. Bosenberg AT, Brock-Utne JG, Gaffin SL, Wells MT, Blake GT. Strenuous exercise causes systemic endotoxemia. *J Appl Physiol.* 1988;65:106-108.
2. Scarpignato C, Hunt RH. Nonsteroidal antiinflammatory drug-related injury to the gastrointestinal tract: clinical picture, pathogenesis, and prevention. *Gastroenterol Clin North Am.* 2010;39:433-464.
3. Nieman DC, Henson DA, Dumke CL, et al. Ibuprofen use, endotoxemia, inflammation, and plasma cytokines during ultramarathon competition. *Brain Behav Immun.* 2006;20:578-584.
4. Lambert GP, Boylan M, Laventure JP, Bull A, Lanspa S. Effect of aspirin and ibuprofen on GI permeability during exercise. *Int J Sports Med.* 2007;28:722-726.

Exercise Intensity and Lymphocyte Subset Apoptosis

Navalta JW, Lyons S, Prestes J, et al (Univ of Nevada, Las Vegas; Western Kentucky Univ, Bowling Green; Catholic Univ of Brasilia, Brazil)
Int J Sports Med 34:268-273, 2013

This investigation assessed the lymphocyte subset response to increasing intensity. Participants completed an exertion test (VO_{2max}), and later performed a 10-min run at 76% VO_{2max} 5-min at 87%, and run to exhaustion at 100% intensity. Blood was sampled at rest, following each intensity, and 1-h post. Cell concentration, apoptosis (annexin V) and migration (CX_3CR1) were evaluated in CD4+, CD8+, and CD19+ subsets. Relative data were analyzed using 1-way ANOVA with significance at $P \le 0.05$. Absolute changes from rest (Δ baseline) were calculated for exercise conditions. CX_3R1 displayed relative changes 1-h post, (CD8+ Pre = 58%, Post = 68%, 1 h-Post = 37%, $P = 0.04$) (CD19+ Pre = 1.9%, Post = 3.2%, 1 h-Post = 5.2%, $P = 0.02$). No relative changes were noted for subsets and annexin V. Absolute changes revealed that CD4+/annexin V+ and CD8+/annexin V+ significantly increased at 76%, ($P < 0.01$). Significant absolute increases were observed in CD4+/CX_3CR1 at 87% VO_{2max} and at 87% and 100% VO_{2max} in CD8+/CX_3CR1 ($P < 0.01$). Subsets respond differently with intensity with respect to cell count, and markers of apoptosis and cell migration. CD4+ and CD8+ appear to be prone to apoptosis with moderate exercise, but significant increases in migration at higher intensities suggests movement of these cells from the vasculature in postexercise measurements (Fig 2).

▶ It has long been known that there are dramatic changes in circulating lymphocyte counts in the first few hours following a bout of exercise,[1,2] and indeed the sudden decline in natural killer cell count has been suggested as one factor increasing vulnerability to upper respiratory infections following a bout of heavy physical activity.[3] Given that only about 1% of lymphocytes are circulating in the blood stream at any given time, the clinical significance of a decline in circulating cell numbers for a few hours after exercise is doubtful. Part of the change is probably from an activation of adhesion molecules as catecholamines are released

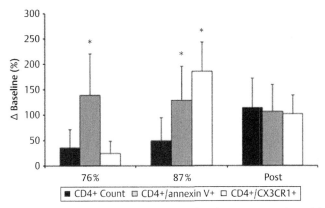

FIGURE 2.—Absolute change from baseline in helper T lymphocytes (CD4+) obtained from subjects (N = 12) following treadmill running at 76% VO_{2max}, 87% VO_{2max}, and to exhaustion (Post). Data is for cell count, apoptosis (annexin V+), and cellular migration (CX3CR1+). *indicates significantly greater than cell count at the given intensity. (Reprinted from Navalta JW, Lyons S, Prestes J, et al. Exercise intensity and lymphocyte subset apoptosis. *Int J Sports Med.* 2013;34:268-273, © 2013, Thieme Medical Publishers, Inc.)

during the exercise. This causes the lymphocytes to undergo a temporary sequestration in reservoir sites. The study of mechanisms underlying this facet of exercise immunology is now helped by the development of markers of apoptosis (annexin V) and cell migration (CX_3CR1). Somewhat surprisingly, moderate exercise (10 minutes of treadmill running at 76% of maximal oxygen intake) was enough to cause a substantial increase in an early marker of apoptosis in relatively obese men (Fig 2), suggesting that a part of the exercise-induced decline in CD4+ (helper T cell) count is due to cell destruction (which could well increase vulnerability to infection). At a higher intensity of effort (87% of maximal oxygen intake), there is also a large increase in the migratory marker, and the authors of the present article suggest this may be an attempt to minimize the apoptotic effect of exercise.

R. J. Shephard, MD (Lond), PhD, DPE

References

1. Kendall A, Hoffman-Goetz L, Houston M, MacNeil B, Arumugam Y. Exercise and blood lymphocyte subset responses: intensity, duration, and subject fitness effects. *J Appl Physiol.* 1990;69:251-260.
2. Simpson RJ, Florida-James GD, Whyte GP, Guy K. The effects of intensive, moderate and downhill treadmill running on human blood lymphocytes expressing the adhesion/activation molecules CD54 (ICAM-1), CD18 (beta2 integrin) and CD53. *Eur J Appl Physiol.* 2006;97:109-121.
3. Nieman DC. Immune response to heavy exertion. *J Appl Physiol.* 1997;82: 1385-1394.

Differential Effects of Acute and Chronic Exercise on Human Neutrophil Functions

Syu G-D, Chen H-I, Jen CJ (Natl Cheng Kung Univ, Tainan, Taiwan)
Med Sci Sports Exerc 44:1021-1027, 2012

Exercise effects on immunity are highly dependent on exercise intensity, duration, and frequency.

Purpose.—Because neutrophils play an essential role in innate immunity, we investigated whether acute severe exercise (ASE) and chronic moderate exercise (CME) differentially regulate human neutrophil functions.

Methods.—Thirteen sedentary young males underwent an initial ASE (pedaling on a bicycle ergometer with increasing loads until exhaustion), and they were subsequently divided into exercise ($n = 8$) and control groups ($n = 5$). The exercise group underwent 2 months of CME (pedaling on the ergometer at a moderate intensity for 30 min each day) followed by 2 months of detraining. The control group was abstained from regular exercise during these 4 months. Additional ASE paradigms were performed every month (in the exercise group) or every 2 months (in the control group). Neutrophils were isolated from blood specimens drawn at rest and immediately after each ASE for assaying chemotaxis, phagocytosis, citrate synthase activity,

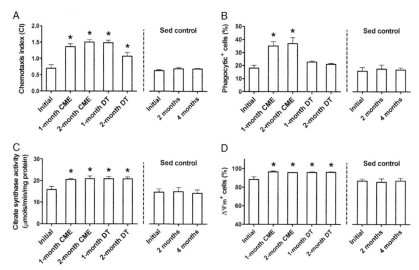

FIGURE 4.—Effects of CME and DT on neutrophil functions. Experiments were carried out using freshly isolated neutrophils obtained from subjects at rest. The initial values were obtained before the execution of any exercise paradigm (the same as before ASE values in Fig. 2) but separated into an exercise group and a sedentary control group. Data were analyzed by one-way ANOVA with repeated measures followed by the Bonferroni posttest. *$P < 0.05$, compared with initial values, $n = 8$. No differences between the exercise ($n = 8$) and sedentary control ($n = 5$) groups were found at the beginning (analyzed by unpaired *t*-tests). There was no time-dependent effect in the sedentary control group. (Reprinted from Syu G-D, Chen H-I, Jen CJ. Differential effects of acute and chronic exercise on human neutrophil functions. *Med Sci Sports Exerc*. 2012;44:1021-1027, with permission from the American College of Sports Medicine.)

and mitochondrial membrane potential ($\Delta\Psi$m). Additional blood specimens were drawn from the exercise group before and immediately after the first bout of CME to determine the acute moderate exercise (AME) effects on neutrophil functions.

Results.—The study's results are the following: 1) the initial ASE enhanced chemotaxis and induced $\Delta\Psi$m depolarization; 2) AME did not influence any measured parameter in neutrophils; 3) CME increased chemotaxis, phagocytosis, citrate synthase activity, and $\Delta\Psi$m; 4) the CME effects remained after detraining except phagocytosis; and 5) the ASE effects disappeared after CME and were partially restored after detraining.

Conclusions.—ASE and CME differentially affected neutrophil functions, whereas AME was ineffective. Moreover, the fact that CME improves neutrophil functions may partially explain why physically active subjects have a low risk of infection (Fig 4).

▶ There is relatively little information about the influence of chronic moderate exercise on the risk of infection, but available reports point to some decrease in the risk of both viral and bacterial infections in regular exercisers.[1,2] The neutrophils play an important role in innate immunity, migrating to sites of infection by a process of chemotaxis and then ingesting the micro-organisms by a process of phagocytosis. Some studies have shown that an acute bout of severe exercise increases these functions, but other studies have seen a decrease in these functions; possibly, this disagreement reflects differences in the severity of the exercise performed relative to the individual's fitness level.

This study demonstrates that in sedentary young men chronic moderate exercise (30 min per day at 60% of maximal work rate for 2 months) increased both neutrophil chemotaxis (with an associated augmentation of the mitochondrial membrane potential) and phagocytosis, with persistence of the enhanced chemotaxis over 2 months of detraining (Fig 4). Given that aging decreases both neutrophil chemotaxis and phagocytosis, it would be interesting to see how far a program of moderate exercise could restore neutrophil function in the elderly, and whether this would then improve their resistance to illness.

R. J. Shephard, MD (Lond), PhD, DPE

References

1. Nieman DC. Exercise, upper respiratory tract infection, and the immune system. *Med Sci Sports Exerc.* 1994;26:128-139.
2. Woods JA, Davis JM, Smith JA, Nieman DC. Exercise and cellular innate immune function. *Med Sci Sports Exerc.* 1999;31:57-66.

High-Intensity Training Reduces CD8⁺ T-cell Redistribution in Response to Exercise

Witard OC, Turner JE, Jackman SR, et al (Univ of Birmingham, Edgbaston, UK; et al)
Med Sci Sports Exerc 44:1689-1697, 2012

Purpose.—We examined whether exercise-induced lymphocytosis and lymphocytopenia are impaired with high-intensity training.

Methods.—Eight trained cyclists ($\dot{V}O_{2max} = 64.2 \pm 6.5$ mL·kg⁻¹·min⁻¹) undertook 1 wk of normal-intensity training and a second week of high-intensity training. On day 7 of each week, participants performed a cycling task, consisting of 120 min of submaximal exercise followed by a 45-min time trial. Blood was collected before, during, and after exercise. CD8⁺ T lymphocytes (CD8TLs) were identified, as well as CD8TL subpopulations on the basis of CD45RA and CD27 expression.

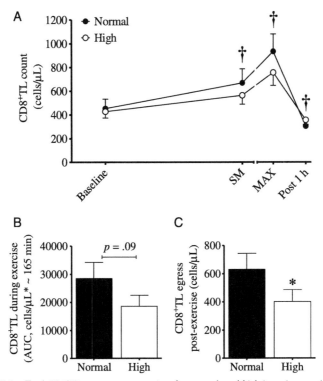

FIGURE 1.—Total CD8⁺TL responses to exercise after normal- and high-intensity exercise training. A. Changes in cell number over time. B. Mobilization of cells expressed as iAUC during the exercise. C. Egress of cells 1 h after exercise. Values are means ± SEM ($n = 8$). †Significantly different from baseline in the corresponding training period ($P < 0.05$). *Significantly different from normal-intensity training ($P < 0.05$). SM, submaximal exercise; MAX, maximal exercise; Post 1 h, 1 h after maximal exercise. (Reprinted from Witard OC, Turner JE, Jackman SR, et al. High-intensity training reduces CD8⁺ T-cell redistribution in response to exercise. *Med Sci Sports Exerc.* 2012;44:1689-1697, with permission from the American College of Sports Medicine.)

Results.—High-intensity training (18,577 ± 10,984 cells per microliter × ~165 min) was associated with a smaller exercise-induced mobilization of CD8$^+$TLs compared with normal-intensity training (28,473 ± 16,163 cells per microliter × ~165 min, $P = 0.09$). The response of highly cytotoxic CD8$^+$TLs (CD45RA$^+$CD27$^-$) to exercise was smaller after 1 wk of high-intensity training (3144 ± 924 cells per microliter × ~165 min) compared with normal-intensity training (6417 ± 2143 cells per microliter × ~165 min, $P < 0.05$). High-intensity training reduced postexercise CD8$^+$TL lymphocytopenia (−436 ± 234 cells per microliter) compared with normal-intensity training (−630 ± 320 cells per microliter, $P < 0.05$). This was driven by a reduced egress of naive CD8$^+$TLs (CD27$^+$CD45RA$^+$). High-intensity training was associated with reduced plasma epinephrine (−37%) and cortisol (−15%) responses ($P < 0.05$).

Conclusions.—High-intensity training impaired CD8$^+$TL mobilization and egress in response to exercise. Highly cytotoxic CD8$^+$TLs were primarily responsible for the reduced mobilization of CD8$^+$TLs, which occurred in parallel with smaller neuroendocrine responses. The reduced capacity for CD8$^+$TLs to leave blood after exercise with high-intensity training was accounted for primarily by naive, and also, highly cytotoxic CD8$^+$TLs. This impaired CD8$^+$TL redistribution in athletes undertaking intensified training may imply reduced immune surveillance (Fig 1).

▶ Exercise immunologists have long studied neutrophil function, NK cell toxicity, and cytokine production, hoping to find an explanation of the increased vulnerability to upper respiratory infection that follows a prolonged bout of endurance exercise or unusually heavy training. However, none of the variables examined have offered a convincing explanation of why the athlete's resistance is impaired.[1] The current consensus is that the problem may lie in a deterioration of mucosal immune function, which normally offers the first line of defense against a viral assault. Witard et al speculates that a further factor may be a reduced trafficking of cytotoxic leukocytes into and out of the circulation after a bout of hard training. Exercise responses of a small group of well-trained male cyclists were compared after a week of normal training and after a week when both the intensity and volume of training had been substantially increased. The week of heavier training decreased leukocyte migration into and out of the circulation in response to the test exercise, with a particularly marked effect on the most cytotoxic cell subtypes (Fig 1). This change could have a direct effect on viral destruction, or alternatively it might reduce extracellular apoptosis of senescent T cells, which again would have an adverse effect on the body's defenses.[2] The explanation of the change in cell migration is less clear. Possibly, the intense training reduced the catecholamine response to the test exercise and thus the extent of cell demargination.[3,4] Cortisol secretion may also have been decreased, and this could have reduced cell egress. This study seems to open a new window upon upper respiratory infections; the need now is to relate immunological changes to well-documented cases of upper respiratory infection.

R. J. Shephard, MD (Lond), PhD, DPE

References

1. MacKinnon LT. Chronic exercise training effects on immune function. *Med Sci Sports Exerc.* 2000;32:S369-S376.
2. Dimitrov S, Lange T, Born J. Selective mobilization of cytotoxic leukocytes by epinephrine. *J Immunol.* 2010;184:503-511.
3. Shephard RJ, Gannon G, Hay JB, Shek PN. Adhesion molecule expression in acute and chronic exercise. *Crit Rev Immunol.* 2000;20:245-266.
4. Simpson RJ. Aging, persistent viral infections, and immunosenescence: can exercise "make space"? *Exerc Sport Sci Rev.* 2011;39:23-33.

Physical Activity and Inflammatory Markers Over 10 Years: Follow-Up in Men and Women From the Whitehall II Cohort Study
Hamer M, Sabia S, Batty GD, et al (Univ College London, UK)
Circulation 126:928-933, 2012

Background.—Inflammatory processes are putative mechanisms underlying the cardioprotective effects of physical activity. An inverse association between physical activity and inflammation has been demonstrated, but no long-term prospective data are available. We therefore examined the association between physical activity and inflammatory markers over a 10-year follow-up period.

Methods and Results.—Participants were 4289 men and women (mean age, 49.2 years) from the Whitehall II cohort study. Self-reported physical activity and inflammatory markers (serum high-sensitivity C-reactive protein and interleukin-6) were measured at baseline (1991) and follow-up (2002). Forty-nine percent of the participants adhered to standard physical activity recommendations for cardiovascular health (2.5 h/wk moderate to vigorous physical activity) across all assessments. Physically active participants at baseline had lower C-reactive protein and interleukin-6 levels, and this difference remained stable over time. Compared with participants who rarely adhered to physical activity guidelines over the 10-year follow-up, the high-adherence group displayed lower $\log_e$ C-reactive protein ($\beta = -0.07$; 95% confidence interval, -0.12 to -0.02) and $\log_e$ interleukin-6 ($\beta = -0.07$; 95% confidence interval, -0.10 to -0.03) at follow-up after adjustment for a range of covariates. Compared with participants who remained stable, those who reported an increase in physical activity of at least 2.5 h/wk displayed lower $\log_e$ C-reactive protein (β coefficient $= -0.05$; 95% confidence interval, -0.10 to -0.001) and loge interleukin-6 (β coefficient $= -0.06$; 95% confidence interval, -0.09 to -0.03) at follow-up.

Conclusions.—Regular physical activity is associated with lower markers of inflammation over 10 years of follow-up and thus may be important in preventing the proinflammatory state seen with aging.

▶ Cross-sectional studies consistently show that systemic inflammation is linked to both body mass index (BMI) and physical activity/fitness.[1] Short-term physical training studies have generally failed to demonstrate changes in inflammation biomarkers independent of change in BMI.[2] This 10-year longitudinal study provides rare information on the long-term influences of physical exercise on systemic inflammation. Prestudy, physically active participants had lower C-reactive protein and interleukin-6 levels, and maintenance or increases of physical activity over the 10-year follow-up period were linked with lower levels of both inflammatory markers. These associations were independent of adiposity and support indications that physical activity is important in preventing the proinflammatory state seen with aging and related diseases such as cardiovascular disease, sarcopenia, neurodegeneration, and depression.

D. C. Nieman, DrPH

References

1. Shanely RA, Nieman DC, Henson DA, Jin F, Knab AM, Sha W. Inflammation and oxidative stress are lower in physically fit and active adults. *Scand J Med Sci Sports*. 2011 Aug 18; http://dx.doi.org/10.1111/j.1600–0838.2011.01373 [Epub ahead of print].
2. Church TS, Earnest CP, Thompson AM, et al. Exercise without weight loss does not reduce C-reactive protein: the INFLAME study. *Med Sci Sports Exerc*. 2010;42:708-716.

Association Between Physical Activity and Risk of Bleeding in Children With Hemophilia

Broderick CR, Herbert RD, Latimer J, et al (Univ of Sydney, Australia; George Inst for Global Health, Sydney, Australia; et al)
JAMA 308:1452-1459, 2012

Context.—Vigorous physical activity is thought to increase risk of bleeds in children with hemophilia, but the magnitude of the risk is unknown.

Objective.—To quantify the transient increase in risk of bleeds associated with physical activity in children with hemophilia.

Design, Setting, and Participants.—A case-crossover study nested within a prospective cohort study was conducted at 3 pediatric hemophilia centers in Australia between July 2008 and October 2010. A total of 104 children and adolescent boys aged 4 through 18 years with moderate or severe hemophilia A or B were monitored for bleeds for up to 1 year. Following each bleed, the child or parent was interviewed to ascertain exposures to physical activity preceding the bleed. Physical activity was categorized according to expected frequency and severity of collisions. The risk of bleeds associated with physical activity was estimated by contrasting exposure to physical activity in the 8 hours before the bleed with exposures in two 8-hour control windows, controlling for levels of clotting factor in the blood.

Main Outcome Measures.—Association of physical activity and factor level with risk of bleeding.

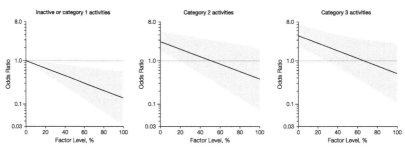

FIGURE 2.—Odds Ratios for Bleeds by Clotting Factor Level and Activity Level. Participants who were inactive or engaged in category 1 activities reported 229 bleeding events; engaged in category 2 activities, 84 events; and engaged in category 3 activities, 16 events. Rates are referenced to the rate of bleeding while inactive or engaging in category 1 activity with a factor level of 0 (horizontal dotted line). The shaded regions represent 95% CIs. The curves and the confidence intervals have been constructed from the conditional logistic regression model. Category 1 includes activities that do not involve expected collisions (eg, swimming); category 2, activities in which significant collisions might occur (eg, basketball); and category 3, activities in which significant collisions are inevitable (eg, wrestling). (Reprinted from Broderick CR, Herbert RD, Latimer J, et al. Association between physical activity and risk of bleeding in children with hemophilia. *JAMA*. 2012;308:1452-1459, Copyright 2012, American Medical Association. All rights reserved.)

Results.—The participants were observed for 4839 person-weeks during which time 436 bleeds occurred. Of these, 336 bleeds occurred more than 2 weeks after the preceding bleed and were used in the primary analysis of risk. Compared with inactivity and category 1 activities (eg, swimming), category 2 activities (eg, basketball) were associated with a transient increase in the risk of bleeding (30.6% of bleed windows vs 24.8% of first control windows; odds ratio, 2.7; 95% CI, 1.7-4.8, $P < .001$). Category 3 activities (eg, wrestling) were associated with a greater transient increase in risk (7.0% of bleed windows vs 3.4% of first control windows; odds ratio, 3.7; 95% CI, 2.3-7.3, $P < .001$). To illustrate absolute risk increase, for a child who bleeds 5 times annually and is exposed on average to category 2 activities twice weekly and to category 3 activities once weekly, exposure to these activities was associated with only 1 of the 5 annual bleeds. For every 1% increase in clotting factor level, bleeding incidence was lower by 2% (95% CI, 1%-3%; $P = .004$).

Conclusions.—In children and adolescents with hemophilia, vigorous physical activity was transiently associated with a moderate relative increase in risk of bleeding. Because the increased relative risk is transient, the absolute increase in risk of bleeds associated with physical activity is likely to be small (Fig 2).

▶ Before the introduction of plasma-derived and recombinant clotting factors, children with hemophilia were generally advised against participation in vigorous physical activity, because this was thought to increase the risk of bleeding.[1] In particular, there was a fear of recurrent bleeding into joints and development of a disabling hemophilic arthropathy.[2] However, the risk of serious bleeding has been greatly reduced by the administration of prophylactic Factor VIII,[3,4] and the study of Broderick and associates makes a useful re-evaluation of the risks of physical activity for affected children, looking retrospectively at parents' recollections of physical activity in 8-hour periods preceding a bleed. Although there was still a measurable increase of risk of bleeds requiring additional doses of clotting factor for an hour or so immediately following activities such as basketball and wrestling (Fig 2), the authors judged the risk as small and that this hazard was outweighed by the other advantages of participation in a reasonable volume of activity. The main limitation of the study is recall bias—when a bleed occurred, the parents probably sought more diligently for an explanatory bout of physical activity than in the control period. However, this would not negate the findings, because an error of this sort would exaggerate the true risk of physical activity. An alternative source of bias, particularly with older children, might be a failure to report a bout of physical activity that preceded a bleed because of a fear that their lives would be further restricted. Finally, subclinical bleeding was not explored, and there remains a need to monitor the effects of such bleeding on joint health.

R. J. Shephard, MD (Lond), PhD, DPE

References

1. Weigel N, Carlson BR. Physical activity and the hemophiliac: yes or no? *Am Correct Ther J*. 1975;29:197-205.
2. Aledort LM, Haschmeyer RH, Pettersson H. A longitudinal study of orthopaedic outcomes for severe factor-VIII-deficient haemophiliacs. The Orthopaedic Outcome Study Group. *J Intern Med*. 1994;236:391-399.
3. Manco-Johnson MJ, Abshire TC, Shapiro AD, et al. Prophylaxis versus episodic treatment to prevent joint disease in boys with severe hemophilia. *N Engl J Med*. 2007;357:535-544.
4. Gringeri A, Lundin B, von Mackensen S, et al. A randomized clinical trial of prophylaxis in children with hemophilia A (the ESPRIT Study). *J Thromb Haemost*. 2011;9:700-710.

Sickle cell trait associated with a RR of death of 37 times in national collegiate athletic association football athletes: a database with 2 million athlete-years as the denominator

Harmon KG, Drezner JA, Klossner D, et al (Univ of Washington, Seattle; Natl Collegiate Athletic Association, Indianapolis, IN; et al)
Br J Sports Med 46:325-330, 2012

Background.—This study examines sickle cell trait (SCT) as a cause of sudden death in National Collegiate Athletic Association (NCAA) athletes and explores the cost-effectiveness of different screening models.

Methods.—The authors reviewed the cause of all cases of sudden death in NCAA student-athletes from January 2004 through December 2008. The authors also explored the cost-effectiveness of screening for this condition in selected populations assuming that identifying athletes with SCT would prevent death.

Results.—There were 273 deaths and a total of 1 969 663 athlete-participant-years. Five (2%) deaths were associated with SCT. In football athletes, there were 72 (26%) deaths. Of these, 52 (72%) were due to trauma unrelated to sports activity and 20 (28%) were due to medical causes; nine

TABLE 3.—Cost-Effectiveness Analysis Sickle Cell Screening for 2004 to 2008 (No Start-Up Costs with $30 Test)

	Black Football Athletes	All Football Athletes	All Black Athletes	All Athletes
Total number of athletes screened in 5 years	20 290	61 609	59 582	398 466
Cost of screening	$30	$30	$30	$30
Cost of screening programme	$608 700	$1 848 270	$1 787 460	$11 953 980
Cost to identify one athlete with SCT	$429	$27 957	$429	$22 047
Cost to prevent one death over 5 years	$121 740	$369 654	$357 492	$2 390 796
Cost per life-year saved	$2435	$7393	$7150	$47 816

SCT, sickle cell trait.

deaths were cardiac (45%), five were associated with SCT (25%). Thirteen of the 20 deaths due to medical causes occurred during exertion; cardiac (6, 46%) SCT associated (5, 39%), and heat stroke unrelated to SCT (2, 15%). All deaths associated with SCT occurred in black Division I football athletes. The risk of exertional death in Division I football players with SCT was 1:827 which was 37 times higher than in athletes without SCT. The cost per case identified varied widely depending on the population screened and the price of the screening test.

Conclusions.—Exertional death in athletes with SCT occurs at a higher rate than previously appreciated. More research is needed to (1) understand the pathophysiology of death in SCT-positive athletes and (2) determine whether screening high-risk populations reduces mortality (Table 3).

▶ Sickle cell trait seems an important cause of death among North American football players[1,2]; this condition affects as many as 14% of black participants. In military personnel, the presence of sickle cell trait increases the risk of sudden death during basic training 28-fold,[3] and as the present study demonstrates, the risk is increased 15-fold for all sports and 37-fold for football players. The risk for black team members is sufficiently high (1 in 827 athletes) that a $30 screening test certainly seems warranted, at least in cost terms, with an expense of only $2435 per life-year saved (Table 3). However, screening also presupposes an effective treatment plan, and available options for the treatment of sickle cell trait are somewhat sketchy; play should not be restricted unduly, and the only likely effective measures are to maintain better hydration and to show greater caution, with thorough acclimatization both at high altitudes and under hot conditions.[4] An interesting side issue is what causes sudden death: does the etiology offer some new possibility for prevention? One recent article suggested that there was a leakage of potassium ions from the damaged red cells, with death from hyperkalemia.[5]

R. J. Shephard, MD (Lond), PhD, DPE

References

1. Mitchell BL. Sickle cell trait and sudden death—bringing it home. *J Natl Med Assoc*. 2007;99:300-305.
2. Scheinin L, Wetli CV. Sudden death and sickle cell trait: medicolegal considerations and implications. *Am J Forensic Med Pathol*. 2009;30:204-208.
3. Kark JA, Posey DM, Schumacher HR, Ruehle CJ. Sickle-cell trait as a risk factor for sudden death in physical training. *N Engl J Med*. 1987;317:781-787.
4. Tripette J, Loko G, Samb A, et al. Effects of hydration and dehydration on blood rheology in sickle cell trait carriers during exercise. *Am J Physiol Heart Circ Physiol*. 2010;299:H908-H914.
5. Loosemore M, Walsh SB, Morris E, et al. Sudden exertional death in sickle cell trait. *Br J Sports Med*. 2012;46:312-314.

5 Metabolism and Obesity, Nutrition and Doping

Nutrition and Ergogenic Aids

Preexercise galactose and glucose ingestion on fuel use during exercise
O'Hara JP, Carroll S, Cooke CB, et al (Leeds Metropolitan Univ, UK; Univ of Hull, UK; et al)
Med Sci Sports Exerc 44:1958-1967, 2012

Purpose.—This study determined the effect of ingesting galactose and glucose 30 min before exercise on exogenous and endogenous fuel use during exercise.

Methods.—Nine trained male cyclists completed three bouts of cycling at 60% W_{max} for 120 min after an overnight fast. Thirty minutes before exercise, the cyclists ingested a fluid formulation containing placebo, 75 g of galactose (Gal), or 75 g of glucose (Glu) to which ^{13}C tracers had been added, in a double-blind randomized manner. Indirect calorimetry and isotope ratio mass spectrometry were used to calculate fat oxidation, total carbohydrate (CHO) oxidation, exogenous CHO oxidation, plasma glucose oxidation, and endogenous liver and muscle CHO oxidation rates.

Results.—Peak exogenous CHO oxidation was significantly higher after Glu (0.68 ± 0.08 g·min^{-1}, $P < 0.05$) compared with Gal (0.44 ± 0.02 g·min^{-1}); however, mean rates were not significantly different (0.40 ± 0.03 vs. 0.36 ± 0.02 g·min^{-1}, respectively). Glu produced significantly higher exogenous CHO oxidation rates during the initial hour of exercise ($P < 0.01$), whereas glucose rates derived from Gal were significantly higher during the last hour ($P < 0.01$). Plasma glucose and liver glucose oxidation at 60 min of exercise were significantly higher for Glu (1.07 ± 0.1 g min^{-1}, $P < 0.05$, and 0.57 ± 0.08 g·min^{-1}, $P < 0.01$) compared with Gal (0.64 ± 0.05 and 0.29 ± 0.03 g·min^{-1}, respectively). There were no significant differences in total CHO, whole body endogenous CHO, muscle glycogen, or fat oxidation between conditions.

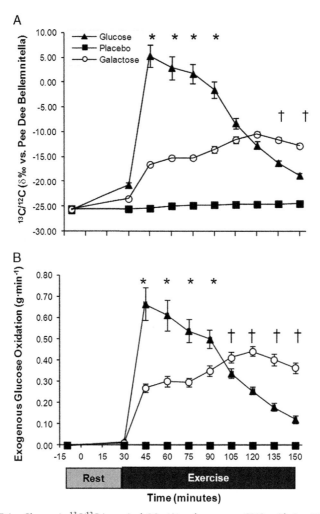

FIGURE 1.—Changes in $^{13}C/^{12}C$ in expired CO_2 (A) and exogenous CHO oxidation (B) at rest and during exercise after the preexercise ingestion of placebo and ^{13}C-labeled glucose (Glu) and galactose (Gal). Values are mean ± SE, $N = 9$. * Glu significantly higher than Gal ($P < 0.05$). † Gal significantly higher than Glu ($P < 0.05$). (Reprinted from O'Hara JP, Carroll S, Cooke CB, et al. Preexercise galactose and glucose ingestion on fuel use during exercise. *Med Sci Sports Exerc.* 2012;44:1958-1967, with permission from the American College of Sports Medicine.)

Conclusion.—The preexercise consumption of Glu provides a higher exogenous source of CHO during the initial stages of exercise, but Gal provides the predominant exogenous source of fuel during the latter stages of exercise and reduces the reliance on liver glucose (Fig 1).

▶ Sports nutritionists have long debated the merits of providing solutions of glucose, galactose, or fructose to endurance competitors. Fructose is now generally avoided, because it is absorbed slowly from the intestine, leading to sensations of gastric discomfort.[1] Glucose and galactose are absorbed by the same sodium co-transport system[2]; however, glucose can be metabolized immediately, whereas the galactose must first be converted to glucose in the liver.[3] In keeping with this biological requirement, O'Hara and colleagues used ^{13}C tracer techniques to show that when carbohydrate is provided 30 minutes before an endurance event, over the first hour glucose provides a greater exogenous source of fuel, but during the second hour galactose provides a better source of carbohydrate (Fig 1). Further, in prolonged events, galactose conserves liver glycogen reserves better than glucose. The choice between the 2 nutrients should thus be guided by the expected duration of an event: glucose if < 1 hour, and galactose if > 1 hour.

R. J. Shephard, MD (Lond), PhD, DPE

References

1. Holdsworth CD, Dawson AM. The absorption of monosaccharides in man. *Clin Sci.* 1964;27:371-379.
2. Turk E, Zabel B, Mundlos S, Dyer J, Wright EM. Glucose/galactose malabsorption caused by a defect in the Na+/glucose cotransporter. *Nature.* 1991;350:354-356.
3. Holden HM, Rayment I, Thoden JB. Structure and function of enzymes of the Leloir pathway for galactose metabolism. *J Biol Chem.* 2003;278:43885-43888.

L-Arginine but not L-glutamine likely increases exogenous carbohydrate oxidation during endurance exercise

Rowlands DS, Clarke J, Green JG, et al (Massey Univ, Wellington, New Zealand; et al)
Eur J Appl Physiol 112:2443-2453, 2012

The addition of L-arginine or L-glutamine to glucose-electrolyte solutions can increase intestinal water, glucose, and sodium absorption in rats and humans. We evaluated the utility of L-arginine and L-glutamine in energy-rehydration beverages through assessment of exogenous glucose oxidation and perceptions of exertion and gastrointestinal distress during endurance exercise. Eight cyclists rode 150 min at 50% of peak power on four occasions while ingesting solutions at a rate of 150 mL 15 min^{-1} that contained ^{13}C-enriched glucose (266 mmol L^{-1}) and sodium citrate ([Na$^+$] 60 mmol L^{-1}), and either: 4.25 mmol L^{-1} L-arginine or 45 mmol L^{-1} L-glutamine, and as controls glucose only or no glucose. Relative to glucose only, L-arginine invoked a likely 12% increase in exogenous glucose oxidation (90% confidence limits: ± 8%); however, the effect of L-glutamine was possibly trivial (4.5 ± 7.3%). L-Arginine also led to very likely small reductions in endogenous fat oxidation rate relative to glucose (12 ± 4%) and L-glutamine (14 ± 4%), and relative to no glucose, likely reductions in exercise oxygen consumption (2.6 ± 1.5%) and plasma lactate concentration (0.20 ± 0.16 mmol L^{-1}). Effects on endogenous and total carbohydrate oxidation were inconsequential. Compared with glucose only, L-arginine and L-glutamine caused likely small-moderate effect size increases in perceptions of stomach fullness, abdominal cramp, exertion, and muscle tiredness

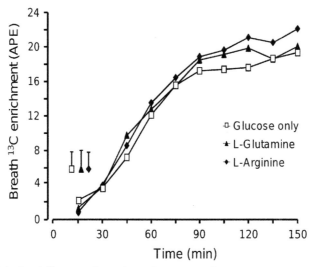

FIGURE 1.—Breath $^{13}CO_2$ enrichment during the 150 min cycling exercise. *Data* are raw means and *bars* are the between-subject standard deviation. (Reprinted from Rowlands DS, Clarke J, Green JG, et al. L-Arginine but not L-glutamine likely increases exogenous carbohydrate oxidation during endurance exercise. *Eur J Appl Physiol.* 2012;112:2443-2453, with kind permission from Springer Science+Business Media.)

during exercise. Addition of L-arginine to a glucose and electrolyte solution increases the oxidation of exogenous glucose and decreases the oxygen cost of exercise, although the mechanisms responsible and impact on endurance performance require further investigation. However, L-arginine also increases subjective feelings of gastrointestinal distress, which may attenuate its other benefits (Fig 1).

▶ One factor contributing to success in a long-distance event is the ability to metabolize exogenous glucose, rather than draw on intramuscular stores of glycogen.[1] The characteristics of the gut wall, particularly epithelial transport, seem to limit the absorption and thus the oxidation of glucose. One way of augmenting carbohydrate uptake has been to drink a mixture of sugars that are absorbed via differing transporter proteins.[2,3] A second line of approach has been to add various amino acids such as arginine to the beverage used in rehydration.[4] L-arginine may help glucose absorption because it is the substrate for nitric oxide synthase; it thus could increase vasodilation of the gut during exercise,[5] and L-arginine may also increase the efficiency of aerobic exercise by releasing nitric oxide elsewhere in the body.[6] Human tests using 13C-enriched glucose here confirm that there was a greater metabolism of exogenous glucose when the drink was enriched by 4.25 mmol/L of L-arginine (Fig 1). The exercise performed (150 minutes of cycle ergometer exercise at 50% of peak power) is unlikely to have exhausted muscle glycogen reserves completely, and even greater benefit might have been seen if subjects had performed a longer or a more vigorous bout of exercise. However, from a tactical point of view, the addition of the arginine or glutamine increased feelings of gastrointestinal distress and fatigue, and in terms of athletic performance, this would probably have offset any benefit from an increased absorption of glucose.[7]

R. J. Shephard, MD (Lond), PhD, DPE

References

1. Jeukendrup AE. Carbohydrate intake during exercise and performance. *Nutrition.* 2004;20:669-677.
2. Jentjens R, Jeukendrup AE. High rates of exogenous carbohydrate oxidation from a mixture of glucose and fructose ingested during prolonged cycling exercise. *Br J Nutr.* 2005;93:485-492.
3. Rowlands DS, Thorburn MS, Thorp RM, et al. Effect of graded fructose coingestion with maltodextrin on exogenous ^{14}C-fructose and ^{13}C-glucose oxidation efficiency and high-intensity cycling performance. *J Appl Physiol.* 2008;104:1709-1719.
4. Wapnir RA, Wingertzahn MA, Teichberg S. L-Arginine in low concentration improves rat intestinal water and sodium absorption from oral rehydration solutions. *Gut.* 1997;40:602-607.
5. Cynober L, Boucher JL, Vasson M-P. Arginine metabolism in mammals. *J Nutr Biochem.* 1995;6:402-413.
6. Lansley KE, Winyard PG, Fulford J, et al. Dietary nitrate supplementation reduces the O_2 cost of walking and running: a placebo-controlled study. *J Appl Physiol.* 2011;110:591-600.
7. O'Brien WJ, Rowlands DS. The fructose: maltodextrin ratio in a carbohydrate—electrolyte solution differentially affects exogenous- carbohydrate oxidation rate, gut comfort and performance. *Am J Physiol Gastrointest Liver Physiol.* 2011; 300:G181-G189.

Effect of volume of milk consumed on the attenuation of exercise-induced muscle damage

Cockburn E, Robson-Ansley P, Hayes PR, et al (Northumbria Univ, Newcastle upon Tyne, UK)
Eur J Appl Physiol 112:3187-3194, 2012

Exercise-induced muscle damage (EIMD) leads to decrements in muscle performance, increases in intramuscular proteins and delayed-onset of muscle soreness (DOMS). Previous research demonstrated that one litre of milk-based protein—carbohydrate (CHO) consumed immediately following muscle damaging exercise can limit changes in markers of EIMD possibly due to attenuating protein degradation and/or increasing protein synthesis. If the attenuation of EIMD is derived from changes in protein metabolism then it can be hypothesised that consuming a smaller volume of CHO and protein will elicit similar effects. Three independent matched groups of 8 males consumed 500 mL of milk, 1,000 mL of milk or a placebo immediately following muscle damaging exercise. Passive and active DOMS, isokinetic muscle performance, creatine kinase (CK), myoglobin and interleukin-6 were assessed immediately before and 24, 48 and 72 h after EIMD. After 72 h 1,000 mL of milk had a likely benefit for limiting decrements in peak torque compared to the placebo. After 48 h, 1,000 mL of milk had a very likely benefit of limiting increases in CK in comparison to the placebo.

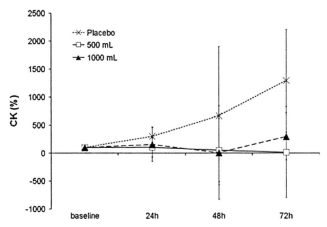

FIGURE 3.—Relative creatine kinase (*CK*) in response to exercise-induced muscle damage in the placebo ($n = 6$), 500 mL ($n = 7$) and 1,000 mL ($n = 7$) groups. Values presented as mean ± standard deviation. (Reprinted from Cockburn E, Robson-Ansley P, Hayes PR, et al. Effect of volume of milk consumed on the attenuation of exercise-induced muscle damage. *Eur J Appl Physiol.* 2012;112:3187-3194, with kind permission from Springer Science+Business Media.)

There were no differences between consuming 500 or 1,000 mL of milk for changes in peak torque and CK. In conclusion, decrements in isokinetic muscle performance and increases in CK can be limited with the consumption of 500 mL of milk (Fig 3).

▶ Muscle soreness, loss of ability to develop force, and structural damage are common problems following eccentric exercise.[1,2] There have been previous suggestions of the value of protein or carbohydrate supplements, with the hypothesis that carbohydrates alter the course of protein metabolism in some way.[3,4] But others have failed to replicate these findings.

This study is quite small in scale, but the beneficial effect of semiskimmed milk (which includes lactose, whey, and casein protein) on the release of creatine kinase (CK) following eccentric or concentric exercise on an isokinetic dynamometer seems dramatic (Fig 3). One weakness in this experimental design is that the subjects drinking the skimmed milk differed from those who had the placebo treatment (1000 mL of water), and it would have been reassuring to see whether the milk drinkers also showed a large CK release if they had not been given milk. It is also a little puzzling that the milk had much less effect on delayed-onset muscle soreness than on CK release. The authors state that there were no intergroup differences in macronutrient intake, but unfortunately they provide no information as to whether the protein intake met recommendations for those performing eccentric training. Further study seems warranted with attention to some of these details.

R. J. Shephard, MD (Lond), PhD, DPE

References

1. MacIntyre DL, Sorichter S, Mair J, Berg A, McKenzie DC. Markers of inflammation and myofibrillar proteins following eccentric exercise in humans. *Eur J Appl Physiol.* 2001;84:180-186.
2. Byrne C, Eston R. The effect of exercise-induced muscle damage on isometric and dynamic knee extensor strength and vertical jump performance. *J Sports Sci.* 2002; 20:417-425.
3. Borsheim E, Aarsland A, Wolfe RR. Effect of an amino acid, protein, and carbohydrate mixture on net muscle protein balance after resistance exercise. *Int J Sport Nutr.* 2004;14:249-265.
4. Tang JE, Manolakos JJ, Kujbida GW, Lysecki PJ, Moore DR, Phillips SM. Minimal whey protein with carbohydrate stimulates muscle protein synthesis following resistance exercise in trained young men. *Appl Physiol Nutr Metab.* 2007;32: 1132-1138.

Metabolism and Hormones

Effect of Statins on Skeletal Muscle: Exercise, Myopathy and Muscle Outcomes

Parker BA, Thompson PD (Hartford Hosp, CT)
Exerc Sport Sci Rev 40:188-194, 2012

Statins are effective in reducing low-density lipoprotein cholesterol and cardiac events but can produce muscle side effects. We have hypothesized that statin-related muscle complaints are exacerbated by exercise and influenced by factors including mitochondrial dysfunction, membrane disruption, and/or calcium handling. The interaction between statins, exercise, and muscle symptoms may be more effectively diagnosed and treated as rigorous scientific studies accumulate (Fig 2).

▶ There has been a growing concern about the overprescription of statins. Although they can induce modest helpful changes in lipid profile and the risks of cardiovascular disease, careful epidemiological studies have also shown that the patient's risk of death is increased by such treatment. Among other adverse effects of statins, there are increased risks of diabetes[1] and of suicide. The underlying basis of such treatment also seems rather weak, because a large fraction of serum cholesterol is of endogenous origin; a high cholesterol level is but 1 expression of an inadequate level of physical activity in relation to intake of food.[2] For the sports physician, a further concern is an adverse impact of statins on muscle function, with myalgia, cramps, and weakness seen in as many as 25% of patients[3] and occasional reports of death from rhabdomyolysis.[4] The review of Parker and Thomson looks at the specific exacerbation of complaints among statin users during and after heavy exercise. There is evidence of increased muscle damage, as shown by an exacerbation of creatine kinase release following both downhill running (Fig 2) and participation in an event such as a marathon run. This is possibly linked to a depletion of intramuscular co-enzyme Q10.[5] Effects seem to be exacerbated by heat stress. Current evidence points to the wisdom in

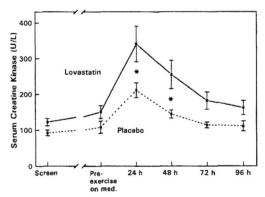

FIGURE 2.—Serum creatine kinase (CK) levels (in units per liter) in men treated with 40 mg·d^{-1} lovastatin (n = 22) or placebo (n = 27) before treatment (screen), after 4 wk of lovastatin or placebo (preexercise on medication), and daily for 4 d after downhill walking. *$P < 0.05$. *Editor's Note*: Please refer to original journal article for full references. (Reprinted from (31). Copyright © 1997 Elsevier. Used with permission.) (Reprinted from Parker BA, Thompson PD. Effect of statins on skeletal muscle: exercise, myopathy and muscle outcomes. *Exerc Sport Sci Rev.* 2012;40:188-194, with permission from the American College of Sports Medicine.)

evaluating very carefully a patient's need for statins, and to consider stopping such treatment for several days if a bout of heavy exercise is contemplated.

R. J. Shephard, MD (Lond), PhD, DPE

References

1. Sattar N, Preiss D, Murray HM, et al. Statins and risk of incident diabetes: a collaborative meta-analysis of randomised statin trials. *Lancet.* 2010;375:735-742.
2. Goode RC, Firstbrook JB, Shephard RJ. Effects of exercise and a cholesterol-free diet on human serum lipids. *Can J Physiol Pharmacol.* 1966;44:575-580.
3. Phillips PS, Haas RH, Bannykh S, et al. Statin-associated myopathy with normal creatine kinase levels. *Ann Intern Med.* 2002;137:581-585.
4. Staffa JA, Chang J, Green L. Cerivastatin and reports of fatal rhabdomyolysis. *N Engl J Med.* 2002;346:539-540.
5. Marcoff L, Thompson PD. The role of coenzyme Q10 in statin-associated myopathy: a systematic review. *J Am Coll Cardiol.* 2007;49:2231-2237.

Associations of Strength Training with Impaired Glucose Metabolism: The AusDiab Study

Minges KE, Magliano DJ, Owen N, et al (Baker IDI Heart and Diabetes Inst, Melbourne, Victoria, Australia; et al)
Med Sci Sports Exerc 45:299-303, 2013

Purpose.—To examine the association of strength training (ST) activity with impaired glucose metabolism (IGM) in Australian adults.

Methods.—On the basis of an oral glucose tolerance test, IGM (which includes impaired fasting glucose, impaired glucose tolerance, or newly diagnosed type 2 diabetes), was assessed in 5831 adults (mean age = 56.0 ± 12.7 yr) without clinically diagnosed diabetes who participated in the

2004–2005 Australian Diabetes, Obesity and Lifestyle Study (AusDiab). Meeting the current ST guideline was based on reporting ST at least two times per week (frequency) or ≥ 40 min·wk^{-1} in total (duration). Multiple logistic regression analyses examined associations of self-reported ST frequency and duration with IGM.

Results.—After adjustment for known confounding factors and total moderate-to vigorous-intensity leisure time exercise, the odds ratio (OR) of IGM was 0.73 (95% confidence interval [CI] = 0.59–0.91, $P \leq 0.005$) in those who met the ST frequency guideline (two or more times per week) and 0.69 (95% CI = 0.55–0.87, $P \leq 0.01$) in those who met the ST duration guideline (≥ 40 min·wk^{-1}). Those who achieved both the recommended frequency and duration of ST had 24% lower odds of IGM. There was also evidence that a moderate frequency (once a week) and duration (10–39 min·wk^{-1}) of ST reduced the odds of IGM (OR frequency = 0.53, 95% CI = 0.51–0.81, $P \leq 0.01$; OR duration = 0.72, 95% CI = 0.52–1.00, $P \leq 0.05$).

Conclusions.—These findings support the importance of including ST activity, at a frequency of at least once per week, within exercise management recommendations for the maintenance of favorable metabolic health, particularly as it may contribute to reducing the risk of developing type 2 diabetes mellitus.

▶ This cross-sectional analysis from the longitudinal Australian Diabetes, Obesity and Lifestyle Study (AusDiab) provides evidence that resistance exercise training (weight lifting) at least 1 day per week was associated with a reduced risk of having impaired glucose metabolism. Approximately 20% of the nearly 5800 participants reported doing resistance exercise 1 day/week or more. This incidence rate is similar to that of the US adult population. If you are caring for patients with impaired glucose metabolism (impaired fasting glucose or glucose intolerance) or type II diabetes mellitus, the following questions from this article could be used to ascertain resistance training behavior: "How many times, in the past week, have you done any activities designed to increase muscle strength or tone, such as lifting weights, pull-ups, push-ups, or sit-ups?" and, if answered affirmatively, "What do you estimate was the total time you spent in these activities in the last week?" A reasonable first goal for patients would be to spend at least 20 minutes in resistance exercise on 1 day per week. A future goal would be to advance to at least 40 minutes on 2 days per week. Because of the cross-sectional study design, it cannot be concluded that this resistance exercise behavior will normalize glucose metabolism or prevent progression to diabetes mellitus. Furthermore, this study provides no recommendation for exercise intensity. An accurate estimate of weight-lifting intensity would be very difficult to obtain from a questionnaire. It's a fair assumption that most middle-aged adults would avoid very high-intensity lifting and therefore the AusDiab study data likely reflect light-to-moderate intensity exercise. The American College of Sports Medicine recommends an intensity of 60% to 70% of the 1-repetition maximum (1-RM) for novice to intermediate exercisers to improve strength, 4% to 50% of the 1-RM for older adults or those who are completely sedentary, 2 to 4 sets of upper and lower body exercises for strength improvement.[1]

C. M. Jankowski, PhD

Reference

1. Garber CE, Blissmer B, Deschenes MR, et al. American College of Sports Medicine position stand. Quantity and quality of exercise for developing and maintaining cardiorespiratory, musculoskeletal, and neuromotor fitness in apparently healthy adults: guidance for prescribing exercise. *Med Sci Sports Exerc.* 2011;43:1334-1359.

Isomaltulose Improves Glycemia and Maintains Run Performance in Type 1 Diabetes

Bracken RM, Page R, Gray B, et al (Swansea Univ, UK; et al)
Med Sci Sports Exerc 44:800-808, 2012

Purpose.—Individuals with type 1 diabetes mellitus (T1DM) are encouraged to reduce rapid-acting insulin and consume CHO to prevent hypoglycemia during or after exercise. However, research comparing the metabolic and performance effects of different CHO is limited. This study compared the alterations in metabolism and fuel oxidation in response to performance running after preexercise ingestion of isomaltulose or dextrose in T1DM.

Methods.—After preliminary testing, on two occasions, seven T1DM individuals consumed $0.6 \text{ g} \cdot \text{kg}^{-1}$ body mass of either dextrose (DEX; glycemic index = 96) or isomaltulose (ISO; glycemic index = 32), 2 h before a discontinuous incremental run to 80% $\dot{V}O_{2peak}$ on a motorized treadmill followed by a 10-min all-out performance test on a nonmotorized treadmill. Blood glucose (BG), acid—base, and cardiorespiratory parameters were measured 2 h before, during, and after both run tests. Data (mean ± SEM) were analyzed using repeated-measures ANOVA.

Results.—Preexercise BG area under the curve was lower under ISO in comparison with DEX (ISO = +4.0 ± 0.3 mmol$\cdot$L$^{-1}\cdot$h^{-1} vs DEX = +7.0 ± 0.6 mmol$\cdot$L$^{-1}\cdot$h^{-1}, $P < 0.01$). Resting blood lactate concentrations and rate of CHO oxidation under ISO were greater than those elicited under DEX ($P < 0.05$). There were no metabolic or cardiorespiratory differences between conditions in response to submaximal exercise despite lower BG concentrations under ISO ($P < 0.05$). T1DM individuals completed the same distance at the same speed during the 10-min run test under both conditions (not significant).

Conclusions.—Consumption of isomaltulose alongside rapid-acting insulin reduction improves BG responses to exercise and produces a similar high-intensity run performance compared with dextrose in T1DM individuals (Fig 1).

▶ Although it is important for patients with type I diabetes mellitus to engage in endurance exercise, maintaining a good control of blood glucose levels during

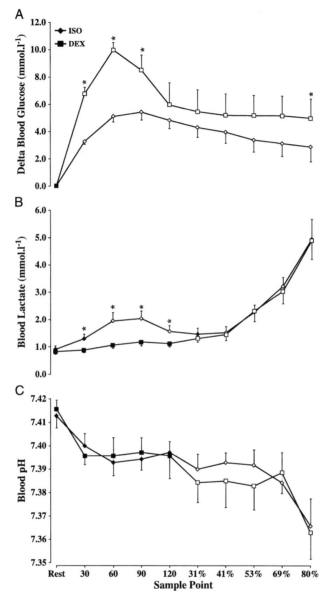

FIGURE 1.—BG (A), lactate (B), and pH (C) responses to ingestion of ISO and DEX. Data are presented as mean ± SEM. *Between-condition difference (*P* < 0.05). *Hollow sample points* indicate a difference from rest (*P* < 0.05). CHO and insulin were administered immediately after the resting sample. Exercise began immediately after the 120-min sample. (Reprinted from Bracken RM, Page R, Gray B, et al. Isomaltulose improves glycemia and maintains run performance in type 1 diabetes. *Med Sci Sports Exerc.* 2012;44:800-808, with permission from the American College of Sports Medicine.)

and particularly after such activity is a continuing challenge.[1-3] One tactic that has attracted recent interest is the administration of a low glycemic index (GI) carbohydrate. This appears to induce less suppression of lipid metabolism than dextrose and thus helps in maintaining blood glucose during and following a bout of endurance exercise.[4] The trial of Bracken et al compared the exercise response of a small group of subjects to isomaltulose and dextrose; in both cases, their dosage of rapid-acting insulin was halved prior to the trial. The isomaltulose gave a much more favorable blood sugar curve than the dextrose, particularly in the 2 hours before beginning exercise (Fig 1), presumably because low GI carbohydrates digest more slowly and cannot cross the intestinal mucosa until they have been broken down to monosaccharides.[5] However, the 2 trials showed no differences in either physical performance. However, in contrast to some previous studies there was no intertrial difference of lipid metabolism during exercise. The results seem sufficiently promising to merit further trials on a larger group of subjects.

R. J. Shephard, MD (Lond), PhD, DPE

References

1. Campaigne BN, Wallberg-Henriksson H, Gunnarsson R. Glucose and insulin responses in relation to insulin dose and caloric intake 12 h after acute physical exercise in men with IDDM. *Diabetes Care.* 1987;10:716-721.
2. MacDonald MJ. Postexercise late-onset hypoglycaemia in insulin dependent diabetic patients. *Diabetes Care.* 1987;10:584-588.
3. Tsalikian E, Maurus N, Beck RW, Janz KF, Chase HP. Impact of exercise on overnight glycemic control in children with type 1 diabetes mellitus. *J Paediatr.* 2005; 147:528-534.
4. West D, Morton R, Stephens JW, et al. Isomaltulose improves post-exercise glycemia by reducing CHO oxidation in T1DM. *Med Sci Sports Exerc.* 2011;43:204-210.
5. Southgate DAT. Digestion and metabolism of sugars. *Am J Clin Nut.* 1995;62: 203s-211s.

Neuromuscular Dysfunction in Diabetes: Role of Nerve Impairment and Training Status

Sacchetti MS, Balducci S, Bazzucchi I, et al ("Foro Italico" Univ, Rome, Italy; "La Sapienza" Univ, Rome, Italy; et al)
Med Sci Sports Exerc 45:52-59, 2013

Purpose.—The purpose of this study was to investigate the effect of diabetes, motor nerve impairment, and training status on neuromuscular function by concurrent assessment of the torque—velocity relationship and muscle fiber conduction velocity (MFCV).

Methods.—Four groups were studied ($n = 12$ each): sedentary patients with diabetes in the first (lower) and fourth (higher) quartile of motor nerve conduction velocity (D1 and D4, respectively), trained diabetic (TD) patients, and nondiabetic sedentary control (C) subjects. Maximal isometric and isokinetic contractions were assessed over a wide range of angular velocities for the elbow flexors and knee extensors to evaluate the

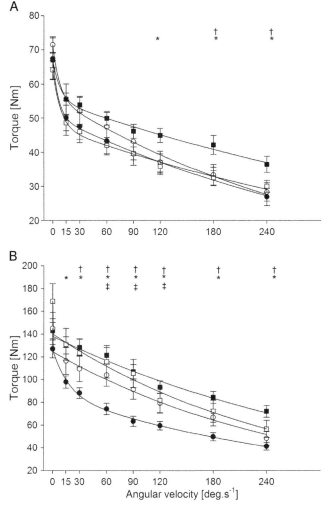

FIGURE 2.—Isokinetic torque during maximal contraction of the EF (A) and KE (B) at different angular velocities in nondiabetic sedentary control subjects (C, *closed squares*), sedentary patients with diabetes in the first (lower) quartile (D1, *closed circles*) and fourth (higher) quartile (D4, *open circles*) of MNCV, and TD patients (*open squares*). $*P < 0.05$ D1 vs C; $^{†}P < 0.05$ D4 vs C; $^{‡}P < 0.05$ D1 vs D4 using Tukey *post hoc* test. (Reprinted from Sacchetti MS, Balducci S, Bazzucchi I, et al. Neuromuscular dysfunction in diabetes: Role of nerve impairment and training status. *Med Sci Sports Exerc.* 2013;45:52-59, with permission from the American College of Sports Medicine.)

torque—velocity relationship. Simultaneously, MFCV was estimated from surface electromyography of the vastus lateralis and biceps brachii.

Results.—Isometric strength was similar among groups. The dynamic strength of elbow flexors was reduced in patients with diabetes at the higher contraction speeds. The strength of knee extensors was lower in sedentary patients with diabetes at all velocities considered, with significantly lower values in D1 than that in D4 at 60°, 90°, and $120° \cdot s^{-1}$, whereas it was similar between TD and C subjects, especially at low contraction velocities. At the vastus lateralis, but not the biceps brachii, MFCV was lower in D1 and D4 as compared with TD and C subjects, showing similar values.

Conclusions.—Muscle weakness in diabetes affects also the upper limb, although to a lower extent than the lower limb, is only partly related to motor nerve impairment, and is dependent on contraction velocity. Exercise training might counteract diabetes-induced alterations in muscle fiber contractile properties and MFCV (Fig 2).

▶ Muscle weakness is a common feature of diabetes mellitus, particularly in patients older than age 60 years[1]; there is not only a reduction of muscle mass,[2] but also a decrease in quality of the remaining muscle, with a poorer force per unit volume of muscle tissue.[3] Part of the problem is due to peripheral neuropathy.[4] The present study demonstrates that the arm muscles are also affected, although to a lesser extent than the legs; the effect is much more marked for dynamic than for static contractions and is dependent on angular velocity of contraction (Fig 2). Changes of muscle contraction properties are possibly associated with abnormalities of sarcolemmal ion channels and a prolonged duration of the action potential. There are 2 practical conclusions: When testing patients with diabetes, it is advisable to use dynamic muscle contractions, and regular exercise can slow the progression of neuropathy[5] and increase muscle strength.[6]

R. J. Shephard, MD (Lond), PhD, DPE

References

1. Gregg EW, Beckles GL, Williamson DF, et al. Diabetes and physical disability among older U.S. adults. *Diabetes Care*. 2000;23:1272-1277.
2. Andreassen CS, Jakobsen J, Ringgaard S, Ejskjaer N, Andersen H. Accelerated atrophy of lower leg and foot muscles—a follow-up study of long-term diabetic polyneuropathy using magnetic resonance imaging (MRI). *Diabetologia*. 2009; 52:1182-1191.
3. Park SW, Goodpaster BH, Strotmeyer ES, et al. Accelerated loss of skeletal muscle strength in older adults with type 2 diabetes: the health, aging, and body composition study. *Diabetes Care*. 2007;30:1507-1512.
4. Andersen H, Nielsen S, Mogensen CE, Jakobsen J. Muscle strength in type 2 diabetes. *Diabetes*. 2004;53:1543-1548.
5. Balducci S, Iacobellis G, Parisi L, et al. Exercise training can modify the natural history of diabetic peripheral neuropathy. *J Diabetes Complications*. 2006;20: 216-223.
6. Colberg SR, Sigal RJ, Fernhall B, et al. Exercise and type 2 diabetes: the American College of Sports Medicine and the American Diabetes Association: joint position statement executive summary. *Diabetes Care*. 2010;33:2692-2696.

Associations of Strength Training with Impaired Glucose Metabolism: The AusDiab Study

Minges KE, Magliano DJ, Owen N, et al (Baker IDI Heart and Diabetes Inst, Melbourne, Victoria, Australia; et al)
Med Sci Sports Exerc 45:299-303, 2012

Purpose.—To examine the association of strength training (ST) activity with impaired glucose metabolism (IGM) in Australian adults.

Methods.—On the basis of an oral glucose tolerance test, IGM (which includes impaired fasting glucose, impaired glucose tolerance, or newly diagnosed type 2 diabetes), was assessed in 5831 adults (mean age = 56.0 ± 12.7 yr) without clinically diagnosed diabetes who participated in the 2004—2005 Australian Diabetes, Obesity and Lifestyle Study (AusDiab). Meeting the current ST guideline was based on reporting ST at least two times per week (frequency) or ≥ 40 min·wk^{-1} in total (duration). Multiple logistic regression analyses examined associations of self-reported ST frequency and duration with IGM.

Results.—After adjustment for known confounding factors and total moderate-to vigorous-intensity leisure time exercise, the odds ratio (OR) of IGM was 0.73 (95% confidence interval [CI] = 0.59—0.91, $P \leq 0.005$) in those who met the ST frequency guideline (two or more times per week) and 0.69 (95% CI = 0.55—0.87, $P \leq 0.01$) in those who met the ST duration guideline (≥ 40 min·wk^{-1}). Those who achieved both the recommended frequency and duration of ST had 24% lower odds of IGM. There was also evidence that a moderate frequency (once a week) and duration (10—39 min·wk^{-1}) of ST reduced the odds of IGM (OR frequency = 0.53, 95% CI = 0.51—0.81, $P \leq 0.01$; OR duration = 0.72, 95% CI = 0.52—1.00, $P \leq 0.05$).

Conclusions.—These findings support the importance of including ST activity, at a frequency of at least once per week, within exercise management recommendations for the maintenance of favorable metabolic health, particularly as it may contribute to reducing the risk of developing type 2 diabetes mellitus.

▶ The prevalence of diabetes is increasing and is associated with significant morbidity and mortality. Strength training improves glycemic control for those with type 2 diabetes and is also linked to prevention and management of sarcopenia, osteoporosis, blood pressure, cardiovascular risk, and musculoskeletal disorders and injuries and reduces susceptibility to falls. The American College of Sports Medicine recommends that strength training be undertaken at least twice per week by those with and without diabetes.[1] The findings from this study show that strength training has favorable effects on metabolic health and thus could reduce the risk of type 2 diabetes. The authors urged that diabetes prevention strategies should give greater emphasis to approaches that incorporate strength training.

D. C. Nieman, DrPH

Reference

1. Colberg SR, Sigal RJ, Fernhall B, et al. Exercise and type 2 diabetes: the American College of Sports Medicine and the American Diabetes Association: joint position statement executive summary. *Diabetes Care.* 2010;33:2692-2696.

A Prospective Study of Weight Training and Risk of Type 2 Diabetes Mellitus in Men

Grnøtved A, Rimm EB, Willett WC, et al (Harvard School of Public Health, Boston, MA; et al)
Arch Intern Med 172:1306-1312, 2012

Background.—The role of weight training in the primary prevention of type 2 diabetes mellitus (T2DM) is largely unknown.

Methods.—To examine the association of weight training with risk of T2DM in US men and to assess the influence of combining weight training and aerobic exercise, we performed a prospective cohort study of 32 002 men from the Health Professionals Follow-up Study observed from 1990 to 2008. Weekly time spent on weight training and aerobic exercise (including brisk walking, jogging, running, bicycling, swimming, tennis, squash, and calisthenics/rowing) was obtained from questionnaires at baseline and biennially during follow-up.

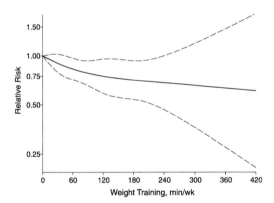

FIGURE 2.—Dose-response relationship between weight training and risk of type 2 diabetes mellitus. Dotted lines represent 95% CIs for the trend obtained from restricted cubic spline regression (4 knots). The model included the following covariates: age (months), aerobic exercise (0, 1-59, 60-149, or ≥ 150 minutes per week), other physical activity of at least moderate intensity (quintiles), television viewing (quintiles), smoking (never, past, or current with cigarette use of 1-14, 15-24, or ≥ 25 per day), alcohol consumption (0, 1-5, 6-10, 11-15, or >15 g/d), coffee intake (0, <1, 1-3, >3-5, >5 cups per day), race (white vs nonwhite), family history of diabetes, intake of total energy, trans fat, polyunsaturated fat to saturated fat ratio, cereal fiber, whole grain, and glycemic load (all dietary factors in quintiles). The analysis was truncated to men reporting no more than 420 minutes per week. P =.59 for the nonlinear relationship. (Reprinted from Archives of Internal Medicine. Grnøtved A, Rimm EB, Willett WC, et al. A prospective study of weight training and risk of type 2 diabetes mellitus in men. *Arch Intern Med.* 2012;172:1306-1312, © 2012, American Medical Association. All rights reserved.)

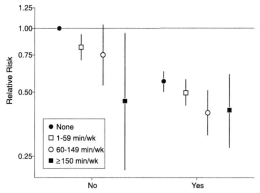

FIGURE 3.—Joint association of weight training and aerobic exercise with the risk of type 2 diabetes mellitus. Data are estimates of relative risk with 95% CIs (vertical line) from multivariable Cox proportional hazards regression models adjusted for age (months), other physical activity of at least moderate intensity (quintiles), television viewing (quintiles), smoking (never, past, or current with cigarette use of 1-14, 15-24, or ≥ 25 per day), alcohol consumption (0, 1-5, 6-10, 11-15, or >15 g/d), coffee intake (0, <1, 1-3, >3-5, or >5 cups per day), race (white vs nonwhite), family history of diabetes, intake of total energy, trans fat, polyunsaturated fat to saturated fat ratio, cereal fiber, whole grain, and glycemic load (all dietary factors in quintiles). Adherence to the recommendations on aerobic exercise is at least 150 minutes per week. (Reprinted from Archives of Internal Medicine. Grnøtved A, Rimm EB, Willett WC, et al. A prospective study of weight training and risk of type 2 diabetes mellitus in men. *Arch Intern Med.* 2012;172:1306-1312, © 2012, American Medical Association. All rights reserved.)

Results.—During 508 332 person-years of follow-up (18 years), we documented 2278 new cases of T2DM. In multivariable-adjusted models, we observed a dose-response relationship between an increasing amount of time spent on weight training or aerobic exercise and lower risk of T2DM ($P < .001$ for trend). Engaging in weight training or aerobic exercise for at least 150 minutes per week was independently associated with a lower risk of T2DM of 34% (95% CI, 7%-54%) and 52% (95% CI, 45%-58%), respectively. Men who engaged in aerobic exercise and weight training for at least 150 minutes per week had the greatest reduction in T2DM risk (59%; 95% CI, 39%-73%).

Conclusions.—Weight training was associated with a significantly lower risk of T2DM, independent of aerobic exercise. Combined weight training and aerobic exercise conferred a greater benefit (Figs 2 and 3).

▶ Regular aerobic physical activity is effective for both prevention and management of type 2 diabetes. Recent studies suggest that resistance exercise improves glycemic control in individuals with type 2 diabetes.[1] However, no previous studies examined whether resistance training can lower the incidence of type 2 diabetes. As summarized in Figs 2 and 3, in this 18-year prospective cohort study, men who engaged in weight training had a reduced risk of type 2 diabetes independent of aerobic exercise. Even modest weight-training regimens seemed to be beneficial.

The risk reduction associated with 150 min/week of weight training (35%) was just below that of comparable amounts of aerobic exercise (50%), and the combination conferred an even greater benefit. These results support guidelines urging adults to engage in a combination of aerobic and resistance training for overall fitness, health, and disease prevention.

D. C. Nieman, DrPH

Reference

1. Umpierre D, Ribeiro PA, Kramer CK, et al. Physical activity advice only or structured exercise training and association with HbA1c levels in type 2 diabetes: a systematic review and meta-analysis. *JAMA*. 2011;305:1790-1799.

Physical Activity and Mortality in Individuals With Diabetes Mellitus: A Prospective Study and Meta-Analysis
Sluik D, Buijsse B, Muckelbauer R, et al (German Inst of Human Nutrition Potsdam-Rehbrücke, Nuthetal, Germany; Charité Univ Med Ctr, Berlin, Germany; et al)
Arch Intern Med 172:1285-1295, 2012

Background.—Physical activity (PA) is considered a cornerstone of diabetes mellitus management to prevent complications, but conclusive evidence is lacking.

Methods.—This prospective cohort study and meta-analysis of existing studies investigated the association between PA and mortality in individuals with diabetes. In the EPIC study (European Prospective Investigation Into Cancer and Nutrition), a cohort was defined of 5859 individuals with diabetes at baseline. Associations of leisure-time and total PA and walking with cardiovascular disease (CVD) and total mortality were studied using multivariable Cox proportional hazards regression models. Fixed- and random-effects meta-analyses of prospective studies published up to December 2010 were pooled with inverse variance weighting.

Results.—In the prospective analysis, total PA was associated with lower risk of CVD and total mortality. Compared with physically inactive persons, the lowest mortality risk was observed in moderately active persons: hazard ratios were 0.62 (95% CI, 0.49-0.78) for total mortality and 0.51 (95% CI, 0.32-0.81) for CVD mortality. Leisure-time PA was associated with lower total mortality risk, and walking was associated with lower CVD mortality risk. In the meta-analysis, the pooled randomeffects hazard ratio from 5 studies for high vs low total PA and all-cause mortality was 0.60 (95% CI, 0.49-0.73).

Conclusions.—Higher levels of PA were associated with lower mortality risk in individuals with diabetes. Even those undertaking moderate amounts of activity were at appreciably lower risk for early death compared with inactive persons. These findings provide empirical evidence supporting the

TABLE 2.—HRs (95% CIs) for Associations Between Total Physical Activity, Leisure-Time Physical Activity, and Walking and Total and CVD Mortality in 5859 Individuals With Diabetes Mellitus

Variable	Inactive	Moderately Inactive	Moderately Active	Active	P Trend
Total Physical Activity[a]					
Total mortality					
Cases/PY	304/15 941	271/17 230	115/10 768	119/9253	
Incidence rate per 1000 PY	19.1	15.7	10.7	12.9	
Sex-adjusted HR (95% CI)[b]	1 [Reference]	0.64 (0.53-0.76)	0.53 (0.42-0.66)	0.62 (0.50-0.78)	<.001
Multivariable HR (95% CI)[c]	1 [Reference]	0.69 (0.57-0.83)	0.62 (0.49-0.78)	0.74 (0.59-0.94)	.001
Multivariable HR (95% CI)[d]	1 [Reference]	0.68 (0.54-0.66)	0.58 (0.43-0.77)	0.81 (0.61-1.08)	.03
CVD mortality					
Cases/PY	99/15 941	61/17 230	27/10 768	25/9253	
Incidence rate per 1000 PY	6.2	3.5	2.5	2.7	
Sex-adjusted HR (95% CI)[b]	1 [Reference]	0.59 (0.43-0.82)	0.40 (0.26-0.63)	0.53 (0.34-0.85)	.001
Multivariable HR (95% CI)[c]	1 [Reference]	0.65 (0.46-0.91)	0.51 (0.32-0.81)	0.62 (0.38-1.01)	.004
Multivariable HR (95% CI)[d]	1 [Reference]	0.46 (0.28-0.74)	0.31 (0.15-0.60)	0.48 (0.25-0.94)	.001
Leisure-Time Physical Activity, MET-h/wk[e]	<45	45-74	75-113	>113	
Total mortality					
Cases/PY	269/14 809	191/11 976	174/12 864	121/13 544	
Incidence rate per 1000 PY	18.2	15.9	13.5	8.9	
Sex-adjusted HR (95% CI)[b]	1 [Reference]	0.80 (0.66-0.98)	0.74 (0.60-0.91)	0.64 (0.50-0.81)	<.001
Multivariable HR (95% CI)[c]	1 [Reference]	0.85 (0.70-1.04)	0.80 (0.64-0.99)	0.73 (0.57-0.93)	.007
Multivariable HR (95% CI)[d]	1 [Reference]	0.77 (0.60-0.99)	0.79 (0.60-1.03)	0.62 (0.46-0.85)	.003
CVD mortality					
Cases/PY	67/14 809	66/11 976	50/12 864	29/13 544	
Incidence rate per 1000 PY	4.5	5.5	3.9	2.1	
Sex-adjusted HR (95% CI)[b]	1 [Reference]	1.09 (0.76-1.57)	0.83 (0.56-1.24)	0.57 (0.35-0.93)	.02
Multivariable HR (95% CI)[c]	1 [Reference]	1.18 (0.81-1.73)	0.90 (0.60-1.37)	0.63 (0.38-1.04)	.06
Multivariable HR (95% CI)[d]	1 [Reference]	0.91 (0.54-1.52)	0.69 (0.39-1.24)	0.30 (0.14-0.64)	.002
Walking, h/wk	<2.0	2.0-4.5	4.6-9.0	>9.0	
Total mortality					
Cases/PY	269/15 930	159/11 778	166/13 302	161/12 183	

(*Continued*)

TABLE 2.—(Continued)

Variable	Inactive	Moderately Inactive	Moderately Active	Active	P Trend
Incidence rate per 1000 PY	16.9	13.5	12.5	13.2	
Sex-adjusted HR (95% CI)[b]	1 [Reference]	0.83 (0.67-1.02)	0.83 (0.67-1.02)	0.95 (0.75-1.19)	.80
Multivariable HR (95% CI)[c]	1 [Reference]	0.88 (0.71-1.09)	0.86 (0.70-1.07)	0.95 (0.75-1.20)	.70
Multivariable HR (95% CI)[d]	1 [Reference]	0.87 (0.67-1.12)	0.76 (0.58-1.00)	0.90 (0.67-1.21)	.24
CVD mortality					
Cases/PY	90/15 930	37/11 778	37/13 302	48/12 183	
Incidence rate per 1000 PY	5.6	3.1	2.8	3.9	
Sex-adjusted HR (95% CI)[b]	1 [Reference]	0.52 (0.35-0.78)	0.49 (0.32-0.75)	0.69 (0.46-1.06)	.21
Multivariable HR (95% CI)[c]	1 [Reference]	0.54 (0.36-0.82)	0.50 (0.32-0.77)	0.64 (0.41-0.98)	.10
Multivariable HR (95% CI)[d]	1 [Reference]	0.40 (0.22-0.74)	0.44 (0.24-0.79)	0.65 (0.35-1.19)	.06

Abbreviations: CVD, cardiovascular disease; HR, hazard ratio; MET, metabolic equivalent; PY, person-years.
[a]Classification of total physical activity level according to the Cambridge Physical Activity Index based on occupational activity and duration of cycling and sports.
[b]Model 1: age and center stratified and adjusted for sex.
[c]Model 2: model 1 additionally adjusted for diabetes medication (no medication, insulin, oral hypoglycemic agents, or both); disease duration; self-reported myocardial infarction, stroke, or cancer; alcohol consumption; smoking behavior; educational attainment; energy; and scores for the first 3 dietary patterns derived from a factor analysis of 16 food groups.
[d]Model 3: excluding participants with self-reported myocardial infarction, stroke, or cancer or follow-up of less than 2 years (n = 5039).
[e]Leisure-time physical activity included walking, cycling, gardening, sports, and household and do-it-yourself activities.

widely shared view that persons with diabetes should engage in regular PA (Table 2).

▶ As with many illnesses, the emphasis of treatment in type 2 diabetes mellitus has tended to be provision of medications to control hypoglycemia,[1] despite evidence that regular physical activity can enhance the control of blood glucose and reduce the need for medication. The consensus recommendation is now that such individuals should have at least 150 minutes of moderate exercise per week,[2,3] and a meta-analysis of 14 controlled trials has shown that such exercise has a beneficial effect on glycemic control.[4]

This article is based on a combined prospective trial of 5859 individuals who had a baseline diagnosis of diabetes (although, unfortunately, this was an unspecified mixture of cases of type 1 and type 2 diabetes) and a meta-analysis of 14 previous trials. At baseline, habitual physical activity was determined by questionnaire. Energy expenditures were summarized as metabolic equivalents per hour per week, with exclusion of 177 individuals who reported implausible levels of physical activity. Study participants were followed for a median period of 9.4 years, with 13% of the sample (755 subjects) dying during this period. Both total mortality and cardiovascular mortality showed a clear inverse relationship to the total reported weekly level of physical activity, leisure activity, and volume of walking (Table 2). Previously published studies suggested a similar level of benefit. It should be emphasized that the physical activity was self-selected, and despite attempts to make statistical adjustments for other risk factors, part of the apparent benefit of exercise could reflect a better-ordered lifestyle among the active individuals or an effect of disease severity upon willingness to participate in an exercise program. Nevertheless, the findings are sufficiently encouraging to warrant further study by means of a prospective intervention.

R. J. Shephard, MD (Lond), PhD, DPE

References

1. Montori VM, Fernéndez-Balsells M. Glycemic control in type 2 diabetes: time for an evidence-based about-face? *Ann Intern Med.* 2009;150:803-808.
2. Buse JB, Ginsberg HN, Bakris GL, et al; American Heart Association; American Diabetes Association. Primary prevention of cardiovascular diseases in people with diabetes mellitus: a scientific statement from the American Heart Association and the American Diabetes Association. *Diabetes Care.* 2007;30:162-172.
3. Sigal RJ, Kenny GP, Wasserman DH, Castaneda-Sceppa C, White RD. Physical activity/exercise and type 2 diabetes: a consensus statement from the American Diabetes Association. *Diabetes Care.* 2006;29:1433-1438.
4. Boulé NG, Haddad E, Kenny GP, et al. Effects of exercise on glycemic control and body mass in type 2 diabetes mellitus: a metaanalysis of controlled clinical trials. *JAMA.* 2001;286:1218-1227.

Obesity

Effects of aerobic and/or resistance training on body mass and fat mass in overweight or obese adults

Willis LH, Slentz CA, Bateman LA, et al (Duke Univ Med Ctr, Durham, NC; et al)
J Appl Physiol 113:1831-1837, 2012

Recent guidelines on exercise for weight loss and weight maintenance include resistance training as part of the exercise prescription. Yet few studies have compared the effects of similar amounts of aerobic and resistance training on body mass and fat mass in overweight adults. STRRIDE AT/RT, a randomized trial, compared aerobic training, resistance training, and a combination of the two to determine the optimal mode of exercise for obesity reduction. Participants were 119 sedentary, overweight or obese adults who were randomized to one of three 8-mo exercise protocols: *1)* RT: resistance training, *2)* AT: aerobic training, and *3)* AT/RT: aerobic and resistance training (combination of AT and RT). Primary outcomes included total body mass, fat mass, and lean body mass. The AT and AT/RT groups reduced total body mass and fat mass more than RT ($P < 0.05$), but they were not different from each other. RT and AT/RT increased lean body mass more than AT ($P < 0.05$). While requiring double the time commitment, a program of combined AT and RT did not result in significantly more fat mass or body mass reductions over AT alone. Balancing time commitments against health benefits, it appears that AT is the optimal mode of exercise for reducing fat mass and body mass, while a program including RT is needed for increasing lean mass in middle-Aged, overweight/obese individuals (Fig 2).

▶ Subjects engaged in substantial amounts of exercise in this study, with resistance training set at 3 days/week, 3 sets/day, 8–12 repetitions/set, and aerobic

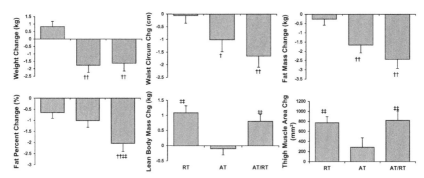

FIGURE 2.—The effect of different modes of exercise on change in measures of body mass and body composition. Error bars indicate SE. ††$P < 0.05$, †$P < 0.10$ Fisher's Post Hoc Test compared with resistance training. ‡‡$P < 0.05$ Fisher's Post Hoc Test compared with aerobic training. (Reprinted from Journal of Applied Physiology. Willis LH, Slentz CA, Bateman LA, et al. Effects of aerobic and/or resistance training on body mass and fat mass in overweight or obese adults. *J Appl Physiol.* 2012;113:1831-1837.)

training achieved through a variety of modes that equaled the energy expenditure of walking/jogging 20 km per week at 65–80% peak volume of oxygen. Perhaps the most important finding of this study, as summarized in Fig 2, is that 8 months of exercise training resulted in a modest improvement in body mass and composition. The real power in body mass loss in overweight individuals is reduction in energy intake.[1] The energy expenditure of exercise training is typically modest for overweight individuals and is often countered by increases in energy intake. Nonetheless, the value of this study is in demonstrating that overweight individuals should concentrate primarily on aerobic training. The fat-free mass of overweight individuals is typically higher than in normal weight individuals. Once the fat mass reaches near-normal levels, resistance training can be added to tone up the fat-free mass that remains.

D. C. Nieman, DrPH

Reference

1. Thomas DM, Bouchard C, Church T, et al. Why do individuals not lose more weight from an exercise intervention at a defined dose? An energy balance analysis. *Obes Rev.* 2012;13:835-847.

Effects of aerobic and/or resistance training on body mass and fat mass in overweight or obese adults

Willis LH, Slentz CA, Bateman LA, et al (Duke Univ Med Ctr, Durham, NC; et al)
J Appl Physiol 113:1831-1837, 2012

Recent guidelines on exercise for weight loss and weight maintenance include resistance training as part of the exercise prescription. Yet few studies have compared the effects of similar amounts of aerobic and resistance training on body mass and fat mass in overweight adults. STRRIDE AT/RT, a randomized trial, compared aerobic training, resistance training,

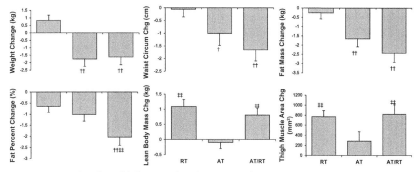

FIGURE 2.—The effect of different modes of exercise on change in measures of body mass and body composition. Error bars indicate SE. ††$P < 0.05$, †$P < 0.10$ Fisher's Post Hoc Test compared with resistance training. ‡‡$P < 0.05$ Fisher's Post Hoc Test compared with aerobic training. (Reprinted from Journal of Applied Physiology. Willis LH, Slentz CA, Bateman LA, et al. Effects of aerobic and/or resistance training on body mass and fat mass in overweight or obese adults. *J Appl Physiol*. 2012;113:1831-1837.)

and a combination of the two to determine the optimal mode of exercise for obesity reduction. Participants were 119 sedentary, overweight or obese adults who were randomized to one of three 8-mo exercise protocols: *1)* RT: resistance training, *2)* AT: aerobic training, and *3)* AT/RT: aerobic and resistance training (combination of AT and RT). Primary outcomes included total body mass, fat mass, and lean body mass. The AT and AT/RT groups reduced total body mass and fat mass more than RT ($P < 0.05$), but they were not different from each other. RT and AT/RT increased lean body mass more than AT ($P < 0.05$). While requiring double the time commitment, a program of combined AT and RT did not result in significantly more fat mass or body mass reductions over AT alone. Balancing time commitments against health benefits, it appears that AT is the optimal mode of exercise for reducing fat mass and body mass, while a program including RT is needed for increasing lean mass in middle-aged, overweight/obese individuals (Fig 2).

▶ The investigators challenged the recommendations that resistance training (RT) should be a part of weight loss—focused exercise behavior. Surprisingly, there had not been a head-to-head comparison of fat loss in response to aerobic training (AT) versus RT or AT plus RT in overweight and obese adults. They found that AT was necessary for a decrease in fat mass and body weight women and men (Fig 2). RT and AT/RT effectively increased lean mass and thigh muscle area. The change in percent of body fat decreased the most in the AT/RT group as a result of both a decrease in fat mass and an increase in lean mass. AT/RT conferred a greater decrease in waist circumference compared with either AT or RT alone, suggesting a unique mechanism for decreasing abdominal fat and, potentially, cardiovascular disease risk. The AT/RT group spent twice as much time exercising per week compared with either the RT or AT groups. These results do not support an independent effect of RT on loss of body fat in overweight and obese adults. Instead, we see a specificity-of-training effect, that is, AT is required for loss of body fat and RT for increases in lean mass. Importantly, lean mass was maintained in response to AT. These results suggest that if loss of fat mass is the outcome of highest priority, then AT should be recommended. Once the desired fat loss is attained, a possible next step would be to shift the emphasis toward maintenance of fat loss and preserving or increasing lean tissue mass.

C. M. Jankowski, PhD

Exercise and diet-induced weight loss attenuates oxidative stress related-coronary vasoconstriction in obese adolescents
Gao Z, Novick M, Muller MD, et al (The Pennsylvania State Univ College of Medicine, Hershey)
Eur J Appl Physiol 113:519-528, 2013

Obesity is a disease of oxidative stress (OS). Acute hyperoxia (breathing 100 % O_2) can evoke coronary vasoconstriction by the oxidative quenching of nitric oxide (NO). To examine if weight loss would alter the hyperoxia-related coronary constriction seen in obese adolescents, we measured the coronary blood flow velocity (CBV) response to hyperoxia using transthoracic Doppler echocardiography before and after a 4-week diet and exercise regimen in 6 obese male adolescents (age 13–17 years, BMI 36.5 ± 2.3 kg/m^2). Six controls of similar age and BMI were also studied. The intervention group lost 9 ± 1 % body weight, which was associated with a reduced resting heart rate (HR), reduced diastolic blood pressure (BP), and reduced RPP (all $P < 0.05$). Before weight loss, hyperoxia reduced CBV by 33 ± 3 %. After weight loss, CBV only fell by 15 ± 3 % ($P < 0.05$). In the control group, CBV responses to hyperoxia were unchanged during the two trials. Thus weight loss: (1) reduces HR, BP, and RPP; and (2) attenuates the OS-related coronary constrictor response seen in obese adolescents. We postulate that: (1) the high RPP before weight loss led to higher myocardial O$_2$ consumption, higher coronary flow and greater NO production, and in turn a large constrictor response to hyperoxia; and (2) weight loss decreased myocardial oxygen demand and NO levels. Under these circumstances, hyperoxia-induced vasoconstriction was attenuated.

▶ This was a small nonrandomized study of the effects of a 4-week weight loss intervention on coronary vascular function in obese male adolescents. Although preliminary in nature, the data suggest that a weight loss of approximately 8% was associated with improved coronary vascular oxidative stress reserve. The summer camp intervention included a dietary intake of 1800 to 2000 kcal/d, with less than 30% of calories from fat and the accumulation of at least 1 hour of structured aerobic activity daily. Age- and body mass index—matched boys served as controls. Nitric oxide—mediated coronary vasoconstriction was measured by transthoracic echo/Doppler ultrasound scan under a baseline condition and after breathing 100% oxygen before and after the camp. In adults, hyperoxia-induced coronary vasoconstriction was caused by the incomplete quenching of free radicals by NO. In the obese teens, vasoconstriction during hypoxia was attenuated after weight loss. This was interpreted as reduced oxidative stress or increased endothelial NO availability. This was the first study to show changes in coronary vascular function in obese adolescents after weight loss. It was beyond the scope of the study to determine the long-term effects of weight change or weight maintenance on vascular function. The chronic oxidative stress of obesity contributes to vascular endothelial dysfunction and obesity-related comorbidities. The vascular insults can start early in life, but this study suggests that vascular function can also be improved before reaching adulthood.

C. M. Jankowski, PhD

Lower Physical Activity Is Associated With Skeletal Muscle Fat Content in Girls

Farr JN, Van Loan MD, Lohman TG, et al (The Univ of Arizona, Tucson; Univ of California Davis)
Med Sci Sports Exerc 44:1375-1381, 2012

Fat contained within skeletal muscle is strongly associated with obesity, type 2 diabetes mellitus, and metabolic syndrome. Physical inactivity may be a risk factor for greater fat infiltration within skeletal muscle during growth.

Purpose.—We sought to examine the relationship between physical activity and skeletal muscle fat content of the calf and thigh in girls.

Methods.—Data from 464 girls, age 8–13 yr, were used to examine the relationship between physical activity and skeletal muscle fat content of the calf and thigh. Calf and thigh muscle density (mg·cm^{-3}), an index of skeletal muscle fat content, was assessed at the 66% tibia and 20% femur sites relative to the respective distal growth plates of the nondominant limb using peripheral quantitative computed tomography. Physical activity level was classified by past-year physical activity questionnaire score.

Results.—Muscle densities of the calf and thigh were inversely correlated with percent total body fat ($r = -0.37$ and -0.48, P values < 0.001) and total body fat mass ($r = -0.33$ and -0.40, P values < 0.001). Multiple linear regression with physical activity, ethnicity, maturity offset, and muscle cross-sectional area as independent variables showed that physical activity was independently associated with muscle densities of the calf ($\beta = 0.14$, $P = 0.002$) and thigh ($\beta = 0.15$, $P < 0.001$). Thus, lower physical activity was associated with higher skeletal muscle fat content.

Conclusions.—Our results suggest that a lower level of physical activity may lead to excess skeletal muscle fat content of the calf and thigh in girls.

▶ This is the first study to demonstrate an association between lower physical activity and greater skeletal muscle fat content in girls, independent of maturity, ethnicity, muscle size, and total body lean mass. The infiltration of fat in muscle is emerging as a hallmark of insulin resistance and the development of type 2 diabetes mellitus. In adults and children with disabilities, low physical activity was associated with greater skeletal muscle fat content. These authors used peripheral quantitative computed tomography to measure muscle density in the calf and thigh regions in 464 healthy girls aged 8 to 13 years. Physical activity over the past year was determined by questionnaire. Approximately 3% of the girls were underweight, 74% were of healthy weight (body mass index within the 5th to 8th percentile), 15% were overweight, and 8% were obese; thus, the sample represented a range of body sizes. One-quarter of the girls achieved the US Centers for Disease Control and Prevention recommendation for children and adolescents of 60 minutes of moderate to vigorous physical activity per day. When the girls were classified by level of physical activity, those in the least active group (9 ± 5 min/day) had significantly more muscle fat than girls in the middle (33 ± 11 min/day) and highest (96 ± 32 min/day) activity groups. This study demonstrated that skeletal muscle fat content begins to accumulate in the peripubertal lifestage in otherwise healthy girls and is related to level of physical activity. It is not known if muscle fat content would be reduced in response to increasing physical activity in youth or whether these changes in behavior and tissue composition would delay the onset or eliminate insulin resistance later in life.

C. M. Jankowski, PhD

Liposuction Induces a Compensatory Increase of Visceral Fat Which Is Effectively Counteracted by Physical Activity: A Randomized Trial

Benatti F, Solis M, Artioli G, et al (Univ of Sao Paulo, Brazil)
J Clin Endocrinol Metab 97:2388-2395, 2012

Context.—Liposuction is suggested to result in long-term body fat regain that could lead to increased cardiometabolic risk. We hypothesized that physical activity could prevent this effect.

Objective.—Our objective was to investigate the effects of liposuction on body fat distribution and cardiometabolic risk factors in women who were either exercise trained or not after surgery.

Design, Setting, and Participants.—Thirty-six healthy normal-weight women participated in this 6-month randomized controlled trial at the University of Sao Paulo, Sao Paulo, Brazil.

Interventions.—Patients underwent a small-volume abdominal liposuction. Two months after surgery, the subjects were randomly allocated into two groups: trained (TR, n = 18, 4-month exercise program) and nontrained (NT, n = 18).

Main Outcome Measures.—Body fat distribution (assessed by computed tomography) was assessed before the intervention (PRE) and 2 months (POST2), and 6 months (POST6) after surgery. Secondary outcome measures included body composition, metabolic parameters and dietary intake, assessed at PRE, POST2, and POST6, and total energy expenditure, physical capacity, and sc adipocyte size and lipid metabolism-related gene expression, assessed at PRE and POST6.

Results.—Liposuction was effective in reducing sc abdominal fat (PRE vs. POST2, $P = 0.0001$). Despite the sustained sc abdominal fat decrement at POST6 ($P = 0.0001$), the NT group showed a significant 10% increase in visceral fat from PRE to POST6 ($P = 0.04$; effect size $= -0.72$) and decreased energy expenditure ($P = 0.01$; effect size $= 0.95$) when compared with TR. Dietary intake, adipocyte size, and gene expression were unchanged over time.

Conclusion.—Abdominal liposuction does not induce regrowth of fat, but it does trigger a compensatory increase of visceral fat, which is effectively counteracted by physical activity (Table 2).

▶ Body fat storage depends on the balance between the intake of food energy and the energy expended, mainly through physical activity. It is thus not surprising that although liposuction appears to give a temporary solution to the

TABLE 2.—Effects of Liposuction Combined with Exercise Training on Body Composition and Energy Expenditure in Adult Women

Variable	TR (n = 18)	NT (n = 18)	Difference (95% CI)	P (TR vs. NT)
Body weight (kg)				
PRE	61.7 (5.4)	59.7 (5.8)	1.9 (−3.8 −7.7)	0.92
POST2[a]	60.8 (5.2)	58.5 (6.1)	2.3 (−3.4−8.1)	0.84
POST6	61.4 (5.7)	58.9 (6.4)	2.5 (−3.2− 8.3)	0.79
Fat mass (kg)				
PRE	17.9 (3.0)	17.6 (3.2)	0.3 (−2.8 −3.4)	0.99
POST2[a]	16.7 (2.7)	16.1 (3.1)	0.6 (−2.5−3.7)	0.99
POST6	16.3 (2.8)[b]	16.6 (3.5)	−0.4 (−3.5−2.7)	0.99
Lean mass (kg)				
PRE	43.9 (3.7)	42.3 (3.9)	1.7 (−2.1−5.4)	0.79
POST2	44.2 (3.7)	42.4 (4.1)	1.8 (−1.9 −5.6)	0.73
POST6	45.1 (3.8)[b,c]	42.2 (4.1)	2.9 (0.2−5.5)	0.03[d]
Abdominal sc fat area (cm^2)				
PRE	246 (42)	244 (52)	2.5 (−45.5−50.6)	1.0
POST2[a]	166 (36)	170 (42)	−3.5 (−42.6−35.6)	0.99
POST6[a]	159 (30)	170 (49)	−11.4 (−51.8−29.0)	0.96
Abdominal visceral fat area (cm^2)				
PRE	42.9 (10.2)	43.1 (14.9)	−0.14 (−13.1−12.8)	1.0
POST2	41.2 (11.0)	42.5 (14.7)	−1.35 (−14.3−11.6)	0.99
POST6	38.1 (9.1)	47.2 (14.2)[b,c]	−9.15 (−18.1 to _0.2)	0.04[d]
Thigh sc fat area (cm^2)				
PRE	173 (26)	164 (32)	8.5 (−22.1−39.2)	0.96
POST2	174 (32)	168 (34)	4.9 (−26.4−36.2)	0.99
POST6	162 (28)[b]	164 (37)	−1.6 (−32.3−29.0)	1.0
Pelvic sc fat area (cm^2)				
PRE	308 (48)	291 (51)	17.0 (−34.1−68.2)	0.90
POST2	310 (61)	293 (52)	19.4 (−30.6−69.6)	0.83
POST6	292 (50)[b]	292 (61)	0.5 (−56.7−57.8)	1.0
Energy expenditure (kcal)				
PRE	2271 (195)	2184 (262)	87.6 (−196.7−372.0)	0.82
POST2				
POST6	2336 (214)	2063 (292)[b]	273.7 (63.9−483.5)	0.01[d]

Data are expressed as mean (SD), estimated mean of differences [95% confidence interval (CI)] and level of significance (P) between TR vs. NT (mixed model for repeated measures). No significant differences were found between groups at baseline.
[a]Main time effect: different from PRE, $P < 0.05$.
[b]Within-group differences: different from PRE, $P < 0.05$.
[c]Within-group differences: different from POST2, $P < 0.05$.
[d]Between-group differences.

accumulation of subcutaneous fat,[1] the body compensates for this by increasing the fat content of visceral fat cells. The epidemiology of this sudden, surgically induced increase of visceral fat is unknown, but if it behaves in the same way as a normal visceral accumulation of fat,[2] the impact on prognosis will be worse than if the subcutaneous fat had remained undisturbed. This small-scale randomized trial demonstrates that a regular exercise program, initiated 2 months after surgery, and performed 3 times per week (both sets of maximum repetition muscle exercise and a substantial 30 to 340 minutes of treadmill exercise at 75% of maximal oxygen intake), can prevent the visceral fat gain (Table 2). The benefit of exercise is to be anticipated, because visceral fat is particularly likely to be mobilized by the secretion of catecholamines.[3]

R. J. Shephard, MD (Lond), PhD, DPE

References

1. Hernandez TL, Kittelson JM, Law CK, et al. Fat redistribution following suction lipectomy: defense of body fat and patterns of restoration. *Obesity (Silver Spring)*. 2011;19:1388-1395.
2. Janiszewski PM, Janssen I, Ross R. Does waist circumference predict diabetes and cardiovascular disease beyond commonly evaluated cardiometabolic risk factors? *Diabetes Care*. 2007;30:3105-3109.
3. Wajchenberg BL. Subcutaneous and visceral adipose tissue: their relation to the metabolic syndrome. *Endocr Rev*. 2000;21:697-738.

Doping

Impact of Changes in Anti-Doping Regulations (WADA Guidelines) on Asthma Care in Athletes

Couto M, Horta L, Delgado L, et al (Centro Hospitalar São João E.P.E., Porto, Portugal; Anti-Doping Authority of Portugal, Lisbon)
Clin J Sport Med 23:74-76, 2013

Objective.—To investigate how changes to the World Anti-Doping Agency (WADA) guidelines on asthma medication requests have impacted the management of asthmatic athletes in Portugal.

Design.—Retrospective analysis of asthma medication requests submitted in 2008 to 2010.

Setting.—Portuguese Anti-Doping Authority database.

Participants.—Athletes requesting the use of inhaled corticosteroids and/or β_2-agonists.

Independent Variables.—Demographic, therapeutic, and diagnostic test data.

Main Outcome Measures.—Yearly changes in number of asthma medication requests and diagnostic procedures.

Results.—We analyzed 326 requests: 173 abbreviated Therapeutic Use Exemptions (TUEs) in 2008 (objective tests not required), 9 Declaration of Use (DoU) and 76 TUEs in 2009, and 39 DoU and 29 TUEs in 2010. Spirometry was performed in 87% and 37% of athletes in 2009 and 2010, respectively; the corresponding figures for bronchoprovocation were 59% and 16%, almost all positive in both years.

Conclusions.—Applications for inhaler use have decreased by approximately half since objective asthma testing became mandatory. Our findings show that WADA guidelines have an impact on asthmatic athletes care: In 2009 a more rigorous screening was possible, leading to withdrawal of unnecessary medication. Constant changes, however, jeopardize this achievement and nowadays introduce safety issues stemming from the unsupervised use of inhaled β_2-agonists (Fig 1).

▶ Symptoms are poor predictors when diagnosing asthma,[1] and I have long wondered how much the reported high incidence of exercise-induced asthma in many sports[2,3] represented an attempt by athletes to obtain access to the supposed ergogenic advantage of inhaled β-2 agonists. A change of regulations

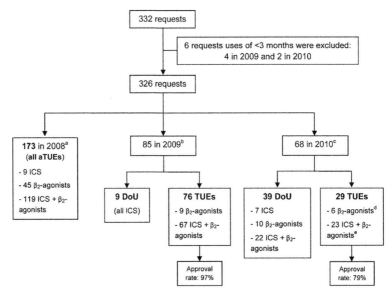

FIGURE 1.—Flow chart showing requests for asthma medication submitted by athletes to the Anti-Doping Authority of Portugal between 2008 and 2010. Notes: [a]In 2008, only an abbreviated TUE was required for ICS and IBAs salbutamol, salmeterol, formoterol, and terbutaline (ie, no objective testing or approval was required). [b]In 2009, salbutamol, salmeterol, terbutaline, and formoterol required a full TUE and ICS required a DoU. [c]In 2010, salbutamol, salmeterol, and ICS required a DoU while terbutaline and formoterol required a full TUE. [d]Three requests for formoterol (of which 2 were not approved), 2 for terbutaline (of which 1 was not approved), and 1 for indacaterol. [e]Twenty-one requests for formoterol (of which 3 were not approved) and 2 requests for salbutamol/terbutaline use. (Reprinted from Couto M, Horta L, Delgado L, et al. Impact of changes in anti-doping regulations (WADA Guidelines) on asthma care in athletes. *Clin J Sport Med.* 2013;23:74-76, with permission from Lippincott Williams & Wilkins.)

by the International Olympic Committee and the World Anti-Doping Agency for therapeutic use exemptions (TUEs) has now allowed some evaluation of overprescription, because objective evidence such as a positive response to a bronchodilator or a bronchial provocation test is now required to obtain such permission.[4,5] A retrospective analysis of TUEs in Portugal shows a dramatic decrease in such requests from 2008 to 2010 (Fig 1), suggesting that before objective testing, there was substantial abuse of this program, a view supported by one analysis of British athletes.[6] Part of the recent decline in TUEs also reflects athletes who have switched to inhaled bronchodilators that simply require a declaration of use.

R. J. Shephard, MD (Lond), PhD, DPE

References

1. Rundell KW, Im J, Mayers LB, et al. Self-reported symptoms and exercise-induced asthma in the elite athlete. *Med Sci Sports Exerc.* 2001;33:208-213.
2. Carlsen KH, Anderson SD, Bjermer L, et al. Exercise-induced asthma, respiratory and allergic disorders in elite athletes: epidemiology, mechanisms and diagnosis: part I of the report from the Joint Task Force of the European Respiratory Society (ERS) and the European Academy of Allergy and Clinical Immunology (EAACI) in cooperation with GA2LEN. *Allergy.* 2008;63:387-403.

3. Cummiskey J, Carlsen K, Kim K, et al. Sports pulmonology. In: Schwellnus MP, ed. *The Olympic Textbook of Medicine in Sport.* Oxford, UK: Wiley-Blackwell; 2008: 268-301.
4. International Olympic Committee. *IOC Consensus Statement on Asthma in 2008.* Lausanne, Switzerland: International Olympic Committee; 2008.
5. World Anti-Doping Agency. http://www.wada-ama.org/en/Science-Medicine/TUE/. Accessed January 28, 2013.
6. Dickinson JW, Whyte GP, McConnell AK, Harries MG. Impact of changes in the IOC-MC asthma criteria: a British perspective. *Thorax.* 2005;60:629-632.

Formoterol Concentrations in Blood and Urine: The World Anti-Doping Agency 2012 Regulations

Eibye K, Elers J, Pedersen L, et al (Bispebjerg Hosp, Copenhagen, Denmark; et al)
Med Sci Sports Exerc 45:16-22, 2013

Introduction.—We examined urinary and serum concentrations of formoterol in asthmatic and healthy individuals after a single dose of 18 μg inhaled formoterol and after repeated inhaled doses in healthy individuals. Results were evaluated using the World Anti-Doping Agency (WADA) 2012 threshold for formoterol.

Methods.—On the day of this open-label, crossover study, 10 asthmatic subjects who regularly used beta2-agonists and 10 healthy participants

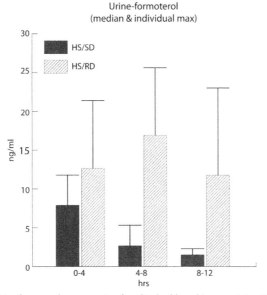

FIGURE 2.—Urine formoterol concentration found in healthy subjects receiving 18 μg formoterol as single-dose inhalation at T_0 (HS/SD) and healthy subjects receiving repetitive doses of 18 μg formoterol at T_0, T_2, T4, and T_6 (HS/RD). Urine was collected from 0 to 4 h, from 4 to 8 h, and from 8 to 12 h. Sticks marking individual maximum. (Reprinted from Eibye K, Elers J, Pedersen L, et al. Formoterol concentrations in blood and urine: the world anti-doping agency 2012 regulations. *Med Sci Sports Exerc.* 2013;45:16-22, with permission from the American College of Sports Medicine.)

with no previous use of beta2-agonists received a single dose of 18 μg formoterol. Further, 10 nonasthmatic participants inhaled 18 μg formoterol every second hour until obtaining a total of 72 μg, which is twice the maximum daily dose (36 μg formoterol) permitted by the WADA. Blood samples were collected at baseline, 30 min, 1, 2, 3, 4, and 6 h after the first inhalation. Urine samples were collected at baseline, 0−4, 4−8, and 8−12 h after the first inhalation.

Results.—Median urine concentration, corrected for specific gravity, after the single-dose administration peaked during 0−4 h after inhalation at a maximum of 7.4 ng·mL^{-1} in asthmatic subjects and 7.9 ng·mL^{-1} in healthy subjects. Median urine concentration after repeated doses peaked during 4−8 h after inhalation of a total of 72 μg formoterol at a maximum of 16.8 ng·mL^{-1} in healthy participants. The maximum individual concentration of 25.6 ng·mL^{-1} was found after inhalation of a total of 72 μg formoterol.

Conclusions.—We found no significant differences in urinary and serum concentrations of formoterol between asthmatic and healthy subjects. We found high interindividual variability in the concentrations in all groups. Our data support the WADA 2012 urinary threshold of 30 ng·mL^{-1} formoterol as being an adverse analytical finding (Fig 2).

▶ Formoterol is a long-acting β2-agonist with a rapid onset of action. The therapeutic use of inhaled salbutamol and salmeterol in international competition has been permitted by antidoping legislation since 2010, but until recently, the use of formoterol by asthmatic athletes has required a therapeutic use exemption (TUE). The regulations changed in 2012, and inhalation of therapeutic doses of formoterol is now permitted to a maximum of 36 μg/d (the normal dose is 4.5−9 μg twice daily). However, urinary concentrations of more than 30 ng/mL are regarded as an adverse finding that requires further investigation. The data of Eibye et al suggest that this is a very reasonable ceiling; even after taking twice the permitted dose, urinary concentrations reached only about 16 ng/mL (Fig 2), with one of 10 subjects peaking at 25.6 ng/mL. Abusers might try to hide their actions by secreting a dilute urine, and future research should provide standards that also take account of urinary-specific gravity. Another possible issue is whether a competitive advantage can be obtained by taking legally permitted amounts of salbutamol and formoterol in combination.

R. J. Shephard, MD (Lond), PhD, DPE

Urine and Serum Concentrations of Inhaled and Oral Terbutaline

Elers J, Hostrup M, Pedersen L, et al (Bispebjerg Hosp, København NV, Denmark; et al)
Int J Sports Med 33:1026-1033, 2012

We examined urine and serum concentrations after *therapeutic* use of single and repetitive doses of inhaled and *supratherapeutic* oral use of terbutaline. We compared the concentrations in 10 asthmatics and 10 healthy

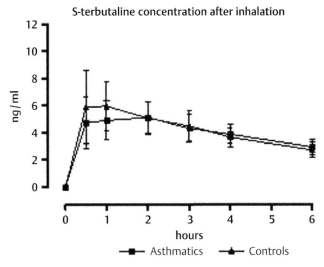

FIGURE 2.—Terbutaline concentrations in serum after inhaled and oral use. (Reprinted from Elers J, Hostrup M, Pedersen L, et al. Urine and serum concentrations of inhaled and oral terbutaline. *Int J Sports Med.* 2012;33:1026-1033, © 2012, Thieme Medical Publishers, Inc.)

subjects in an open-label, cross-over study with 2 mg *inhaled* and 10 mg *oral* terbutaline on 2 study days. Further, 10 healthy subjects were administered 1 mg *inhaled* terbutaline in 4 repetive doses with total 4 mg. Blood samples were collected at baseline and during 6 h after the first inhalations. Urine samples were collected at baseline and during 12 h after the first inhalations. Median (IQR) urine concentrations peaked in the period 0–4 h after inhalation with *Cmax* 472 (324) ng/mL in asthmatics and 661 (517) ng/mL in healthy subjects, and 4–8 h after oral use with *Cmax* 666 (877) ng/mL in asthmatic and 402 (663) ng/mL in healthy subjects. In conclusion we found no significant differences in urine and serum concentrations between asthmatic and healthy subjects. We compared urine and serum concentrations after *therapeutic* inhaled doses and *supratherapeutic* oral doses and observed significant statistical diffences in both groups but found it impossible to distinguish between therapeutic and prohibited use based on doping tests with urine and blood samples (Fig 2).

▶ The problem of complaints of asthma in athletes continues to vex sports physicians, and the situation became yet more complicated in 2012 with permission to use terbutaline if the athlete is given a "therapeutic use exemption." Although there have been studies of urine and blood concentrations allowing laboratories to distinguish the permitted inhalation from the prohibited oral administration of salbutamol,[1-3] such data are as yet lacking for terbutaline. The present study thus collected serum and urine data from both asthmatics and healthy subjects after inhalation of 2 mg and oral administration of 10 mg of terbutaline; it also looked at responses to repeated doses, as might be likely with an asthmatic individual. Responses were very similar in healthy and asthmatic individuals, and the disappointing conclusion was reached that at present neither serum nor urine testing was adequate to distinguish the therapeutic use of terbutaline from doping (Fig 2). There remains scope to examine how far vigorous exercise modifies the uptake and metabolism of orally administered terbutaline. Here is 1 more problem for antidoping experts to confront!

R. J. Shephard, MD (Lond), PhD, DPE

References

1. Bergés R, Segura J, Ventura R, et al. Discrimination of prohibited oral use of salbutamol from authorized inhaled asthma treatment. *Clin Chem.* 2000;46:1365-1375.
2. Elers J, Pedersen L, Henninge J, et al. Blood and urinary concentrations of salbutamol in asthmatic subjects. *Med Sci Sports Exerc.* 2010;42:244-249.
3. Schweizer C, Saugy M, Kamber M. Doping test reveals high concentrations of salbutamol in a Swiss track and field athlete. *Clin J Sport Med.* 2004;14:312-315.

A polymerase chain reaction-based methodology to detect gene doping
Carter A, Flueck M (Univ of Manchester, UK)
Eur J Appl Physiol 112:1527-1536, 2012

The non-therapeutic use of genes to enhance athletic performance (gene doping) is a novel threat to the World of Sports. Skeletal muscle is a prime target of gene therapy and we asked whether we can develop a test system to produce and detect gene doping. Towards this end, we introduced a plasmid (pCMV-FAK, 3.8 kb, 50 μg) for constitutive expression of the chicken homologue for the regulator of muscle growth, focal adhesion kinase (FAK), via gene electro transfer in the anti-gravitational muscle, *m. soleus, or gastrocnemius medialis* of rats. Activation of hypertrophy signalling was monitored by assessing the ribosomal kinase p70S6K and muscle

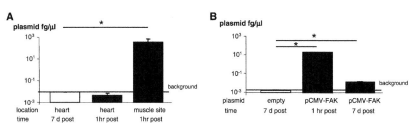

FIGURE 5.—Time course for PCR detection of exogenous FAK in serum of transfected rats. Calculated amount of pCMV-FAK plasmid in blood serum (a) and muscle samples (b) from *soleus* muscles of transfected and non-transfected rats. Serum samples were collected close to the site of pCMV-FAK plasmid injection ('muscle site') or the left ventricle ('heart') 1 day or 7 days after plasmid injection. *Asterisk* indicates $p < 0.05$ based on a *T* test. (Reprinted from Carter A, Flueck M. A polymerase chain reaction-based methodology to detect gene doping. *Eur J Appl Physiol.* 2012;112:1527-1536, with kind permission from Springer Science+Business Media.)

fibre cross section. Detectability of the introduced plasmid was monitored with polymerase chain reaction in deoxyribonucleic acids (DNA) from transfected muscle and serum. Muscle transfection with pCMV-FAK elevated FAK expression 7- and 73-fold, respectively, and increased mean cross section by 52 and 16% in targeted muscle fibres of *soleus* and *gastrocnemius* muscle 7 days after gene electro transfer. Concomitantly p70S6K content was increased in transfected *soleus* muscle (+110%). Detection of the exogenous plasmid sequence was possible in DNA and cDNA of muscle until 7 days after transfection, but not in serum except close to the site of plasmid deposition, 1 h after injection and surgery. The findings suggest that the reliable detection of gene doping in the immoral athlete is not possible unless a change in the current practice of tissue sampling is applied involving the collection of muscle biopsy close to the site of gene injection (Fig 5).

▶ It is unclear whether gene doping has yet become a reality in top international sports,[1] but nevertheless there have been calls to develop methods capable of detecting this potential abuse.[2,3] Certainly, there have been reports of dramatic responses to gene manipulation in rats, and the same gains could theoretically be achieved in human athletes. There are many possible targets for genetic manipulation, including muscle hypertrophy induced by variants of insulin-like growth factor-1 or blockade of myostatin, increase of hematocrit through use of erythropoietin, angiogenesis induced by vascular endothelial growth factors and changes in muscle phenotype.[3] The polymerase chain reaction is probably the method of choice for detecting gene doping, because it amplifies the DNA sequence of any vector that has been introduced.[4] The studies of Cater and Flueck were conducted on rats; the authors were able to detect doping in muscle-biopsy specimens for up to 7 days, but unfortunately they were less successful with the blood specimens that would normally be available to those controlling for doping (Fig 5). Plainly, much more research is needed if there is good evidence that athletes are engaging in this type of abuse.

R. J. Shephard, MD (Lond), PhD, DPE

References

1. Andersen JL, Schjerling P, Saltin B. Muscle, genes and athletic performance. *Sci Am*. 2000;283:48-55.
2. Gassmann M, Rusconi S, Flueck M. *Observatorium Gene Doping*. Geneva, Switzerland: Bundesamt für Sport (BASPO); 2005.
3. Haisma HJ, de Hon O. Gene doping. *Int J Sports Med*. 2006;27:257-266.
4. Baoutina A, Coldham T, Bains GS, Emslie KR. Gene doping detection: evaluation of approach for direct detection of gene transfer using erythropoietin as a model system. *Gene Ther*. 2010;17:1022-1032.

Hemoglobin Mass and Biological Passport for the Detection of Autologous Blood Doping

Pottgiesser T, Echteler T, Sottas P-E, et al (Univ Hosp of Freiburg, Germany; Swiss Anti-Doping Laboratory, Epalinges, Switzerland)
Med Sci Sports Exerc 44:835-843, 2012

Purpose.—The most promising attempt to reveal otherwise undetectable autologous blood doping is the Athlete Biological Passport enabling a longitudinal monitoring of hematological measures. Recently, the determination of hemoglobin mass (tHb) was suggested to be incorporated in the adaptive model of the Athlete Biological Passport. The purpose therefore was to evaluate the performance of tHb as part of the adaptive model for the detection of autologous blood transfusions in a longitudinal blinded study.

Methods.—Twenty-one subjects were divided into a doped group ($n = 11$) and a control group ($n = 10$). During the time course of a simulated cycling season (42 wk) including three major competitions (Classics, Grand Tour, World Championships), multiple autologous transfusions of erythrocyte concentrates were assigned in the doped group. A blinded investigator ordered up to 10 tHb measurements (carbon monoxide rebreathing) per subject, mimicking an intelligent doping testing approach in obtaining hematological data (tHb, OFFmass (novel marker including reticulocytes), and respective sequences) for the adaptive model.

Results.—The final analysis included 199 of 206 overall tHb measurements. The use of tHb, OFFmass, and their sequences as markers of the adaptive model at the 99% specificity level allowed identification of 10 of 11 doped subjects (91% sensitivity) including one false positive in the control group. At the 99.9% specificity level, 8 of 11 subjects were identified without false positives (73% sensitivity).

Conclusions.—It seems that the problems of tHb determination by carbon monoxide rebreathing limit the application of this method in antidoping. Because of its potential to detect individual abnormalities associated with autologous blood transfusions shown in this study, a method for tHb determination that is compatible with today's standards of testing should be the focus of future research.

▶ The detection of autologous blood transfusions remains a challenge for anti-doping agencies, with athlete "passports" recording changes in such parameters as hemoglobin concentrations, reticulocyte counts, and various red cell indices.[1] Indices involving hemoglobin concentrations and reticulocyte counts are dependent on variations in plasma volume, so there is some virtue in supplementing this information by an estimate of total hemoglobin mass (tHb), which is independent of plasma volume. However, the usefulness of tHb data has been evaluated only once,[2] following a known autologous transfusion. In this controlled and blinded 42-week longitudinal study, the authors evaluate success in detecting repeated 1-unit or 2-unit autologous blood transfusions by repeated carbon monoxide rebreathing assessments of tHb and of a statistic similar to the OFF-hr,[3] previously used in some detection procedures. OFFmass was calculated as tHb $-200\sqrt{(\%}$ reticulocytes). The combination of tHb and OFFmass detected 10 of 11 cases of doping. Unfortunately, not only does the inhaled carbon monoxide have some toxicity, but like so many tests, it is also possible for the unscrupulous athlete to manipulate the results of rebreathing by allowing leakage of carbon monoxide in some of their tests. For this reason, these authors are forced to the conclusion that although the tHb method has potential in a cooperative subject, it cannot be used in doping control until an alternative method of determining tHb is developed.

R. J. Shephard, MD (Lond), PhD, DPE

References

1. World Anti-Doping Code. *Athlete Biological Passport Operating Guidelines and Compilation of Required Elements Version 2.1.* World Anti-Doping Agency; 2010. http://www.wada-ama.org. Accessed July 20, 2012.
2. MØrkeberg J, Sharpe K, Belhage B, et al. Detecting autologous blood transfusions: a comparison of three passport approaches and four blood markers. *Scand J Med Sci Sports.* 2011;21:235-243.
3. Gore CJ, Parisotto R, Ashenden MJ, et al. Second-generation blood tests to detect erythropoietin abuse by athletes. *Haematologica.* 2003;88:333-344.

Spurious Hb Mass Increases Following Exercise
Gough CE, Eastwood A, Saunders PU, et al (Australian Inst of Sport, Canberra, Australia; South Australian Sports Inst, Adelaide, Australia; Australian Inst of Sport, Belconnen, Australia; et al)
Int J Sports Med 33:691-695, 2012

Sensitivity of the Athlete Blood Passport for blood doping could be improved by including total haemoglobin mass (Hb$_{mass}$), but this measure may be unreliable immediately following strenuous exercise. We examined the stability of Hb$_{mass}$ following ultra-endurance triathlon (3.8 km swim, 180 km bike, 42.2 km run). 26 male sub-elite triathletes, 18 Racers and

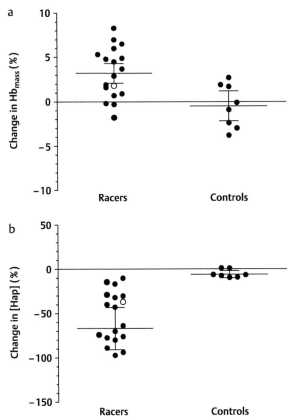

FIGURE 1.—Scatter plot showing individual values for percent change in **a** Hb_{mass} and **b** [Hap] for Racers and Controls. Horizontal lines represent group mean changes ± 90% CL. Open circles indicate one individual with a trace of haemoglobin detected in the urine post-race. (Reprinted from Gough CE, Eastwood A, Saunders PU, et al. Spurious Hb mass increases following exercise. *Int J Sports Med.* 2012;33:691-695, with permission from Georg Thieme Verlag KG Stuttgart.)

8 Controls, were tested for Hb_{mass} using CO re-breathing, twice 1−5 days apart. Racers were measured before and 1−3 h after the triathlon. Controls did no vigorous exercise on either test day. Serum haptoglobin concentration and urine haemoglobin concentration were measured to assess intravascular haemolysis. There was a 3.2% ($p < 0.01$) increase in Racers' Hb_{mass} from pre-race (976 g ± 14.6%, mean ± % coefficient of variation) to post-race (1 007 g ± 13.8%), as opposed to a −0.5% decrease in Controls (pre-race 900 g ± 13.9%, post-race 896 g ± 12.4%). Haptoglobin was −67% ($p < 0.01$) reduced in Racers (pre-race 0.48 g/L ± 150%, post-race 0.16 g/L ± 432%), compared to −6% reduced in Controls (pre-race 1.08 g/L ± 37%, post-race 1.02 g/L ± 37%). Decreased serum haptoglobin concentration in Racers, which is suggestive of mild intravascular blood loss, was contrary to the apparent Hb_{mass} increase post-race. Ultra-endurance triathlon racing may confound the accuracy of post-exercise

Hb$_{mass}$ measures, possibly due to splenic contraction or an increased rate of CO diffusion to intramuscular myoglobin (Fig 1).

▶ The measurement of total hemoglobin mass has been proposed as a useful component of an athlete's antidoping passport[1,2] because it is a value that is independent of the individual's state of hydration. Resting determinations of total hemoglobin mass by the rebreathing of carbon monoxide apparently remain stable throughout the year,[2] although the impact of a bout of very strenuous exercise on the data is less well-established. Potential problems include intravascular hemolysis and artifacts in the carbon monoxide rebreathing technique. It is important to be able to make measurements of hemoglobin levels immediately after an event, because dishonest competitors have been known to draw off the equivalent of an autologous transfusion immediately after completing a race.[3] The present observations were obtained before and 1 to 3 hours after an ultra-endurance triathlon. Surprisingly, the total hemoglobin mass showed a 3% increase after the event (Fig 1). The authors of the present report postulate either a contraction of the spleen, with expulsion of additional red cells into the circulation, or a problem with the carbon monoxide rebreathing technique immediately after exercise. The first explanation is not very likely, because most studies of humans have suggested the human spleen cannot function in this way. However, those examining the question previously may not have used an exercise bout as severe as an ultra-marathon; one study did find the spleen expelling 100 mL of blood during hypoxic stress,[4] and this would be sufficient to boost the total hemoglobin by 3%. The alternative explanation is that an increased proportion of carbon monoxide is absorbed by myoglobin, either because myoglobin has leaked into the circulation or because muscle perfusion remains greatly increased during the postexercise period. Whatever the cause, the 3% increase in hemoglobin gives the mistaken impression that a bag of blood has been infused, making post-race measurements of total hemoglobin of little value in preventing blood doping.

R. J. Shephard, MD (Lond), PhD, DPE

References

1. Pottgiesser T, Umhau M, Ahlgrim C, et al. Hb mass measurement suitable to screen for illicit autologous blood transfusions. *Med Sci Sports Exerc.* 2007;39:1748-1756.
2. Prommer N, Sottas PE, Schoch C, et al. Total hemoglobin mass—a new parameter to detect blood doping? *Med Sci Sports Exerc.* 2008;40:2112-2118.
3. Schumacher YO, Wenning M, Robinson N, et al. Diurnal and exercise-related variability of haemoglobin and reticulocytes in athletes. *Int J Sports Med.* 2010; 31:225-230.
4. Stewart IB, McKenzie DC. The human spleen during physiological stress. *Sports Med.* 2002;32:361-369.

Anti-"negative-doping" testing: a new perspective in anti-doping research?
Lippi G, Sanchis-Gomar F, Banfi G (Azienda Ospedaliero-Universitaria di Parma, Italy; Univ of Valencia, Spain; IRCCS Galeazzi and Univ of Milan, Italy)
Eur J Appl Physiol 112:2383-2384, 2012

Background.—The World Anti-Doping Agency (WADA) promotes, coordinates, and monitors drug abuse in sport. Doping has two primary objectives: to win, which involves enhancing physiologic performance, or to lose, which is less usual. Generally doping to lose has occurred in horse-racing, when large doses of opioids, neuroleptics, or tranquilizers are illicitly administered to horses to decrease their performance and allow others to have an unfair advantage. Evidence indicates that doping to lose, or negative doping, is now occurring in sports. The World Anti-Doping Code has instituted an anti-doping program to protect athletes' fundamental right to participate in a doping-free sport and to promote health and fairness of competition.

Regulated Substances.—The doping agents and methods usually used are classified according to their biologic action. The major categories are non-approved substances; anabolic agents; peptide hormones, growth factors, and related substances; beta-2 agonists; hormone antagonists and modulators; and diuretics and other masking agents. Strategies such as adding performance-decreasing substances are not included in this listing and are not regulated.

All benzodiazepines cause a dose-related central nervous system depressant activity, but some do not appreciably alter the recovery of subjective, physiologic, and performance measures. Flunitrazepam can significantly lower values for maximal isometric force and cardiovascular parameters, negatively affecting some strength characteristics and cardiovascular parameters during physical exercise. Benzodiazepines are available in many legally prescribed formats but are also widely abused.

Negative Doping.—Manipulating foods and/or beverages with substances to diminish performance is not a typical form of doping but might be done to influence the outcome of athletic performances. It is reported that beta-blockers can diminish performance and allow an athlete to better control the stress that can be experienced before or during competition. The development of new methods to detect such agents is crucial to curbing negative doping. Several pre-analytical and analytical challenges have hampered current anti-doping testing. In addition, to place a substance on the prohibited list requires (1) scientific evidence or experience showing it has the potential to enhance or actually enhances sport performance; (2) medical evidence or experience that suggests it represents an actual or potential health risk to the athlete; and (3) evidence the use of the substance or method violates the spirit of sport. In the case of using performance-diminishing substances, at least two of these criteria are applicable.

Conclusions.—The objectives of WADA are to keep athletes healthy and ensure the fairness of competitions. It is important that efforts be made to revise the prohibited list to include agents and methods that decrease athletic performance.

▶ All of the efforts of the antidoping networks to date have been directed against the possibility that an athlete may have taken some prohibited substance in an attempt to enhance performance. However, as these authors point out, there is also a risk (particularly in games such as soccer, where large amounts of money are wagered on the outcome of a match) that someone may attempt to reduce the performance of a key player. Such interference has been well recognized in horse-racing circles for a long time. This brief article describes a situation where 5 Italian first-division soccer players experienced varying degrees of sickness, and a testing of their urine disclosed the presence of the short-acting benzodiazepine lormetazepam. This drug is a central nervous system depressant, with the potential to cause an impairment of mental performance critical to the outcome of a match. There seems a need to revise doping regulations to make deliberate attempts to depress performance just as illegal as attempts to enhance the abilities of an athlete.

R. J. Shephard, MD (Lond), PhD, DPE

6 Cardiorespiratory Disorders

Acute Cardiac Problems

Focused Transthoracic Echocardiography by Sports Medicine Physicians: Measurements Relevant to Hypertrophic Cardiomyopathy
Yim ES, Gillis EF, Ojala K, et al (Children's Hosp Boston, MA; New England Baptist Hosp, Boston, MA; Northeastern Univ, Boston, MA)
J Ultrasound Med 32:333-338, 2013

Objectives.—The purpose of this study was to investigate whether sports medicine physicians can use portable echocardiography to obtain measurements pertinent to hypertrophic cardiomyopathy.

Methods.—Thirty male collegiate athletes, aged 18 to 21 years, were prospectively enrolled. Focused portable echocardiography was performed by a board-certified sports medicine physician and a resident physician, followed by comprehensive echocardiography within 2 weeks by a registered diagnostic cardiac sonographer. A left parasternal long-axis view was acquired to measure 3 dimensions: (1) end-diastolic interventricular septal thickness (IVSd), (2) end-diastolic left ventricular internal diameter (LVIDd), and (3) end-diastolic left ventricular posterior wall thickness (LVPWd).

Results.—Intraclass correlation coefficients between the sports medicine physician and the sonographer were strong: 0.77 for IVSd, 0.73 for LVIDd, and 0.64 for LVPWd. Intraclass correlation coefficients between measurements by the resident physician and sonographer were strong to moderate: 0.61 for IVSd, 0.62 for LVIDd, and 0.63 for LVPWd. Across all 3 readers, intraclass correlation coefficient calculations were 0.77 for IVSd, 0.81 LVIDd, and 0.75 for LVPWd, which indicated strong inter-rater reliability.

Conclusions.—Sports medicine physicians are able to obtain measurements relevant to the diagnosis of hypertrophic cardiomyopathy with focused portable echocardiography that are consistent with comprehensive echocardiography by a registered sonographer (Table 1).

▶ There is a growing desire by sports physicians to screen athletes for hypertrophic cardiomyopathy, because this is one of the more frequently cited causes of sudden death of young competitors during exercise, at least in North America.[1] In

TABLE 1.—Measurements by 3 Readers

Parameter	Sports Medicine Physician	Resident Physician	Registered Sonographer
IVSd, mm	10.0 ± 1.3	10.1 ± 0.8	9.5 ± 1.0
LVIDd, mm	53 ± 4.6	53 ± 4.7	53 ± 3.0
LVPWd, mm	9.1 ± 0.8	9.9 ± 0.9	9.5 ± 0.9

Values are mean ± SD.

Europe, the common approach to athletic screening is to undertake a resting electrocardiogram (ECG) recording. However, the inevitable difficulty with this approach stems from Bayes theorem—one is looking for a very rare pathology, and the screening procedure yields a large number of false positive test results. The athlete must thus either be advised (wrongly) against sport participation, or there will be a need for further, potentially costly, laboratory investigations on those unfortunate individuals who are classed as "abnormal" following an ECG evaluation. The most common ancillary form of investigation is echocardiography. Yim et al examine whether a sports physician or resident can obtain the necessary echo measurements using a portable echocardiograph instead of referring the athlete to a major cardiology center. In a small sample of healthy individuals, the values obtained by the sports physician with the portable equipment were compared with the findings of a sonographer using the latest hospital equipment. The means look fairly comparable for the 3 basic measures traditionally used in an echocardiographic diagnosis of hypertrophic cardiomyopathy (Table 1), and the authors of the present article take comfort from this. However, they must advise the individual athlete—and here the situation is less satisfactory (correlations of 0.64–0.77, indicating only a moderate correlation of individual data points); sonographers can obtain greater inter-rater consistency.[2] A further issue is that the modern diagnosis of hypertrophic cardiomyopathy rests less on these static measurements and more on the dynamic patterns of movement seen in the left ventricle. I have yet to be convinced that there is practical value in attempting such screening in athletes with no family history or symptoms. But for those who wish to go this route, it seems that detailed evaluations in a well-equipped cardiology department will still be needed to weed out a large number of false-positive diagnoses.

R. J. Shephard, MD (Lond), PhD, DPE

References

1. Maron BJ, Shirani J, Poliac LC, et al. Sudden death in young competitive athletes. Clinical, demographic, and pathological profiles. *JAMA*. 1996;276:199-204.
2. Vignola PA, Bloch A, Kaplan AD, et al. Interobserver variability in echocardiography. *J Clin Ultrasound*. 1977;5:238-242.

Head-to-head comparison between echocardiography and cardiac MRI in the evaluation of the athlete's heart

Prakken NHJ, Teske AJ, Cramer MJ, et al (Univ Med Ctr Utrecht, The Netherlands)
Br J Sports Med 46:348-354, 2012

Objective.—Echocardiographic cut-off values are often used for cardiac MRI in athletic persons. This study investigates the difference between echocardiographic and cardiac MRI measurements of ventricular and atrial dimensions and ventricular wall thickness, and its effect on volume and wall mass prediction in athletic subjects compared with non-athletic controls.

Methods.—Healthy non-athletic (59), regular athletic (59) and elite athletic (63) persons, aged 18—39 years and training 2.5 ± 1.9, 13.0 ± 3.0 and 25.0 ± 5.4 h/week, respectively ($p < 0.001$), underwent echocardiography and cardiac MRI consecutively. Left ventricular (LV) and right ventricular (RV) dimensions were measured on both modalities. LV and RV end-diastolic and end-systolic volumes and LV wall mass were determined on cardiac MRI. Echocardiographic M-mode LV volumes (Teichholz formula) and LV wall mass (American Society of Echocardiography formula) were calculated.

Results.—LV and RV dimensions were smaller on echocardiography ($p < 0.001$), and although the correlation with the cardiac MRI volume was good ($p < 0.01$), the difference in volume was large (LV end-diastolic volume difference 93 ± 32 g, $p < 0.001$). LV wall thickness and calculated wall mass were significantly ($p < 0.001$) larger on echocardiography (wall mass difference -101 ± 34 g, $p < 0.001$). Differences in absolute dimensions did not change significantly between non-athletic and athletic persons; however, the difference in echocardiographic estimations of LV volumes and wall mass did increase significantly with the larger athlete's heart, requiring possible correction of the standard echocardiographic formulas.

Conclusions.—Echocardiography shows systematically smaller atrial and ventricular dimensions and volumes, and larger wall thickness and mass, compared with cardiac MRI. Correction for the echocardiographic formulas can facilitate better intertechnique comparability. These findings should be taken into account in the interpretation of cardiac MRI findings in athletic subjects in whom cardiomyopathy is suspected on echocardiography (Fig 2).

▶ One of the immediate concomitants of electrocardiogram (ECG) screening of the athlete is the need to rule out a false-positive response by a determination of ventricular dimensions, using echocardiography or magnetic resonance imaging (MRI) screening. Proponents of ECG screening often make the assumption that echocardiography provides an unequivocal answer in regard to a false positive ECG, readily confirmed by MRI data.[1-4] There has long been discussion of appropriate cut-off points for detecting a pathological cardiac enlargement.[5] The article

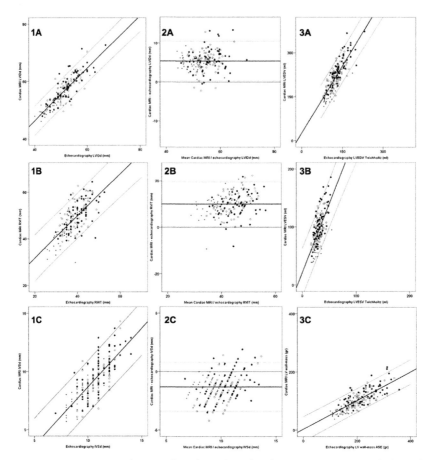

FIGURE 2.—Comparison between echocardiographic and cardiac MRI measurements and calculated echocardiographic left ventricle (LV) volume and wall mass versus cardiac MRI. (1) Echocardiograpic measurements plotted against cardiac MRI. Solid line indicates the linear regression, dashed line the 95% CI; (2) Bland–Altman plot, solid line indicates the bias and the dashed lines the 1.96 SD; LV long-axis internal diameter at end-diastole (LVIDd) (A), RVIT, right ventricle inflow tract diameter at end-diastole (B) and the septal and wall thickness (IVSd) (C) are shown. Stars, non-athletic; open circles, regular athletic; solid circles, elite athletic subjects. (3) LV end-diastolic volume (LVEDV) (A), end-systolic volume (LVESV) (B), and LV mass (C) calculated for the parasternal long-axis view on echocardiography plotted against the calculated volumes and wall mass on cardiac MRI. Note the increase in bias with larger volumes/mass. ASE, American Society of Echocardiography. (Reprinted from Prakken NHJ, Teske AJ, Cramer MJ, et al. Head-to-head comparison between echocardiography and cardiac MRI in the evaluation of the athlete's heart. *Br J Sports Med.* 2012;46:348-354, with permission from BMJ Publishing Group Ltd.)

of Prakken and associates makes 2 very important additional points. Not only is there a large systematic difference between echocardiographic and MRI findings, but there are also very large inter-individual differences in this bias, even if the 2 measurements are made on the same day (Fig 2).

R. J. Shephard, MD (Lond), PhD, DPE

References

1. Corrado D, Pelliccia A, Bjornstad HH, et al; Cardiovascular preparticipation screening of young competitive athletes for prevention of sudden death: proposal for a common European protocol. Consensus Statement of the Study Group of Sport Cardiology of the Working Group of Cardiac Rehabilitation and Exercise Physiology and the Working Group of Myocardial and Pericardial Diseases of the European Society of Cardiology. *Eur Heart J.* 2005;26:516-524.
2. Lai WW, Gauvreau K, Rivera ES, et al. Accuracy of guideline recommendations for two-dimensional quantification of the right ventricle by echocardiography. *Int J Cardiovasc Imaging.* 2008;24:691-698.
3. Guo YK, Yang ZG, Ning G, et al. Sixty-four-slice multidetector computed tomography for preoperative evaluation of left ventricular function and mass in patients with mitral regurgitation: comparison with magnetic resonance imaging and echocardiography. *Eur Radiol.* 2009;19:2107-2116.
4. Grothues F, Smith GC, Moon JC, et al. Comparison of interstudy reproducibility of cardiovascular magnetic resonance with two-dimensional echocardiography in normal subjects and in patients with heart failure or left ventricular hypertrophy. *Am J Cardiol.* 2002;90:29-34.
5. Shephard RJ. The athlete's heart: is big beautiful? *Br J Sports Med.* 1996;30:5-10.

Accuracy of ECG interpretation in competitive athletes: the impact of using standardised ECG criteria

Drezner JA, Asif IM, Owens DS, et al (Univ of Washington, Seattle; et al)
Br J Sports Med 46:335-340, 2012

Background.—Interpretation of ECGs in athletes is complicated by physiological changes related to training. The purpose of this study was to determine the accuracy of ECG interpretation in athletes among different physician specialties, with and without use of a standardised ECG criteria tool.

Methods.—Physicians were asked to interpret 40 ECGs (28 normal ECGs from college athletes randomised with 12 abnormal ECGs from individuals with known cardiovascular pathology) and classify each ECG as (1) 'normal or variant — no further evaluation and testing needed' or (2) 'abnormal — further evaluation and testing needed.' After reading the ECGs, participants received a two-page ECG criteria tool to guide interpretation of the ECGs again.

Results.—A total of 60 physicians participated: 22 primary care (PC) residents, 16 PC attending physicians, 12 sports medicine (SM) physicians and 10 cardiologists. At baseline, the total number of ECGs correctly interpreted was PC residents 73%, PC attendings 73%, SM physicians 78% and cardiologists 85%. With use of the ECG criteria tool, all physician groups significantly improved their accuracy ($p < 0.0001$): PC residents 92%, PC attendings 90%, SM physicians 91% and cardiologists 96%. With use of the ECG criteria tool, specificity improved from 70% to 91%, sensitivity improved from 89% to 94% and there was no difference comparing cardiologists versus all other physicians ($p = 0.053$).

TABLE 3.—Statistical Measures of Performance Before and After Criteria Tool

Physician Groups	Sensitivity (Before)	Sensitivity (After)	Specificity (Before)	Specificity (After)
Cardiologists	94.2%	98.3%	81.1%	94.6%
Sports medicine	91.0%	94.4%	72.3%	89.6%
Primary-care attendings	87.0%	95.3%	66.7%	87.7%
Primary-care residents	87.9%	91.3%	66.1%	91.6%
All physicians	89.3%	94.2%	70.0%	90.7%

Conclusions.—Providing standardised criteria to assist ECG interpretation in athletes significantly improves the ability to accurately distinguish normal from abnormal findings across physician specialties, even in physicians with little or no experience (Table 3).

▶ Italian cardiologists have argued for a number of years that the risk of sudden death during sport can be reduced by mandatory annual electrocardiogram (ECG) screening of athletes.[1] The evidence supporting this claim is debatable,[2-4] and the big objection to this approach is that many of the test results are false positives. As Bayes theorem demonstrates, it is difficult to avoid this problem when applying a fallible test to detect a very rare condition. In consequence, much money is spent on additional cardiological examinations, athletes are unnecessarily excluded from competition, and unnecessary fears are generated in those who receive false-positive reports. The problem can be reduced if more specific criteria are developed to evaluate the ECG of athletes, and the Italian investigators are now using a more restrictive protocol for ECG interpretation,[5] apparently reducing false positives from 7% to 15% of athletes to a still substantial 2% to 5%,[6] although the implications of this change in protocol for the supposed reduction in incidents of sudden deaths has yet to be clarified. The other big question is the level of competency required for ECG interpretation, and the study of Drezner et al demonstrates a substantial narrowing of the interpretation gap between cardiologists and primary care physicians when using the standardized criteria (Table 3). It would be interesting to add to this table figures for evaluation by exercise physiologists trained in ECG interpretation. However, one can still question whether the incidence of sudden death during sport is sufficient to contemplate the potential disqualification of 5% of athletes.

R. J. Shephard, MD (Lond), PhD, DPE

References

1. Corrado D, Basso C, Pavei A, et al. Trends in sudden cardiovascular death in young competitive athletes after implementation of a preparticipation screening program. *JAMA.* 2006;296:1593-1601.
2. Shephard RJ. Mass ECG screening of athletes. *Br J Sports Med.* 2008;42:707-708.
3. Shephard RJ. How strong is "new evidence" for mandatory ECG screening of athletes? *BMJ.* 2010;341.
4. Shephard RJ. Is electrocardiogram screening of North American athletes now warranted? *Clin J Sports Med.* 2011;21:189-191.
5. Corrado D, Pelliccia A, Heidbuchel H, et al. Recommendations for interpretation of 12-lead electrocardiogram in the athlete. *Eur Heart J.* 2010;31:243-259.

6. Marek J, Bufalino V, Davis J, et al. Feasibility and findings of large-scale electrocardiographic screening in young adults: data from 32, 561 subjects. *Heart Rhythm.* 2011;8:1555-1559.

Cardiovascular Risk of High- Versus Moderate-Intensity Aerobic Exercise in Coronary Heart Disease Patients

Rognmo Ø, Moholdt T, Bakken H, et al (Norwegian Univ of Science and Technology (NTNU), Trondheim, Norway; Røros Rehabilitation Ctr, Norway; et al)
Circulation 126:1436-1440, 2012

Background.—Exercise performed at higher relative intensities has been found to elicit a greater increase in aerobic capacity and greater cardioprotective effects than exercise at moderate intensities. An inverse association has also been detected between the relative intensity of physical activity and the risk of developing coronary heart disease, independent of the total volume of physical activity. Despite that higher levels of physical activity are effective in reducing cardiovascular events, it is also advocated that vigorous exercise could acutely and transiently increase the risk of sudden cardiac death and myocardial infarction in susceptible persons. This issue may affect cardiac rehabilitation.

Methods and Results.—We examined the risk of cardiovascular events during organized high-intensity interval exercise training and moderate-intensity training among 4846 patients with coronary heart disease in 3 Norwegian cardiac rehabilitation centers. In a total of 175 820 exercise training hours during which all patients performed both types of training, we found 1 fatal cardiac arrest during moderate-intensity exercise (129 456 exercise hours) and 2 nonfatal cardiac arrests during high-intensity interval exercise (46 364 exercise hours). There were no myocardial infarctions in the data material. Because the number of high-intensity training hours was 36% of the number of moderate-intensity hours, the rates of complications to the number of patient-exercise hours were 1 per 129 456 hours of moderate-intensity exercise and 1 per 23 182 hours of high-intensity exercise.

Conclusions.—The results of the current study indicate that the risk of a cardiovascular event is low after both high-intensity exercise and moderate-intensity exercise in a cardiovascular rehabilitation setting. Considering the significant cardiovascular adaptations associated with high-intensity exercise, such exercise should be considered among patients with coronary heart disease (Table 1).

▶ Studies in which the total exercise energy expenditure has been held constant have shown a greater cardio-protective effect when the intensity of exercise is moderately high.[1,2] It thus seems logical to recommend vigorous rather than moderate exercise to coronary rehabilitation programs, although fears have sometimes been raised regarding a resultant increased risk of cardiac incidents during

TABLE 1.—The Number of Patients, Exercise-Hours, and the Corresponding Number of Cardiovascular Events Associated With Moderate- and High-Intensity Exercise, Respectively

Center	Patients, n	Total Training, h	Moderate Intensity, h	High Intensity, h
Ålesund	775	25 720 (1)	15 232	10 488 (1)
Feiring	2629	85 208 (2)	63 032 (1)	22 176 (1)
Røros	1442	64 892	51 192	13 700
Total	4846	175 820	129 456	46 364
Event rates				
Cardiac arrest, fatal			1	0
Cardiac arrest, nonfatal			0	2
Myocardial infarction			0	0
Risk of events		1/58 607	1/129 456	1/23 182

The numbers in parentheses indicate the number of events in each center according to intensity.

the rehabilitation class. It is difficult to determine the precise risk because the incidence with any type of program is very low. Although the study of Rognmo et al was based on 175 820 hours of rehabilitation, they observed only 1 fatal and 2 nonfatal cardiac arrests and no myocardial infarcts (Table 1). The high-intensity program involved interval training, with 4-minute bursts at 85% to 90% of peak heart rate and active recovery intervals, whereas the moderate exercise was at 60% to 70% of peak heart rate, with exercise performed on the treadmill, cycle ergometer, and outdoors (walking and cross-country skiing). Although the numbers suggest a trend to a greater immediate risk with the higher intensity program, the number of incidents is clearly insufficient to be sure of this; a worldwide registry of cardiac rehabilitation programs is needed to get valid statistics. Against the possibility of greater risk, one must set the greater increase of peak oxygen intake seen with the interval program, because peak oxygen intake is a good marker of long-term prognosis.[3,4] Moreover, vigorous exercise seems needed to reverse pathological changes in the ventricle.[5,6] Finally, the most important message from this study is that the risk is extremely low with either program, and is plainly outweighed by the long-term benefits of rehabilitation.

R. J. Shephard, MD (Lond), PhD, DPE

References

1. Swain DP, Franklin BA. Comparison of cardioprotective benefits of vigorous versus moderate intensity aerobic exercise. *Am J Cardiol.* 2006;97:141-147.
2. Wen CP, Wai JP, Tsai MK, et al. Minimum amount of physical activity for reduced mortality and extended life expectancy: a prospective cohort study. *Lancet.* 2011; 378:1244-1253.
3. Kavanagh T, Mertens DJ, Hamm LF, et al. Prediction of long-term prognosis in 12 169 men referred for cardiac rehabilitation. *Circulation.* 2002;106:666-671.
4. Kavanagh T, Mertens DJ, Hamm LF, et al. Peak oxygen intake and cardiac mortality in women referred for cardiac rehabilitation. *J Am Coll Cardiol.* 2003;42:2139-2143.
5. Wisloff U, Stoylen A, Loennechen JP, et al. Superior cardiovascular effect of aerobic interval training versus moderate continuous training in heart failure patients: a randomized study. *Circulation.* 2007;115:3086-3094.
6. Amundsen BH, Rognmo O, Hatlen-Rebhan G, et al. High intensity aerobic exercise improves diastolic function in coronary artery disease. *Scand Cardiovasc J.* 2008;42:110-117.

Improving the Positive Predictive Value of Exercise Testing in Women for Coronary Artery Disease

Levisman JM, Aspry K, Amsterdam EA (Univ of California (Davis) Med Ctr, Sacramento)
Am J Cardiol 110:1619-1622, 2012

The exercise treadmill test (ETT) in women has been limited by a low positive predictive value (PPV) for coronary artery disease (CAD). However, the reliability of previous studies was unsatisfactory because of the inclusion of younger women with a low prevalence of CAD. To further evaluate the diagnostic properties of the ETT in women, we evaluated a group of women with chest pain who had a positive ETT result and subsequent coronary angiography. Of the 111 women, 56 had significant CAD on angiogram, yielding a PPV of 51% for the group. However, inclusion in the analysis of several pretest attributes and specific exercise test responses improved the PPV of the ETT. Age had a major effect, with the youngest group (35 to 50 years old) having a PPV of 36% compared to 68% in the oldest group (>65 years old). Several specific exercise responses (ST-segment depression >2 mm and delayed ST-segment recovery >3.0 minutes) further separated true from false positives across all age groups, increasing the PPV to approximately 80%. Onset of ischemia at a relatively low cardiac workload of <80% maximum predicted heart rate was not a significant predictor. In conclusion, the standard ETT should remain the test of choice in ambulatory women with chest pain and no significant abnormalities on baseline electrocardiogram especially in those >65 years of age (Fig 3).

▶ Physicians commonly order laboratory tests without any very clear idea of the likelihood that the procedure they have ordered will add to the probability of correct diagnosis. One such relatively expensive investigation is an exercise stress test, commonly requested for younger female patients. Several reports[1-3] have suggested that such testing has little practical value. Part of the problem is that the individual undergoing testing has a low probability of having myocardial vascular disease; thus, according to Bayes' theorem there is a strong likelihood of many false-positive and false-negative results. The diagnostic value of the test increases in samples in which the prevalence of the disease is higher (in other words, in older patients). This effect is very evident in the study of Levisman et al. They looked at the treadmill test results in a sample of 111 women presenting with chest pain, where coronary disease had also been assessed by coronary angiogram. In those women aged 30 to 50 years, the positive predictive value of an ST depression of 1 mm was only 17%, but the value rose to 56% in those aged > 65 years (Fig 3). But even in the younger women, an ST depression > 2 mm yielded a positive predictive value of 69%. Three points emerge from this study. First, the idea that the exercise electrocardiogram is a poor predictor of myocardial ischemia in women probably arose because test outcomes in women were compared with samples of men of similar age, but with a greater prevalence of myocardial ischemia. Second, the exercise stress test does provide useful information in women who are older than 65 years. Finally, if such testing is

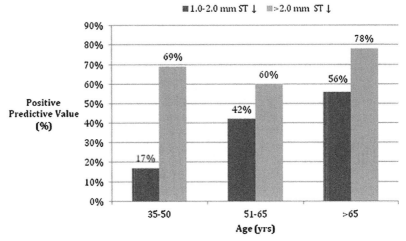

FIGURE 3.—Effect of 1.0- to 2.0-mm (*black bars*) and ≥2.0-mm (*gray bars*) ST-segment depression on the positive predictive value of the exercise treadmill test in women by age group ($p < 0.01$ in 35- to 50-year-old group). (Reprinted from Levisman JM, Aspry K, Amsterdam EA. Improving the positive predictive value of exercise testing in women for coronary artery disease. *Am J Cardiol.* 2012;110:1619-1622, Copyright 2012, with permission from Elsevier.)

applied to younger women, it is important to look for substantial ST segmental depression (2 mm rather than 1 mm).

R. J. Shephard, MD (Lond), PhD, DPE

References

1. Weiner DA, McCabe CH, Ryan TJ. Exercise testing for the diagnosis of coronary artery disease. *Am Heart J.* 1980;99:811-812.
2. Guiteras P, Chaitman BR, Waters DD, et al. Diagnostic accuracy of exercise ECG lead systems in clinical subsets of women. *Circulation.* 1982;65:1465-1474.
3. Kwok Y, Kim C, Grady D, Segal M, Redberg R. Meta-analysis of exercise testing to detect coronary artery disease in women. *Am J Cardiol.* 1999;83:660-666.

Chronic Cardiac Problems

Exercise-induced arrhythmogenic right ventricular cardiomyopathy: fact or fallacy?

Sharma S, Zaidi A (St Georges Univ of London, UK)
Eur Heart J 33:938-940, 2012

Background.—Exercise is considered a potent and cost-effective way to manage adverse risk profiles for generalized atherosclerosis. Persons who exercise regularly have an average life expectancy 7 years longer than sedentary counterparts. Relatively modest levels of exercise are sufficient for these benefits. The concept that intense exercise may be detrimental for persons with normal hearts is rarely considered. Most highly trained athletes exercise intensively for several hours a day, creating workloads of 200 to 300 metabolic equivalents (METS) per week, which are five to 10 times greater than the levels recommended for preventing coronary atherosclerosis. Interestingly, the past 30 years have witnessed an increase in obesity and cardiac morbidity because of a lack of habitual exercise along with a rise in the number of persons engaging in grueling ultra-endurance events that greatly exceed usual exercise recommendations. Studies that investigate the effects of extreme exercise were summarized.

Alterations in Cardiac Status of Athletes.—Athletes often have modestly increased heart size but preserved indices of systolic and diastolic function and high functional capacity. The few adverse cardiac events in athletes are mostly related to hereditary or congenital cardiac abnormalities. Thus exercise may be beneficial at all doses.

Transient increases in serum concentrations of biomarkers of cardiac damage are noted, often with impaired left ventricular (LV) myocardial relaxation. Up to 50% of marathon runners have elevated serum cardiac troponin concentrations. The meaning of these temporary phenomenon is unknown, but athletes tested after racing tend to be free of myocardial inflammation. Veteran endurance athletes have a fivefold increase in the prevalence of atrial fibrillation, suggesting that too much exercise may be cardiotoxic in predisposed persons. Reports of sinoatrial disease, heart block, and complex ventricular arrhythmias in seemingly healthy athletes support this suggestion. Cardiac enlargements tend to remain even years after retiring from competitive sports, which may indicate adverse cardiac remodeling. The focus is usually on the LV, with the right ventricle (RV) often ignored, although it undergoes the same preload during exercise. Exercise-induced pulmonary artery pressures over 80 mm Hg can be produced, which may adversely affect electrical and structural remodeling of the RV.

Evidence.—Studies of intensive exercisers show that enlarged RV dimensions are related to impaired systolic function after strenuous exercise. Biomarkers of cardiac damage correlate with RV but not LV systolic function. Race duration correlates with level of RV dysfunction. Nearly all cardiac function parameters return to normal within a week of racing. Complex RV arrhythmias are found in symptomatic athletes taking part in endurance activities, predominantly cycling. About a fourth of these persons had RV structural abnormalities after RV angiography, about half had RV structural abnormalities on magnetic resonance imaging (MRI), and about 90% fulfilled the diagnostic criteria for arrhythmogenic right ventricular cardiomyopathy (ARVC). An "exercise-induced ARVC" has been postulated, which would be phenotypically identical to the familial disorder but produced by training rather than genetic features.

Conclusions.—Many features remain to be evaluated before exercise-induced chronic RV damage can be clearly linked to extreme exercising behaviors. Increases in genetic and biochemical markers of fibrogenesis during exercise may represent a form of physiologic super-compensation.

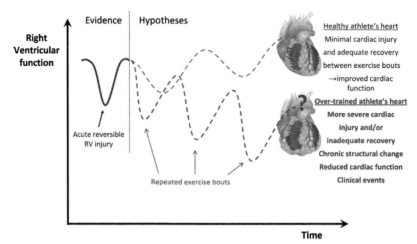

FIGURE 1.—Potential impact of repeated bouts of ultra-endurance exercise on right ventricular structure and function. (Reprinted from Sharma S, Zaidi A. Exercise-induced arrhythmogenic right ventricular cardiomyopathy: fact or fallacy? *Eur Heart J.* 2012;33:938-940, with permission The Author.)

The results of the various studies provide many opportunities for further study (Fig 1).

▶ During the past year, much media attention has been attracted by reports such as that of La Gerche and associates, who suggested that repeated marathon running can lead to myocardial scarring, electrocardiographic abnormalities, and a worsening of prognosis relative to more sedentary individuals. One investigation noted that late gadolinium enhancement is evidence of fibrosis that is associated with the number of years spent training and the number of competitive marathons and ultraendurance marathons completed.[1] A study in rats subjected to equivalent levels of stress for 16 weeks[2] also found evidence of eccentric cardiac hypertrophy with diastolic dysfunction, atrial dilation, collagen deposition in the right ventricle, and messenger RNA and protein expression of fibrosis markers in both atria and right ventricle. Ventricular tachycardia could also be induced in 5 of 12 exercise rats (42%) compared with only 1 of 16 sedentary rats (6%). However, in the rats, these findings were reversed within 8 weeks of ceasing the bouts of prolonged exercise. La Gerche et al also found an immediate deterioration of right ventricular function that was correlated with serum markers of myocardial injury (Fig 1). There was a short-term recovery, but chronic structural change with impairment of ventricular function later became apparent in some of the most practiced veteran athletes. These observations are in contrast with the optimism that once allowed "postcoronary" patients to participate in the Boston marathon,[3] and they may offer a note of caution to runners such as the 68-year-old who recently boasted of running 148 561 miles over a 43-year running career.[4] For a few people, marathon participation may indeed provide a stimulus to regular training, but for most people, it is probably preferable to commend the type of activity for which we have been anthropologically prepared—long distance but moderately intense physical activity.

R. J. Shephard, MD (Lond), PhD, DPE

References

1. Wilson M, O'Hanlon R, Prasad S, et al. Diverse patterns of myocardial fibrosis in lifelong, veteran endurance athletes. *J Appl Physiol.* 2011;110:1622-1626.
2. Benito B, Gay-Jordi G, Serrano-Mollar A, et al. Cardiac arrhythmogenic remodeling in a rat model of long-term intensive exercise training. *Circulation.* 2011;123: 13-22.
3. Kavanagh T, Shephard RH, Pandit V. Marathon running after myocardial infarction. *JAMA.* 1974;229:1602-1605.
4. Wilson MG, Whyte GP. Is life-long exercise damaging to the heart? *Br J Sports Med.* 2012;46:623-624.

Rehabilitation after myocardial infarction trial (RAMIT): multi-centre randomised controlled trial of comprehensive cardiac rehabilitation in patients following acute myocardial infarction

West RR, Jones DA, Henderson AH (Univ of Wales College of Medicine, Cardiff, UK; Univ of Wales College of Medicine, Cardiff, UK)
Heart 98:637-644, 2012

Background.—It is widely believed that cardiac rehabilitation following acute myocardial infarction (MI) reduces mortality by approximately 20%. This belief is based on systematic reviews and meta-analyses of mostly small trials undertaken many years ago. Clinical management has been transformed in the past 30–40 years and the findings of historical trials may have little relevance now.

Objectives.—The principal objective was to determine the effect of cardiac rehabilitation, as currently provided, on mortality, morbidity and health-related quality of life in patients following MI. The secondary objectives included seeking programmes that may be more effective and characteristics of patients who may benefit more.

Design, Setting, Patients, Outcome Measures.—A multi-centre randomised controlled trial in representative hospitals in England and Wales compared 1813 patients referred to comprehensive cardiac rehabilitation programmes or discharged to 'usual care' (without referral to rehabilitation). The primary outcome measure was all-cause mortality at 2 years. The secondary measures were morbidity, health service use, health-related quality of life, psychological general well-being and lifestyle cardiovascular risk factors at 1 year. Patient entry ran from 1997 to 2000, follow-up of secondary outcomes to 2001 and of vital status to 2006. A parallel study compared 331 patients in matched 'elective' rehabilitation and 'elective' usual care (without rehabilitation) hospitals.

Results.—There were no significant differences between patients referred to rehabilitation and controls in mortality at 2 years (RR 0.98, 95% CI 0.74 to 1.30) or after 7–9 years (0.99, 95% CI 0.85 to 1.15), cardiac events,

TABLE 1.—Comparison of Patients Randomised to Rehabilitation or Control or in Rehabilitation or Control Hospital, at Baseline

Characteristic/Medical History/ Lifestyle Habit	Randomised Controlled Trial		Elective Hospitals	
	Rehabilitation, n=903	Control, n=910	Rehabilitation, n=197	Control, n=134
Age	Mean (SD)			
	64.2 (11.2)	64.7 (10.9)	63.1 (11.8)	64.9 (12.1)
Gender	Number (%)			
Men	656 (72.6)	677 (74.4)	157 (79.7)	95 (70.9)
Women	247 (27.4)	233 (25.6)	40 (20.3)	39 (29.1)
Previous myocardial infarction	102 (11.6)	116 (13.0)	29 (15.3)	23 (19.2)
Previous angina	224 (25.4)	226 (25.5)	29 (15.6)	29 (23.8)
Previous hypertension treated	222 (25.1)	216 (24.3)	46 (24.5)	28 (23.3)
Untreated	49 (5.5)	38 (4.3)	10 (5.3)	6 (5.0)
Previous diabetes				
Insulin dependent	19 (2.1)*	36 (4.0)*	4 (2.1)	2 (1.6)
Non-insulin dependent	78 (8.8)	69 (7.7)	23 (12.2)†	5 (3.9)†
Smoking	364 (40)	374 (41)	80 (41)	42 (31)
Alcohol (moderate and heavy)	145 (16)	159 (18)	33 (17)	19 (14)
Diet (eating fresh fruit daily)	455 (50)	461 (51)	107 (54)	64 (48)
Physical exercise (>100 kcal/day)	100 (11)	120 (13)	30 (15)	26 (18)

*Significant difference between randomised groups p<0.05.
†Significant difference between elective groups p<0.05.

seven of eight domains of the health-related quality of life scale ('Short Form 36', SF36) or the psychological general well-being scale. Rehabilitation patients reported slightly less physical activity. No differences between groups were reported in perceived overall quality of cardiac aftercare. Data from the 'elective' hospitals comparison concurred with these findings.

Conclusion.—In this trial, comprehensive rehabilitation following MI had no important effect on mortality, cardiac or psychological morbidity, risk factors, health-related quality of life or activity. This finding is consistent with systematic reviews of all trials reported since 1983. The value of cardiac rehabilitation as practised in the UK is open to question (Table 1).

▶ No benefit from cardiac rehabilitation! This article will be perceived as rank heresy by many exercise-oriented cardiologists. The issue was seemingly settled in the 1980s, when a number of substantial meta-analyses of well-controlled trials[1-3] demonstrated a 20% reduction of mortality (but little change of recurrence rates) in those receiving formal cardiac rehabilitation. However, there were dissident voices, even in the early history of cardiac rehabilitation. Postmortem studies did not suggest any great regression of atheromatous plaques, and one of the larger early multicenter trials found no advantage of graded aerobic exercise relative to a placebo treatment of light recreational activity and the other ancillaries of coronary rehabilitation.[4] The study of Rechnitzer illustrated one of the difficulties in conducting a meaningful controlled trial of this issue: attending a rehabilitation center for recreational activity encouraged the controls to become more active, to the point where some of the controls were undertaking more activity than the less compliant experimental subjects. When data were reanalyzed, examining the prospects of those who increased their fitness relative to those who did not, a health benefit was seen in the active group,[5] although statisticians might argue that they were able to exercise because their infarct was less severe. A more recent Cochrane review found a reduction of all-cause mortality in 12 "exercise only" trials, but not in 28 more comprehensive trials.[6] West and associates argue that the findings of early trials should in any case be reevaluated, because the nonexercise components of treatment have changed so dramatically in the past 30 years. They organized a substantial randomized trial, with experimental subjects following Grade 3 programs as recommended by the British Heart Association, usually led by nurses, once or twice per week for 6-8 weeks, to a total of 20 hours. Controls received all of the treatments with the exception of supervised exercise. Primary assessment was based on all-cause mortality at 2 years. However, both the initial amount of exercise and its leadership seem somewhat suspect, and this is borne out by looking at one-year data, when fewer experimental subjects were exercising than controls (Table 1). In such circumstances, it is hardly surprising that the exercise component of treatment was ineffective; the answer seems not to reject exercise, but rather to find a more effective way of delivering it. It is worth underlining that the highly effective Toronto Rehabilitation Center program was based not on a total of 20 hours of exercise, but on 1 hour of activity at progressively increasing intensities performed daily for 1 or more years.

R. J. Shephard, MD (Lond), PhD, DPE

References

1. May GS, Furberg CD, Eberlin KA, et al. Secondary prevention after myocardial infarction: a review of long-term trials. *Progr Cardiovasc Dis.* 1983;24:335-359.
2. Oldridge NB, Guyatt G, Fischer M, et al. Randomized controlled trials of cardiac rehabilitation: combined experience of randomized clinical trials. *JAMA.* 1988; 260:245-250.
3. Shephard RJ. Exercise in the tertiary prevention of ischemic heart disease: experimental proof. *Can J Sports Sci.* 1989;14:74-84.
4. Rechnitzer PA, Sangal S, Cunningham D, et al. A controlled prospective study of the effect of endurance training on the recurrence rate of myocardial infarction. *Am J Epidemiol.* 1975;102:358-365.
5. Cunningham DA, Rechnitzer PA, Jones NL, et al. The issue of poor compliance in exercise trials: a place for post-hoc analyses? *Sports Train Med Rehab.* 1990;2:131-139.
6. Jolliffe JA, Rees K, Taylor RS, et al. Exercise-based rehabilitation for coronary heart disease. *Cochrane Database Syst Rev.* 2000;(4):CD001800.

Determination of the Effectiveness of Accelerometer Use in the Promotion of Physical Activity in Cardiac Patients: A Randomized Controlled Trial
Izawa KP, Watanabe S, Hiraki K, et al (St. Marianna Univ School of Medicine Hosp, Kawasaki, Japan; et al)
Arch Phys Med Rehabil 93:1896-1902, 2012

Objective.—To investigate the effect of the self-monitoring of physical activity by hospitalized cardiac patients attending phase I cardiac rehabilitation (CR).

TABLE 3.—Physical Activity Between Groups

Variable	Group A (n=52) t1	t2	Group B (n=51) t1	t2	Interaction F	P
Average daily number of steps	4588.0±2056.3	8609.6±3064.5*	5155.2±2424.5	5512.9±2571.8[†]	54.5	<.0001
Average daily energy expenditure (kcal)	128.6±77.8	242.6±111.5*	140.0±86.2	155.9±135.4[†]	23.6	<.0001

*P<.05 within terms (t1 vs t2)
[†]P<.05 between groups (group A vs group B).

Design.—Randomized controlled trial.

Setting.—University hospital CR program.

Participants.—CR patients (N = 126) with a mean age of 59.1 years.

Interventions.—Patients were randomly assigned to the self-monitoring group (group A, n = 63) or the control group (group B, n = 63). Along with CR, group A patients performed self-monitoring of their physical activity at the beginning of a phase I CR program (acute in-hospital phase for inpatients) and ending just before they began a phase II CR program (postdischarge recovery phase for outpatients).

Main Outcome Measures.—Physical activity (averages of daily number of steps taken and daily energy expenditure for 1 wk) as measured by accelerometer was assessed in both groups at baseline (t1) and before the beginning of phase II CR (t2).

Results.—Although there were no significant differences in physical activity values between groups A and B at t1, values of group A at t2 were significantly higher than those of group B (8609.6 vs 5512.9 steps, $P < .001$; 242.6 vs 155.9kcal, $P < .001$).

Conclusions.—Self-monitoring of patient physical activity from phase I CR might effectively increase the physical activity level in preparation for entering a phase II CR program. Results of the present study could contribute to the development of new strategies for the promotion of physical activity in cardiac patients (Table 3).

▶ The activity level of many patients at the beginning of Phase II cardiac rehabilitation is understandably quite low[1,2]; more than half were taking less than 5000 steps/day,[1] which reflects a very limited level of activity. There is also growing recognition of the potential of wearing a simple and inexpensive pedometer/accelerometer as a means of stimulating habitual physical activity.[3] Izawa and associates here demonstrate what seem substantial benefits in those wearing a Kenz Lifecorder uniaxial accelerometer and recording data on an exercise calendar during Phase I cardiac rehabilitation (Table 3). The activity levels of the patients wearing the accelerometer apparently moved into the training zone, whereas those of the controls showed little change from initial values. However, there remains scope for further research. It is unfortunate that no comparisons of functional capacity were made between the 2 groups of patients, and this will be something to evaluate in further studies. It is also not completely clear how far the large advantage of the experimental group was due to wearing an accelerometer, because a physiotherapist provided these individuals with detailed instruction on monitoring and recording data; this attention may have been at least as important as the instrumentation. A future investigation should ensure equal attention is provided to experimental and control groups.

R. J. Shephard, MD (Lond), PhD, DPE

References

1. Savage PD, Ades PA. Pedometer step counts predict cardiac risk factors at entry to cardiac rehabilitation. *J Cardiopulm Rehabil Prev.* 2008;28:370-377.
2. Ayabe M, Brubaker PH, Dobrosielski D, et al. The physical activity patterns of cardiac rehabilitation program participants. *J Cardiopulm Rehabil.* 2004;24:80-86.
3. Bravata DM, Smith-Spangler C, Sundaram V, et al. Using pedometers to increase physical activity and improve health: a systematic review. *JAMA.* 2007;298:2296-2304.

A novel cardiopulmonary exercise test protocol and criterion to determine maximal oxygen uptake in chronic heart failure
Bowen TS, Cannon DT, Begg G, et al (Univ of Leeds, UK)
J Appl Physiol 113:451-458, 2012

Cardiopulmonary exercise testing for peak oxygen uptake $(\dot{V}o_{2peak})$ can evaluate prognosis in chronic heart failure (CHF) patients, with the peak respiratory exchange ratio (RER_{peak}) commonly used to confirm maximal effort and maximal oxygen uptake $(\dot{V}o_{2max})$. We determined the precision of RER_{peak} in confirming $\dot{V}o_{2max}$, and whether a novel ramp-incremental (RI) step-exercise (SE) (RISE) test could better determine $\dot{V}o_{2max}$ in CHF. Male CHF patients ($n = 24$; NYHA class I–III) performed a symptom-limited RISE-95 cycle ergometer test in the format: RI (4–18 W/min; ~10 min); 5 min recovery (10 W); SE (95% peak RI work rate). Patients ($n = 18$) then performed RISE-95 tests using slow (3–8 W/min; ~15 min) and fast (10–30 W/min; ~6 min) ramp rates. Pulmonary gas exchange was measured breath-by-breath. $\dot{V}o_{2peak}$ was compared within patients by unpaired t-test of the highest 12 breaths during RI and SE phases to confirm $\dot{V}o_{2peak}$ and its 95% confidence limits (CI_{95}). RER_{peak} was significantly influenced by ramp rate (fast, medium, slow: 1.21 ± 0.1 vs. 1.15 ± 0.1 vs. 1.09 ± 0.1; $P = 0.001$), unlike $\dot{V}o_{2peak}$ (mean $n = 18$; 14.4 ± 2.6 ml·kg^{-1}·min^{-1}; $P = 0.476$). Group $\dot{V}o_{2peak}$ was similar between RI and SE ($n = 24$; 14.5 ± 3.0 vs. 14.7 ± 3.1 ml·kg^{-1}·min^{-1}; $P = 0.407$); however, within-subject comparisons confirmed $\dot{V}o_{2max}$ in only 14 of 24 patients (CI_{95} for $\dot{V}o_{2max}$ estimation averaged 1.4 ± 0.8 ml·kg^{-1}·min^{-1}). The RER_{peak} in CHF was significantly influenced by ramp rate, suggesting its use to determine maximal effort and $\dot{V}o_{2max}$ be abandoned. In contrast, the RISE-95 test had high precision for $\dot{V}o_{2max}$ confirmation with patient-specific CI_{95} (without secondary criteria), and showed that $\dot{V}o_{2max}$ is

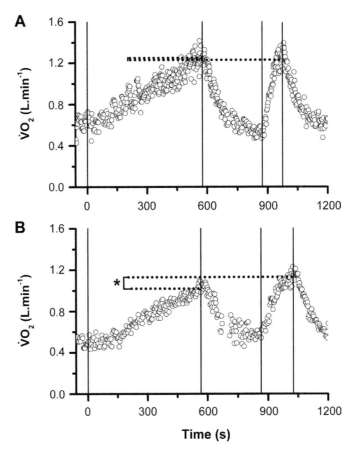

FIGURE 2.—Breath-by-breath pulmonary oxygen uptake ($\dot{V}_{O_2}$) dynamics in two CHF patients in response to the ramp-incremental (RI) step-exercise (SE) at 95% peak RI work rate (i.e., RISE-95) test. In the patients presented, one confirmed maximal oxygen uptake ($\dot{V}_{O_2max}$; A), while the other did not ($\dot{V}_{O_2peak}$; B). Our within-patient analysis confirmed $\dot{V}_{O_2max}$ in patients by statistically comparing the highest 12 breaths during exercise in the RI and SE phases, with values of $P > 0.05$ confirming $\dot{V}_{O_2max}$. Dotted lines are presented to highlight the differences in the values of $\dot{V}_{O_2peak}$ between the RI and SE phases. *$P < 0.05$. (Reprinted from Bowen TS, Cannon DT, Begg G, et al. A novel cardiopulmonary exercise test protocol and criterion to determine maximal oxygen uptake in chronic heart failure. *J Appl Physiol.* 2012;113:451-458, with permission from the American Physiological Society.)

commonly underestimated in CHF. The RISE-95 test was well tolerated by CHF patients, supporting its use for $\dot{V}_{O_2max}$ confirmation (Fig 2).

▶ Cardiorespiratory assessment of peak oxygen intake is commonly undertaken in patients with congestive heart failure in order to assess the progress of rehabilitation, to determine prognosis, and to decide the timing of cardiac transplantation.[1] Values less than 14 mL/kg/minute are a key factor in priority listing of patients. However, the usefulness of this index can be questioned, because many patients with chronic cardiac failure cease treadmill or cycle ergometer exercise because of muscle weakness, breathlessness, or fatigue without reaching a purely cardiac limitation of oxygen transport.[2] In healthy individuals, a secondary criterion of a true maximal cardiac effort is a respiratory gas exchange ratio (RER) greater than 1.15, although even in healthy subjects the value that is observed tends to vary according to the ramp exercise testing protocol that is being used. It is commonly recommended that a progressive maximal exercise test should last 8 to 10 minutes.[3]

This article shows that in patients with chronic heart failure there was a large difference of RER if the test duration was allowed to vary between 5 and 15 minutes. Nevertheless, the peak oxygen intake remained relatively comparable over this range, and it thus seems a fairly stable criterion. I view with some skepticism the authors' claim that their new double ramp test (Fig 2) can detect a true cardiac limit of oxygen transport in patients with a peak oxygen intake of around 14 ml/kg/minute; probably, those who are dealing with chronic congestive failure will need to be content to base their judgments on the peak value that a patient can achieve (and on clinical as well as physiological assessment).

R. J. Shephard, MD (Lond), PhD, DPE

References

1. Mancini DM, Eisen H, Kussmaul W, Mull R, Edmunds LH Jr, Wilson JR. Value of peak exercise oxygen consumption for optimal timing of cardiac transplantation in ambulatory patients with heart failure. *Circulation.* 1991;83:778-786.
2. Wagner PD. Determinants of maximal oxygen transport and utilization. *Annu Rev Physiol.* 1996;58:21-50.
3. Howley ET, Bassett DR Jr, Welch HG. Criteria for maximal oxygen uptake: review and commentary. *Med Sci Sports Exerc.* 1995;27:1292-1301.

Testosterone therapy during exercise rehabilitation in male patients with chronic heart failure who have low testosterone status: A double-blind randomized controlled feasibility study
Stout M, Tew GA, Doll H, et al (Univ Hosp of South Manchester, Wythenshawe, Manchester, UK; Sheffield Hallam Univ, UK; Univ of East Anglia, Norwich, UK; et al)
Am Heart J 164:893-901, 2012

Background.—This study assessed the feasibility of a 12-week program of exercise, with and without intramuscular testosterone supplementation, in male patients with chronic heart failure (CHF) and low testosterone status and collected preliminary data for key health outcomes.

Methods.—Male patients with CHF (n = 41, age 67.2 years, range 51-84 years) with mean ± SD testosterone levels of 10.7 ± 2.6 nmol/L (309 ± 76 ng/dL) were randomly allocated to exercise with testosterone or placebo groups. Feasibility was assessed in terms of recruitment, intervention compliance, and attrition. Outcomes included an incremental shuttle walk test, peak oxygen uptake, muscular strength, echocardiographic measures, N-terminal pro—brain natriuretic peptide, inflammatory markers, depression (Beck Depression Inventory), and health-related

TABLE 2.—Maximum Walking Distance, Aerobic Exercise Performance, Quadriceps, and Grip Strength at Baseline and End Point

| | Testosterone (n = 15) | | Placebo (n = 13) | | |
	Baseline	End Point	Baseline	End Point	P
Shuttle walk distance (m)	418.7 ± 153.7	492.7 ± 215.3*	556.2 ± 112.1	661.5 ± 158.8*	.68
Incremental cycle ergometer test					
Peak Vo_2 (mL kg^{-1} min^{-1})	15.0 ± 4.4	18.2 ± 4.8†	17.4 ± 3.6	18.8 ± 3.4	.42
Peak power output (W)	88.3 ± 20.8	103.3 ± 31.1*	94.2 ± 23.2	105.8 ± 20.8*	.79
Peak quadriceps torque production (Nm)					
Knee extension 60°/s (1 rad/s)	122.2 ± 51.7	134.0 ± 44.7*	141.6 ± 42.1	145.0 ± 40.9	.63
Knee extension 180°/s (3 rad/s)	78.5 ± 30.5	83.5 ± 31.4	89.0 ± 25.2	96.0 ± 33.0	.64
Knee extension 300°/s (5.3 rad/s)	67.5 ± 24.9	70.7 ± 23.2	73.3 ± 22.6	80.1 ± 24.2	.42
Knee flexion 60°/s (1 rad/s)	50.3 ± 21.5	62.9 ± 22.0*	64.2 ± 23.8	62.9 ± 19.0	.22
Knee flexion 180°/s (3 rad/s)	46.5 ± 20.8	55.3 ± 24.6*	49.8 ± 18.6	56.4 ± 13.8	.86
Knee flexion 300°/s (5.3 rad/s)	53.1 ± 25.6	56.2 ± 28.9	52.3 ± 17.0	57.8 ± 12.9	.81
Handgrip strength (kg)	38.6 ± 8.6	40.7 ± 7.1	44.5 ± 7.6	47.0 ± 9.0*	.50

Data are presented as mean ± SD. P value for ANCOVA is shown in the right hand column.
*$P < .05$.
$^{\dagger}P < .01$ indicates significance of group difference from baseline (paired t test).

quality of life (Minnesota Living with Heart Failure Questionnaire and Medical Outcomes Study Short-Form).

Results.—Attrition was 30% but with 100% compliance to exercise and injections in patients who completed the study. Similar improvements in shuttle walk test (18% vs 19%), body mass (−1.3 kg vs −1.0 kg), and hand grip strength (2.1 kg vs 2.5 kg) from baseline were observed in both groups. The exercise with testosterone group showed improvements from baseline in peak oxygen uptake ($P < .01$), Beck Depression Inventory ($P < .05$), leg strength ($P < .05$), and several Medical Outcomes Study Short-Form quality of life domains ($P < .05$), which were generally not apparent in the exercise with placebo group. Echocardiographic measures, N-terminal pro–brain natriuretic peptide, and inflammatory markers were mostly unchanged.

Conclusions.—This study shows for the first time that testosterone supplementation during a program of exercise rehabilitation is feasible and can positively impact on a range of key health outcomes in elderly male patients with CHF who have a low testosterone status (Table 2).

▶ It is now generally accepted that exercise rehabilitation is helpful for patients who have stable congestive heart failure.[1] However, several studies of such patients have found that a substantial part of their disability is caused by a weakness of the skeletal muscles, and it is thus logical to include muscle strengthening exercises in the rehabilitation program. The practical issue when implementing such a policy is that many of the patients are elderly and lack the levels of testosterone needed for muscle hypertrophy.[2,3] Stout et al have now carried out a small-scale randomized, controlled trial of the benefits of including testosterone therapy in a 12-week exercise program for elderly patients with congestive heart failure. All had low total testosterone levels (< 15 nmol/L), commonly accepted as the threshold of androgen deficiency.[4] The exercise program was held twice per week, and it included aerobic interval training on a cycle ergometer and resistance exercise for the quadriceps, hamstrings, pectorals, latissimus dorsi, and deltoid muscles. The experimental group also received intramuscular testosterone (100 mg once per fortnight for 12 weeks). Unfortunately, experimental and control groups were not very well matched. On some tests, such as the shuttle walk, the experimental group showed no greater improvement than controls, but on other measures, including peak oxygen intake, leg strength, and mood state, gains were larger in those receiving the testosterone (Table 2). Possibly, benefits would be greater with larger doses of testosterone, but this might also increase the risk of cardiovascular side effects. Further larger-scale studies seem warranted, using various doses of testosterone and continuing the supplements for longer than 12 weeks.

R. J. Shephard, MD (Lond), PhD, DPE

References

1. Piña IL, Apstein CS, Balady GJ, et al. Exercise and heart failure: a statement from the American Heart Association Committee on exercise, rehabilitation, and prevention. *Circulation.* 2003;107:1210-1225.
2. Kontoleon PE, Anastasiou-Nana MI, Papapetrou PD, et al. Hormonal profile in patients with congestive heart failure. *Int J Cardiol.* 2003;87:179-183.
3. Malkin CJ, Pugh PJ, West JN, van Beek EJ, Jones TH, Channer KS. Testosterone therapy in men with moderate severity heart failure: a double-blind randomized placebo controlled trial. *Eur Heart J.* 2006;27:57-64.
4. Vermeulen A. Androgen replacement therapy in the aging male—a critical evaluation. *J Clin Endocrinol Metab.* 2001;86:2380-2390.

10-Year Exercise Training in Chronic Heart Failure: A Randomized Controlled Trial

Belardinelli R, Georgiou D, Cianci G, et al (Lancisi Heart Inst, Ancona, Italy; Columbia Univ, NY)
J Am Coll Cardiol 60:1521-1528, 2012

Objectives.—This study investigated the effect of a very long-term exercise training program is not known in chronic heart failure (CHF) patients.

Background.—We previously showed that long-term moderate exercise training (ET) improves functional capacity and quality of life in New York Heart Association class II and III CHF patients.

Methods.—We studied 123 patients with CHF whose condition was stable over the previous 3 months. After randomization, a trained group (T group, n = 63) underwent a supervised ET at 60% of peak oxygen consumption (Vo_2), 2 times weekly for 10 years, whereas a nontrained group (NT group, n = 60) did not exercise formally. The ET program was supervised and performed mostly at a coronary club with periodic control sessions twice yearly at the hospital's gym.

Results.—In the T group, peak Vo_2 was more than 60% of age- and gender-predicted maximum Vo_2 each year during the 10-year study ($p < 0.05$ vs. the NT group). In NT patients, peak Vo_2 decreased progressively

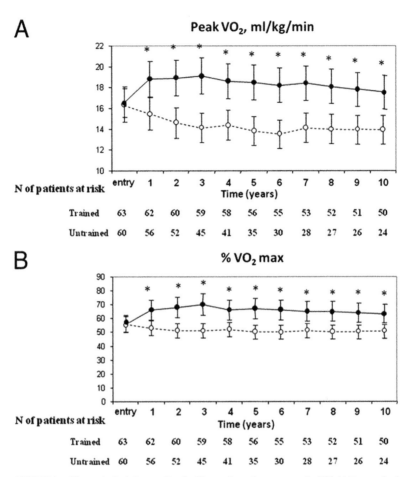

A   Peak VO₂, ml/kg/min

N of patients at risk	entry	1	2	3	4	5	6	7	8	9	10
Trained	63	62	60	59	58	56	55	53	52	51	50
Untrained	60	56	52	45	41	35	30	28	27	26	24

B   % VO₂ max

N of patients at risk	entry	1	2	3	4	5	6	7	8	9	10
Trained	63	62	60	59	58	56	55	53	52	51	50
Untrained	60	56	52	45	41	35	30	28	27	26	24

FIGURE 1.—Changes in Peak Oxygen Uptake Changes in peak oxygen uptake (VO₂) (**A**) as an absolute value and (**B**) as relative to maximum VO_2 (VO_{2max}) in trained patients (**solid lines**) and controls (**empty circles, dotted lines**) during the study period. $*p < 0.01$. For details, see text. (Reprinted from the Journal of the American College of Cardiology. Belardinelli R, Georgiou D, Cianci G, et al. 10-year exercise training in chronic heart failure: a randomized controlled trial. *J Am Coll Cardiol.* 2012;60:1521-1528, Copyright 2012, with permission from the American College of Cardiology Foundation.)

with an average of $52 \pm 8\%$ of maximum VO_2 predicted. Ventilation relative to carbon dioxide output (VE/VcO_2) slope was significantly lower (35 ± 9) in T patients versus NT patients (42 ± 11, $p < 0.01$). Quality-of-life score was significantly better in the T group versus the NT group (43 ± 12 vs. 58 ± 14, $p < 0.05$). During the 10-year study, T patients had a significant lower rate of hospital readmission (hazard ratio: 0.64, $p < 0.001$) and cardiac mortality (hazard ratio: 0.68, $p < 0.001$) than controls. Multivariate analysis selected peak VO_2 and resting heart rate as independent predictors of events.

Conclusions.—Moderate supervised ET performed twice weekly for 10 years maintains functional capacity of more than 60% of maximum Vo_2 and confers a sustained improvement in quality of life compared with NT patients. These sustained improvements are associated with reduction in major cardiovascular events, including hospitalizations for CHF and cardiac mortality (Fig 1).

▶ As our cardiac rehabilitation program in Toronto expanded during the 1970s and 1980s, there was an increasing number of referrals of patients who had varying degrees of congestive heart failure, and through cautious experimentation we established that the immediate prognosis of those with stable congestive heart failure was enhanced by a program of moderate exercise, aimed at restoring not only poor cardiac function but peripheral muscular limitation.[1] Other authors also confirmed the short-to-moderate-term benefit of rehabilitation programs.[2,3] The study of Belardinelli et al adds a small-scale randomized trial over a 10-year period, with assessment of outcome in terms of such hard end-points as peak oxygen intake, recurrence, and death. The patients had moderate and stable congestive failure, with a ventricular ejection fraction < 40%. The exercise program was supervised, ensuring good adherence; sessions were held twice a week at a "coronary club," with sessions at 70% of peak oxygen intake lasting for up to 1 hour; exercise responses were monitored at the hospital every 6 months. Those exercising twice per week had a consistently higher peak oxygen intake than the controls (Fig 1), and their quality of life was greater. The numbers were rather small to comment accurately on recurrences and mortality, but nevertheless there were 35 events in the controls versus 12 events in the experimental group; the exercisers had both fewer readmissions for acute heart failure and also fewer deaths than the control subjects. These findings compare with the previously reported unsupervised Heart Failure: A Controlled Trial Investigation Outcomes of Exercise Training study, in which crossover of exercise patterns may have occurred and no benefit was seen.[4] It thus appears that an appropriately supervised long-term moderate exercise program is both safe and beneficial for cardiac patients with stable congestive heart failure. However, further trials of clinical outcomes are desirable on a larger patient sample. Furthermore, Belardinelli et al do not appear to have incorporated any specific exercises directed to the peripheral muscles, and it would be also helpful to have information on long-term responses to such therapy.

R. J. Shephard, MD (Lond), PhD, DPE

References

1. Shephard RJ. Exercise for patients with congestive heart failure. *Sports Med.* 1997; 23:75-92.
2. Belardinelli R, Georgiou D, Cianci G, Purcaro A. Randomized, controlled trial of long-term moderate exercise training in chronic heart failure: effects on functional capacity, quality of life, and clinical outcome. *Circulation.* 1999;99:1173-1182.
3. Smart N, Marwick TH. Exercise training for patients with heart failure: a systematic review of factors that improve mortality and morbidity. *Am J Med.* 2004;116:693-706.
4. O'Connor CM, Whellan DJ, Lee KL, et al. HF-ACTION Investigators. Efficacy and safety of exercise training in patients with chronic heart failure: HF-ACTION randomized controlled trial. *JAMA.* 2009;301:1439-1450.

Exercise training improves exercise capacity in adult patients with a systemic right ventricle: a randomized clinical trial

Winter MM, van der Bom T, de Vries LCS, et al (Academic Med Ctr, Amsterdam, The Netherlands; et al)
Eur Heart J 33:1378-1385, 2012

Objective.—To assess whether exercise training in adult patients with a systemic right ventricle (RV) improves exercise capacity and quality of life and lowers serum N-terminal prohormone brain natriuretic peptide (NT-proBNP) levels.

Design.—Multi-centre parallel randomized controlled trial.

Participants.—Patients with a systemic RV due to congenitally or surgically corrected transposition of the great arteries.

Methods.—Fifty-four adult patients with a systemic RV, were randomized using unmarked opaque envelopes to an intervention group ($n = 28$) with three training sessions per week for 10 consecutive weeks, and a control group ($n = 26$). Randomization was stratified by participating centre. At baseline, and follow-up, we determined maximal exercise capacity ($V'O_{2peak}$), serum NT-proBNP levels, and quality of life by means of the SF-36, and the TAAQOL Congenital Heart Disease questionnaires. The final analysis was performed by linear regression, taking into account the stratified randomization.

Results.—Forty-six patients were analysed (male 50%, age 32 ± 11 years, intervention group $n = 24$, control group $n = 22$). Analysis at 10 weeks showed a significant difference in $V'O_{2peak}$ (3.4 mL/kg/min, 95% CI: 0.2 to 6.7; $P = 0.04$) and resting systolic blood pressure (-7.6 mmHg, 95% CI: -14.0 to -1.3; $P = 0.03$) in favour of the exercise group. No significant changes were found in serum NT-proBNP levels or quality of life in the intervention group or in the control group nor between groups. None of the patients in the intervention group had to discontinue the training programme due to adverse events.

Conclusion.—In adult patients with a systemic RV exercise training improve exercise capacity. We recommend to revise restrictive guidelines, and to encourage patients to become physically active. (Trial registration: The study was registered at http://trialregister.nl. Identifier: NTR1909.) (Table 2).

▶ Adults with a systemic right ventricle are commonly cautioned against exercising, due primarily to a lack of data on outcomes in sedentary versus active adults.[1,2] This is unfortunate, because their effort tolerance is usually poor,[3,4] and there is evidence that in children and adolescents with this type of condition a program of exercise is beneficial.[5] The present small-scale randomized trial compared usual treatment versus the response to 10 weeks of training (home-based stepping exercise, with 5 × 4-minute sessions of exercise at 75% rising to 90% of maximal heart rate performed 3 times per week, with compliance reinforced by weekly e-mail contact). At the end of the 10 weeks, the experimental group showed about a 10% advantage of peak aerobic power relative to controls

TABLE 2.—Exercise Response

Characteristics	Intervention		Control		Difference (95% CI) at 10 weeks	P-value
	Baseline	Follow-up	Baseline	Follow-up		
Cardiopulmonary exercise testing						
$V'O_{2peak}$ (mL/kg/min)	27 ± 7	29 ± 7	26 ± 9	26 ± 8	3.4 (0.2 to 6.7)	0.04
$V'O_{2peak}$ (mL/min)	2043 ± 558	2219 ± 547	1973 ± 740	1920 ± 650	283 (22 to 544)	0.03
$V'O_{2peak}$ (% pred)	70 ± 18	76 ± 20	73 ± 18	74 ± 19	5.2 (−0.9 to 11.5)	0.10
$V'E/V'CO_2$ slope	30 ± 5	30 ± 4	31 ± 8	31 ± 8	−1.3 (−4.9 to 2.4)	0.48
OUES	1931 ± 431	2101 ± 452	2203 ± 855	2193 ± 594	94 (−229 to 417)	0.55
Haemodynamics						
Systolic blood pressure, rest (mmHg)	115 ± 12	109 ± 7	120 ± 15	119 ± 14	−7.6 (−14.0 to −1.3)	0.02
Systolic blood pressure, max (mmHg)	159 ± 21	163 ± 24	159 ± 23	165 ± 27	−0.9 (−15.2 to 13.4)	0.90
Heart rate, rest (beats/minute)	75 ± 15	70 ± 12	79 ± 10	77 ± 14	−6.6 (−15.0 to 1.8)	0.12
Heart rate, max (b.p.m.)	155 ± 28	160 ± 29	147 ± 37	148 ± 32	5.5 (−3.3 to 14.2)	0.21
Laboratory testing						
NT-proBNP (ng/L)	166 (25−2816)	183 (29−2778)	227 (25−1696)	222 (5−1521)	109 (−6 to 224)	0.06
Quality of life						
SF-36						
Mental health component	−0.04 ± 0.85	−0.16 ± 0.8	0.07 ± 0.86	0.16 ± 0.72	−0.2 (−0.5 to 0.1)	0.17
Physical health component	0.08 ± 0.81	0.21 ± 0.68	−0.24 ± 0.95	−0.25 ± 0.99	0.2 (−0.1 to 0.5)	0.20
CHD-TAAQOL						
Symptoms	89 (69−100)	91 (58−100)	88 (53−100)	86 (60−100)	2.0 (−2.0 to 6.1)	0.31
Worries	80 (60−100)	84 (40−100)	92 (60−100)	92 (54−100)	−3.3 (−9.6 to 3.0)	0.30
Impact	89 (71−97)	85 (69−97)	87 (60−100)	86 (69−100)	−0.2 (−3.8 to 3.4)	0.91

Data are mean ± standard deviation or median (range); 95% CI, 95% confidence interval; L/min, litre per minute; mL/kg/min, millilitre per kilogram per minute; mL/min, millilitre per minute; % pred, percentage of predicted; ng/L, nanogram per litre; OUES, oxygen uptake efficiency slope.

and a substantial (average 7.6 mm Hg) drop in resting systolic blood pressure (Table 2). Moreover, the exercise program did not give rise to any adverse events (including chest pain, palpitations, dizziness, or other symptoms) over the 10 weeks of observation. The main need before generalizing the findings might seem a longer-term follow-up on a larger sample of patients to be certain of the safety of such exercise; however, most laboratories would find it difficult to accumulate a sample of more than 50 cases of systemic right ventricle willing to be randomized for such a trial.

R. J. Shephard, MD (Lond), PhD, DPE

References

1. Hirth A, Reybrouck T, Bjarnason-Wehrens B, Lawrenz W, Hoffmann A. Recommendations for participation in competitive and leisure sports in patients with congenital heart disease: a consensus document. *Eur J Cardiovasc Prev Rehabil.* 2006;13:293-299.
2. Pelliccia A, Fagard R, Bjørnstad HH, et al. Recommendations for competitive sports participation in athletes with cardiovascular disease: a consensus document from the Study Group of Sports Cardiology of the Working Group of Cardiac Rehabilitation and Exercise Physiology and the Working Group of Myocardial and Pericardial Diseases of the European Society of Cardiology. *Eur Heart J.* 2005;26:1422-1445.
3. Engelfriet P, Boersma E, Oechslin E, et al. The spectrum of adult congenital heart disease in Europe: morbidity and mortality in a 5 year follow-up period. The Euro Heart Survey on adult congenital heart disease. *Eur Heart J.* 2005;26:2325-2333.
4. Winter MM, Bouma BJ, Groenink M, et al. Latest insights in therapeutic options for systemic right ventricular failure: a comparison with left ventricular failure. *Heart.* 2009;95:960-963.
5. Fredriksen PM, Kahrs N, Blaasvaer S, et al. Effect of physical training in children and adolescents with congenital heart disease. *Cardiol Young.* 2000;10:107-114.

Physical Activity, High-Sensitivity C-Reactive Protein, and Total and Cardiovascular Disease Mortality in Type 2 Diabetes
Vepsäläinen T, Soinio M, Marniemi J, et al (Univ of Turku and Turku Univ Hosp, Finland; Natl Inst forHealth and Welfare, Turku, Finland; et al)
Diabetes Care 34:1492-1496, 2011

Objective.—Physical activity reduces high-sensitivity C-reactive protein (hs-CRP), cardiovascular disease (CVD), and total mortality in type 2 diabetic patients. However, it is not known whether the effects of physical activity on mortality depend on the levels of hs-CRP in patients with type 2 diabetes.

Research Design and Methods.—We prospectively followed-up on 569 type 2 diabetic patients, aged 45–64 years, who were free of CVD at baseline. Participants were stratified according to the level of hs-CRP (<1.0, 1.0–3.0, or >3.0 mg/L) and the degree of physical activity (0–4 metabolic equivalent tasks [METs] or >4 METs). The Cox proportional hazards model was used to estimate the joint association between physical activity and hs-CRP levels and the risk of mortality.

Results.—During an 18-year follow-up, 356 patients died, 217 of whom died of CVD. Those who were physically more active had significantly reduced total, CVD and coronary heart disease (CHD) mortality among patients with elevated hs-CRP levels (>3 mg/L). These findings persisted in multivariable analyses. However, in patients with an hs-CRP level <1 mg/L or between 1 and 3 mg/L, there was no statistically significant relationship between physical activity and CVD or CHD mortality.

Conclusions.—Physical activity reduces total, CVD, and CHD mortality in type 2 diabetic patients with elevated hs-CRP levels. This suggests that the anti-inflammatory effect of physical activity may counteract increased CVD and CHD morbidity and mortality associated with high CRP levels.

▶ The persistent increase in inflammation biomarkers is defined as chronic or systemic inflammation and is linked with multiple disorders and diseases, including atherosclerosis and cardiovascular disease (CVD), the metabolic syndrome, diabetes mellitus, sarcopenia, arthritis, osteoporosis, chronic obstructive pulmonary disease, dementia, depression, and various types of cancers.[1] C-reactive protein (CRP) is the most frequently measured inflammatory biomarker, and individuals with CRP values in the upper tertile of the adult population (> 3.0 mg/L) have a 2-fold increase in CVD risk compared with those with a CRP concentration below 1.0 mg/L.[2] In this study, physical activity reduced cardiovascular and total mortality in middle-aged type 2 diabetic subjects with elevated CRP levels (Fig 1 in the original article). Thus the protective effect of physical activity against CVD may be most apparent in patients with systemic inflammation.

D. C. Nieman, DrPH

References

1. Devaraj S, Valleggi S, Siegel D, Jialal I. Role of C-reactive protein in contributing to increased cardiovascular risk in metabolic syndrome. *Curr Atheroscler Rep.* 2010;12:110-118.
2. Pearson TA, Mensah GA, Alexander RW, et al. Markers of inflammation and cardiovascular disease: application to clinical and public health practice: a statement for healthcare professionals from the Centers for Disease Control and Prevention and the American Heart Association. *Circulation.* 2003;107:499-511.

Vascular Problems and Hypertension

Comparison of the acute impact of maximal arm and leg aerobic exercise on arterial stiffness

Ranadive SM, Fahs CA, Yan H, et al (Univ of Illinois at Urbana-Champaign)
Eur J Appl Physiol 112:2631-2635, 2012

Acute aerobic exercise decreases arterial stiffness based on the intensity of the exercise and the arterial segment studied. Arm exercise may differentially affect arterial stiffness compared to leg exercise but this has not been studied. We hypothesized that maximal aerobic exercise would reduce local peripheral pulse wave velocity i.e. femoral-dorsalis pedis (LPWV)

TABLE 1.—Comparison of Variables Between Arm and Leg Ergometry

Variable	Arm		Leg	
	Pre	Post	Pre	Post
APWV (m/s)[#]	6.95 (0.24)	6.03 (0.26)[@,*]	6.59 (0.25)	6.44 (0.30)
LPWV (m/s)	9.07 (0.49)	8.13 (0.55)	8.71 (0.50)	7.56 (0.40)*
CPWV (m/s)	5.54 (0.25)	5.70 (0.33)	5.58 (0.32)	5.53 (0.24)

Values are mean ± SEM.
APWV Brachial pulse wave velocity, *LPWV* leg pulse wave velocity.
[#]$p < 0.05$ denotes interaction between conditions.
[*]$p < 0.05$ denotes a main effect of time.
[@]$p < 0.05$ from pre.

following leg exercise and carotid-radial (APWV) following arm exercise without any crossover effect. The main purpose of the study is to compare the effects of maximal arm versus leg aerobic exercise on peripheral and central arterial stiffness. Fifteen healthy participants (9 males and 6 females, 25 ± 5 years) performed maximal arm-ergometer and leg-ergometer exercise in a randomized, crossover design. Peripheral and central pulse wave velocities (PWV) were obtained using applanation tonometry before and 10 min after each maximal exercise bout. 2×2 repeated measures analysis of variance was used to detect differences between conditions. There was a significant interaction in the APWV between the two exercise modes. However, there was no condition or interaction effect on LPWV following maximal arm versus leg exercise. There was no significant difference in central PWV between conditions or with time. There was no change in MAP (75 ± 6–77 ± 3) after maximal arm exercise as compared to the maximal leg exercise (73 ± 6–80 ± 2). Arm exercise produced a more generalized effect on arterial stiffness than leg exercise. The prescription of upper limb exercise may be considered for purposes of eliciting post-exercise systemic changes in arterial stiffness (Table 1).

▶ Ranadive and associates show that a bout of exhausting aerobic exercise performed with the arms has a greater impact on arterial stiffness in the nonexercised limbs than does an equivalent amount of exercise performed with the legs (Table 1). They thus suggest that arm exercise may have greater therapeutic value than leg exercise for individuals with arterial stiffening. This idea certainly merits further exploration, but in the present study arterial stiffness was assessed only once: 10 minutes after exercise. It is doubtful if the change in stiffness at this stage has any great significance for long-term prognosis. What would be of greater interest would be a comparison of the relative long-term antihypertensive effects of arm and leg exercise. Certainly, the fact that the immediate post-exercise blood pressures were the same with the 2 modes of exercise indicates the likelihood of differential benefit. Further, most people have access to some form of leg exercise, whether treadmill, cycle ergometer, or walking, but an arm ergometer would be less readily available to most patients.

R. J. Shephard, MD (Lond), PhD, DPE

Physical Activity Reduces Salt Sensitivity of Blood Pressure: The Genetic Epidemiology Network of Salt Sensitivity Study

Rebholz CM, for the GenSalt Collaborative Research Group (Tulane Univ, New Orleans, LA; et al)
Am J Epidemiol 176:S106-S113, 2012

Salt sensitivity of blood pressure (BP) is influenced by genetic and environmental factors. A dietary feeding study was conducted from October 2003 to July 2005 that included a 7-day low-sodium intervention (51.3 mmol sodium/day) followed by a 7-day high-sodium intervention (307.8 mmol sodium/day) among 1,906 individuals who were 16 years of age or older and living in rural northern China. Salt sensitivity of BP was defined as mean BP change from the low-sodium intervention to the high-sodium intervention. Usual physical activity during the past 12 months was assessed at baseline using a standard questionnaire. The multivariable-adjusted means of systolic BP responses to high-sodium intervention were 5.21 mm Hg (95% confidence interval (CI): 4.55, 5.88), 4.97 mm Hg (95% CI: 4.35, 5.59), 5.02 mm Hg (95% CI: 4.38, 5.67), and 3.96 mm Hg (95% CI: 3.29, 4.63) among participants from the lowest to the highest quartiles of physical activity, respectively ($P = 0.003$ for linear trend). The multivariable-adjusted odds ratio of high salt sensitivity of systolic BP was 0.66 (95% CI: 0.49, 0.88) for persons in the highest quartile of physical activity compared with those in the lowest quartile. Physical activity is significantly, independently, and inversely related to salt sensitivity of BP and may be particularly effective in lowering BP among salt-sensitive individuals (Table 2).

▶ The control of plasma sodium, although an important health measure,[1] is an annoying problem for patients with hypertension, given the tendency of commercial enterprises to add ever more salt to the products they market. People are known to vary in their sensitivity to an excess of salt, depending on age, sex, race, body weight, alcohol intake, genetic factors, and the presence of hypertension.[2-5] This article makes the interesting observation that salt sensitivity is also associated with a person's level of habitual physical activity (Table 2). The association remains largely unchanged by multivariate analysis, and it seems in line with the known beneficial effects of physical activity on hypertension. Nevertheless, experimental studies are needed to prove a causal relationship. Possible mechanisms remain to be explored. The authors suggest effects on insulin resistance, endothelial function, and sympathetic nerve activity. High-sodium and low-sodium interventions were also short-lived (7 days), and it remains to be seen whether the beneficial effects of exercise are persistent. Finally, in terms of practical application of the observations, the reported duration of physical activity among study participants (3.3 hours of vigorous activity and 4.6 hours of moderate activity per day) would be hard to attain in a North American population.

R. J. Shephard, MD (Lond), PhD, DPE

TABLE 2.—Mean Absolute and Percentage Blood Pressure Responses to the High-Sodium Intervention by Physical Activity Levels, Genetic Epidemiology Network of Salt Sensitivity Study, China, 2003–2005

Physical Activity Level, MET-Hours per Day	Age- and Sex-Adjusted				Multivariable-Adjusted[a]				Multivariable-Adjusted[b]			
	Systolic		Diastolic		Systolic		Diastolic		Systolic		Diastolic	
	Mean	95% CI	Mean	95% CI	Mean	95% CI	Mean	95% CI	Mean	95% CI	Mean	95% CI
Absolute Blood Pressure Responses, mm Hg												
<15.1	5.30	4.73, 5.87	2.34	1.85, 2.82	5.26	4.60, 5.93	2.20	1.63, 2.76	5.21	4.55, 5.88	2.15	1.59, 2.71
15.1–22.9	5.21	4.71, 5.70	2.23	1.74, 2.72	5.13	4.50, 5.77	2.07	1.49, 2.66	4.97	4.35, 5.59	2.00	1.41, 2.58
23.0–34.4	5.12	4.56, 5.67	2.11	1.63, 2.58	5.09	4.43, 5.74	1.97	1.38, 2.57	5.02	4.38, 5.67	1.92	1.33, 2.51
>34.4	3.94	3.40, 4.48	1.35	0.81, 1.88	3.92	3.24, 4.61	1.19	0.56, 1.82	3.96	3.29, 4.63	1.21	0.59, 1.84
P for trend	0.0009		0.006		0.001		0.007		0.003		0.01	
Percentage Blood Pressure Responses												
<15.1	4.81	4.28, 5.34	3.48	2.76, 4.20	4.79	4.17, 5.41	3.28	2.47, 4.09	4.76	4.14, 5.39	3.24	2.43, 4.05
15.1–22.9	4.67	4.22, 5.11	3.37	2.65, 4.10	4.62	4.05, 5.19	3.16	2.31, 4.01	4.53	3.97, 5.10	3.10	2.25, 3.96
23.0–34.4	4.65	4.14, 5.15	3.19	2.49, 3.89	4.62	4.03, 5.22	2.98	2.09, 3.86	4.59	4.00, 5.18	2.94	2.06, 3.83
>34.4	3.65	3.15, 4.13	2.27	1.48, 3.07	3.61	2.99, 4.23	2.01	1.08, 2.94	3.63	3.02, 4.25	2.02	1.09, 2.95
P for trend	0.002		0.02		0.002		0.02		0.004		0.03	

Abbreviations: CI, confidence interval; MET, metabolic equivalent.
[a]Multivariable model A included age, sex, body mass index, educational level, cigarette smoking, alcohol consumption, and baseline urinary excretion of sodium and potassium.
[b]Multivariable model A plus baseline systolic or diastolic blood pressure.

References

1. Elliott P, Stamler J, Nichols R, et al. Intersalt revisited: further analyses of 24 hour sodium excretion and blood pressure within and across populations: Intersalt Cooperative Research Group. *BMJ*. 1996;312:1249-1253.
2. Weinberger MH. Salt sensitivity of blood pressure in humans. *Hypertension*. 1996; 27:481-490.
3. Vollmer WM, Sacks FM, Ard J, et al. Effects of diet and sodium intake on blood pressure: subgroup analysis of the DASH-sodium trial. *Ann Intern Med*. 2001;135: 1019-1028.
4. He J, Gu D, Chen J, et al. Gender difference in blood pressure responses to dietary sodium intervention in the GenSalt study. *J Hypertens*. 2009;27:48-54.
5. Morris RC, Sebastian A, Forman A, et al. Normotensive salt sensitivity: effects of race and dietary potassium. *Hypertension*. 1999;33:18-23.

Exercise Capacity and Progression From Prehypertension to Hypertension
Faselis C, Doumas M, Kokkinos JP, et al (Veterans Affairs Med Ctr and George Washington Univ School of Medicine and Health Sciences, DC; et al)
Hypertension 60:333-338, 2012

Prehypertension is likely to progress to hypertension. The rate of progression is determined mostly by age and resting blood pressure but may also be attenuated by increased fitness. A graded exercise test was performed in 2303 men with prehypertension at the Veterans Affairs Medical Centers in Washington, DC. Four fitness categories were defined, based on peak metabolic equivalents (METs) achieved. We assessed the association between exercise capacity and rate of progression to hypertension (HTN). The median follow-up period was 7.8 years (mean ($\pm$SD) 9.2 $\pm$ 6.1 years). The incidence rate of progression from prehypertension to hypertension was 34.4 per 1000 person-years. Exercise capacity was a strong and independent predictor of the rate of progression. Compared to the High-Fit individuals (>10.0 METs), the adjusted risk for developing HTN was 66% higher (hazard ratio, 1.66; 95% CI, 1.2 to 2.2; $P = 0.001$) for the Low-Fit and, similarly, 72% higher (hazard ratio, 1.72; 95% CI, 1.2 to 2.3; $P = 0.001$) for the Least-Fit individuals, whereas it was only 36% for the Moderate-Fit (hazard ratio, 1.36; 95% CI, 0.99 to 1.80; $P = 0.056$). Significant predictors for the progression to HTN were also age (19% per 10 years), resting systolic blood pressure (16% per 10 mm Hg), body mass index (15.3% per 5 U), and type 2 diabetes mellitus (2-fold). In conclusion, an inverse, S-shaped association was shown between exercise capacity and the rate of progression from prehypertension to hypertension in middle-Aged and older male veterans. The protective effects of fitness were evident when exercise capacity exceeded 8.5 METs. These findings emphasize the importance of fitness in the prevention of hypertension (Fig 1).

▶ Approximately 42 million men and 28 million women (37% of the adult US population) have prehypertension, and 40% of them will progress to hypertension within 2 years.[1,2] As shown in Fig 1, the risk for developing hypertension was

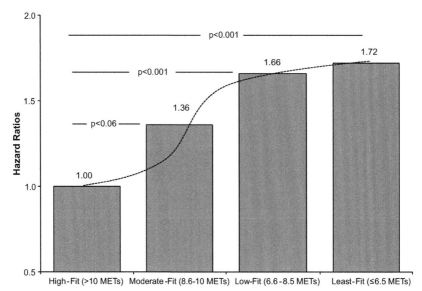

FIGURE 1.—Risk of progression from prehypertension to hypertension, according to fitness categories. Hazard ratios were adjusted for age, body mass index, resting systolic blood pressure, diabetes mellitus, and smoking. (Reprinted from Faselis C, Doumas M, Kokkinos JP, et al. Exercise capacity and progression from prehypertension to hypertension. *Hypertension*. 2012;60:333-338, with permission from American Heart Association, Inc.)

progressively higher as exercise capacity decreased. The most pronounced increase in risk occurred in the 2 lowest-fit categories (66% and 72% higher risk), supporting what the authors perceived was an "S-shaped association between fitness and rate of progression to hypertension." The most important practical finding from this study is that a moderate increase in exercise capacity was enough to attenuate the progression from prehypertension to hypertension. This can be attained by moderate intensity physical activities such as brisk walking for 20 to 40 minutes per session on most days of the week.

D. C. Nieman, DrPH

References

1. Qureshi AI, Suri MF, Kirmani JF, Divani AA. Prevalence and trends of prehypertension and hypertension in United States: National Health and Nutrition Examination Surveys 1976 to 2000. *Med Sci Monit*. 2005;11:CR403-CR409.
2. Julius S, Nesbitt SD, Egan BM, et al. Trial of Preventing Hypertension (TROPHY) Study Investigators. Feasibility of treating prehypertension with an angiotensin-receptor blocker. *N Eng J Med*. 2006;354:1685-1697.

Calf muscle oxygen saturation and the effects of supervised exercise training for intermittent claudication

Beckitt TA, Day J, Morgan M, et al (Bristol Royal Infirmary, UK)
J Vasc Surg 56:470-475, 2012

Objective.—The mechanisms underlying the symptomatic improvement witnessed as a result of exercise training in intermittent claudication remain unclear. There is no reproducible evidence to support increased limb blood flow resulting from neovascularization. Changes in oxygenation of active muscles as a result of blood redistribution are hypothesized but unproven. This study sought evidence of improved gastrocnemius oxygenation resulting from exercise training.

Methods.—The study recruited 42 individuals with claudication. After an initial control period of exercise advice, participants undertook a 3-month supervised exercise program. Spatially resolved near-infrared spectroscopy monitored calf muscle oxygen saturation (Sto_2) during exercise and after a period of cuff-induced ischemia. Comparison was made with 14 individuals undergoing angioplasty for calf claudication. Clinical outcomes of claudication distance and maximum walking distance were measured by treadmill assessment.

Results.—Significant increases occurred in mean [interquartile range] claudication disease (57 [38-78] to 119 [97-142] meters; $P = .01$) and maximum walking distance (124 [102-147] to 241 [193-265] meters; $P = .02$) after supervised exercise but not after the control period. No change occurred in resting Sto_2 at any interval. Angioplasty (27% [21-34] to 19% [13-29]; $P = .02$) but not exercise training (26% [21-32] *vs* 23% [20-31]; $P > .20$) resulted in a reduced Sto_2 desaturation in response to submaximal exercise and an increased hyperemic hemoglobin oxygen recovery rate after ischemia (0.48 [0.39-0.55] to 0.63 [0.52-0.69] s^{-1}; $P = .01$). However supervised exercise reduced the Sto_2 recovery half-time by 17% (82 [64-101] to 68 [55-89] seconds; $P = .02$).

Conclusions.—Supervised exercise training is not associated with increased gastrocnemius muscle oxygenation during exercise or increased hyperemic hemoglobin flow after a model of ischemia. This suggests that the symptomatic improvement witnessed is not the result of increased oxygen delivery to the active muscle. The enhanced recovery after exercise training therefore reflects a combination of enhanced metabolic economy and increased oxidative capacity, suggesting that exercise training helps reverse an acquired metabolic myopathy.

▶ An exercise training program frequently improves walking ability in patients with intermittent claudication, and many people have assumed that exercise somehow improves leg blood flow, possibly by opening up anastomotic collateral blood vessels. However, the endpoint is subjective and could be affected by many things, from a greater mechanical efficiency of walking or an increase of muscle enzyme activity to a form of placebo effect. The issue is of some practical clinical importance, since pharmacologic treatments are not particularly effective and surgical procedures such as angioplasty are not without risk, with a limited duration of benefit.[1,2] Does exercise provide a valid alternative therapy? Although there is much symptomatic benefit, there is little direct evidence of increased blood flow to the limbs; one report suggested an increased washout of xenon-133 from the gastrocnemius muscle.[3]

This study was based on near-infrared spectroscopy, which allows a continuous monitoring of muscle oxygen saturation.[4] The article reports that 12 weeks of supervised exercise (five 8-minute stations that included step-ups, wobble-board, cycling, toe walking, and heel raises, performed at least 3 times per week) had no effect on the development of oxygen desaturation in muscle (in contrast with angioplasty, where benefit was observed). Nevertheless, as in other studies, exercise training almost doubled the walking distance. Some mechanism other than revascularization must be involved.

R. J. Shephard, MD (Lond), PhD, DPE

References

1. Creasy TS, McMillan PJ, Fletcher EW, et al. Is percutaneous transluminal angioplasty better than exercise for claudication? Preliminary results from a prospective randomised trial. *Eur J Vasc Surg.* 1990;4:135-140.
2. Whyman MR, Fowkes FG, Kerracher EM, et al. Randomised controlled trial of percutaneous transluminal angioplasty for intermittent claudication. *Eur J Vasc Endovasc Surg.* 1996;12:167-172.
3. Alpert JS, Larsen OA, Lassen NA. Exercise and intermittent claudication Blood flow in the calf muscle during walking studied by the xenon-133 clearance method. *Circulation.* 1969;39:353-359.
4. Camerota AJ, Throm RC, Kelly P, Jaff M. Tissue (muscle) oxygen saturation (StO2): a new measure of symptomatic lower-extremity arterial disease. *J Vasc Surg.* 2003;38:724-729.

Aggravation of Exercise-Induced Intestinal Injury by Ibuprofen in Athletes
Van Wijck K, Lenaerts K, Van Bijnen AA, et al (Top Inst Food and Nutrition, Wageningen, The Netherlands; Maastricht Univ Med Ctr+, The Netherlands)
Med Sci Sports Exerc 44:2257-2262, 2012

Introduction.—Nonsteroidal anti-inflammatory drugs are commonly used by athletes to prevent anticipated exercise-induced pain, thereby putatively improving physical performance. However, these drugs may have potentially hazardous effects on the gastrointestinal (GI) mucosa during strenuous physical exercise. The aim of the current study was to determine the effect of oral ibuprofen administration before exercise on GI integrity and barrier function in healthy individuals.

Methods.—Nine healthy, trained men were studied on four different occasions: 1) 400 mg ibuprofen twice before cycling, 2) cycling without ibuprofen, 3) 400 mg ibuprofen twice at rest, and 4) rest without ibuprofen intake. To assess small intestinal injury, plasma intestinal fatty acid binding protein (I-FABP) levels were determined, whereas urinary excretion of orally

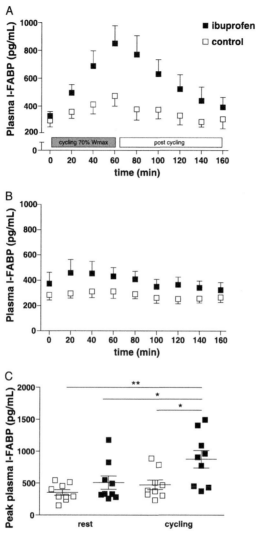

FIGURE 1.—Ibuprofen significantly increases plasma I-FABP levels in rest and during cycling. A. Plasma I-FABP levels in athletes during and after cycling with prior intake of ibuprofen compared with cycling without ibuprofen ($P < 0.0001$). *Squares* represent mean data, with the SEM as *black lines*. B. Plasma I-FABP levels after intake of ibuprofen compared with control (i.e., no ibuprofen) in athletes at rest ($P = 0.0003$). Squares represent mean data, with the SEM as *black lines*. C. Peak plasma I-FABP levels in healthy athletes during rest and cycling conditions with or without ibuprofen. Squares represent individual data, with the mean ± SEM depicted as *black lines* (*$P < 0.05$, **$P \leq 0.001$). (Reprinted from Van Wijck K, Lenaerts K, Van Bijnen AA, et al. Aggravation of exercise-induced intestinal injury by ibuprofen in athletes. *Med Sci Sports Exerc*. 2012;44:2257-2262, with permission from the American College of Sports Medicine.)

ingested multisugar test probes was measured using liquid chromatography and mass spectrometry to assess GI permeability.

Results.—Both ibuprofen consumption and cycling resulted in increased I-FABP levels, reflecting small intestinal injury. Levels were higher after cycling with ibuprofen than after cycling without ibuprofen, rest with ibuprofen, or rest without ibuprofen (peak I-FABP, 875 ± 137, 474 ± 74, 507 ± 103, and 352 ± 44 pg·mL, respectively, $P < 0.002$). In line, small intestinal permeability increased, especially after cycling with ibuprofen (0–2 h urinary lactulose/rhamnose ratio, 0.08 (0.04–0.56) compared with 0.04 (0.00–0.20), 0.05 (0.01–0.07), and 0.01 (0.01–0.03), respectively), reflecting loss of gut barrier integrity. Interestingly, the extent of intestinal injury and barrier dysfunction correlated significantly ($R_S = 0.56$, $P < 0.001$).

Conclusion.—This is the first study to reveal that ibuprofen aggravates exercise-induced small intestinal injury and induces gut barrier dysfunction in healthy individuals. We conclude that nonsteroidal anti-inflammatory drugs consumption by athletes is not harmless and should be discouraged (Fig 1).

▶ It has been recognized for years that during prolonged exercise, the diversion of blood flow from the viscera to the working muscles can cause a local ischemia of the intestines, allowing toxins to traverse the gut wall and enter the bloodstream.[1] It is also recognized that the nonsteroidal anti-inflammatory drugs that are so widely used by athletes often cause gastrointestinal pathologies, including bleeding, ulceration, and perforation.[2,3] Van Wijck et al have now put together these 2 ideas, showing that the administration of ibuprofen compounds the increase in permeability of the gut wall during exercise. The experiment was on a small scale (9 healthy male cyclists or triathletes, with the subjects serving as their own controls). The dose of ibuprofen was modest relative to the consumption of many athletes (just two 400-mg tablets over the preceding 24 hours), and the task was only an hour of cycling at 70% of maximal power output, but this combination was sufficient to provoke a substantial increase of gut permeability, as assessed by blood levels of intestinal fatty acid binding protein (I-FABP),[4] a 15-kDa cytosolic protein present in the mature enterocytes of the small intestine (Fig 1). The finding is certainly a warning against the overuse of ibuprofen, and it was linked with abnormal urinary sugar permeability ratios. However, levels of I-FABP returned to normal with an hour of recovery from exercise, and it is not clear what levels of this marker are associated with a pathologic leakage of endotoxins into the bloodstream.

R. J. Shephard, MD (Lond), PhD, DPE

References

1. van Wijck K, Lenaerts K, van Loon LJ, Peters WH, Buurman WA, Dejong CH. Exercise-induced splanchnic hypoperfusion results in gut dysfunction in healthy men. *PLoS One.* 2011;6:e22366.
2. Wallace JL. Prostaglandins, NSAIDs, and gastric mucosal protection: why doesn't the stomach digest itself? *Physiol Rev.* 2008;88:1547-1565.

3. Allison MC, Howatson AG, Torrance CJ, Lee FD, Russell RI. Gastrointestinal damage associated with the use of nonsteroidal antiinflammatory drugs. *N Engl J Med.* 1992;327:749-754.
4. Derikx JP, Matthijsen RA, de Bruine AP, et al. Rapid reversal of human intestinal ischemia-reperfusion induced damage by shedding of injured enterocytes and ree-pithelialisation. *PLoS One.* 2008;3:e3428.

Abdominal symptoms during physical exercise and the role of gastrointestinal ischaemia: a study in 12 symptomatic athletes

ter Steege RWF, Geelkerken RH, Huisman AB, et al (Univ Med Centre Groningen, The Netherlands; Med Spectrum Twente, Enschede, The Netherlands)
Br J Sports Med 46:931-935, 2012

Background.—Gastrointestinal (GI) symptoms during exercise may be caused by GI ischaemia. The authors report their experience with the diagnostic protocol and management of athletes with symptomatic exercisein-duced GI ischaemia. The value of prolonged exercise tonometry in the diagnostic protocol of these patients was evaluated.

Methods.—Patients referred for GI symptoms during physical exercise underwent a standardised diagnostic protocol, including prolonged exercise tonometry. Indicators of GI ischaemia, as measured by tonometry, were related to the presence of symptoms during the exercise test (S+ and S− tests) and exercise intensity.

Results.—12 athletes were specifically referred for GI symptoms during exercise (five males and seven females; median age 29 years (range 15–46 years)). Type of sport was cycling, long-distance running and triathlon. Median duration of symptoms was 32 months (range 7–240 months). Splanchnic artery stenosis was found in one athlete. GI ischaemia was found in six athletes during submaximal exercise. All athletes had gastric and jejunal ischaemia during maximum intensity exercise. No significant difference was found in gastric and jejunal Pco_2 or gradients between S+ and S− tests during any phase of the exercise protocol. In S+ tests, but not in S− tests, a significant correlation between lactate and gastric gradient was found. In S+ tests, the regression coefficients of gradients were higher than those in S− tests. Treatment advice aimed at limiting GI ischaemia were successful in reducing complaints in the majority of the athletes.

Conclusion.—GI ischaemia was present in all athletes during maximum intensity exercise and in 50% during submaximal exercise. Athletes with GI symptoms had higher gastric gradients per mmol/l increase in lactate, suggesting an increased susceptibility for the development of ischaemia during exercise. Treatment advice aimed at limiting GI ischaemia helped the majority of the referred athletes to reduce their complaints. Our results suggest an important role for GI ischaemia in the pathophysiology of their complaints (Fig 1).

▶ Gastrointestinal symptoms are common in endurance athletes, both during[1] and following[2-4] a sporting event. It is also known that the blood flow to the

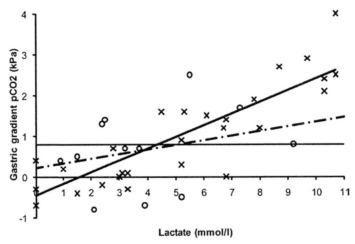

Lactate (mmol/l)

FIGURE 1.—The relationship between lactate and gastric gradient during exercise tonometry in S+ tests (crosses and continuous thick line) and S− tests (circles and dotted line). Regression coefficient for S+ tests was 0.29 (95% CI 0.22 to 0.36, p<0.001); regression coefficient for S− tests was 0.11 (95% CI −0.16 to 0.39, p=0.38). (Reprinted from ter Steege RWF, Geelkerken RH, Huisman AB, et al. Abdominal symptoms during physical exercise and the role of gastrointestinal ischaemia: a study in 12 symptomatic athletes. *Br J Sports Med.* 2012;46:931-935, with permission from the BMJ Publishing Group Ltd.)

viscera is greatly reduced during sustained competition, and there have been reports suggesting that local ischemia can cause a penetration of the gut wall by intestinal endotoxins.[5] However, it is less clear how large a proportion of gastrointestinal problems in the athlete are caused by impaired blood flow to the gut.[1,6] The diagnostic approach used by these authors involves the determination of gas partial pressure gradients between the gut and arterial blood in relation to the intensity of exercise as determined by blood lactate levels (Fig 1). Following this screening, ultrasound or angiography was undertaken. The determination of carbon dioxide pressure gradients did not distinguish between symptomatic and asymptomatic patients, and at the end of the article I was unclear whether this elaborate and presumably expensive protocol offered any great advantage over commonsense advice, such as a small reduction in the intensity of effort and avoidance of nonsteroidal anti-inflammatory drugs if there is gastrointestinal bleeding.

R. J. Shephard, MD (Lond), PhD, DPE

References

1. Moses FM. Exercise-associated intestinal ischemia. *Curr Sports Med Rep.* 2005;4: 91-95.
2. Heer M, Repond F, Hany A, Sulser H, Kehl O, Jäger K. Acute ischaemic colitis in a female long distance runner. *Gut.* 1987;28:896-899.
3. Sullivan SN, Wong C, Heidenheim P. Does running cause gastrointestinal symptoms? A survey of 93 randomly selected runners compared with controls. *N Z Med J.* 1994;107:328-331.
4. Peters HP, Bos M, Seebregts L, et al. Gastrointestinal symptoms in long-distance runners, cyclists, and triathletes: prevalence, medication, and etiology. *Am J Gastroenterol.* 1999;94:1570-1581.

5. Bosenberg AT, Brock-Utne SL, Gaffin MTB, Wells MT, Blake GT. Strenuous exercise causes systemic endotoxemia. *J Appl Physiol.* 1988;65:106-108.
6. Rowell LB, Blackmon JR, Bruce RA. Indocyanine green clearance and estimated hepatic blood flow during mild to maximal exercise in upright man. *J Clin Invest.* 1964;43:1677-1790.

Chronic Respiratory Problems

Airway injury during high-level exercise

Kippelen P, Anderson SD (Brunel Univ, Uxbridge, UK; Royal Prince Alfred Hosp, Camperdown, Australia)
Br J Sports Med 46:385-390, 2012

Airway epithelial cells act as a physical barrier against environmental toxins and injury, and modulate inflammation and the immune response. As such, maintenance of their integrity is critical. Evidence is accumulating to suggest that exercise can cause injury to the airway epithelium. This seems the case particularly for competitive athletes performing high-level exercise, or when exercise takes place in extreme environmental conditions such as in cold dry air or in polluted air. Dehydration of the small airways and increased forces exerted on to the airway surface during severe hyperpnoea are thought to be key factors in determining the occurrence of injury of the airway epithelium. The injury-repair process of the airway epithelium may contribute to the development of the bronchial hyper-responsiveness that is documented in many elite athletes.

▶ The possibility that exposure to extreme environmental conditions could cause pulmonary damage was raised many years ago in connection with Inuit hunting expeditions.[1] Studies in the far north suggested that a combination of mouth breathing and repeated exposure to air temperatures as low as −55°C causes poor lung function and increased hilar markings and signs of pulmonary hypertension, including right bundle branch block (RBBB), in frequent trappers. We estimated a 5% prevalence of RBBB in the Nunavuk community of Igloolik,[2] where many of the residents still engaged in long winter hunting trips.

Similar problems have been described in deep sea divers who have experienced rapid respiratory heat loss because of breathing heliox gas mixtures.[3] More recently, the phenomenon of damage to the respiratory lining has undergone more sophisticated analysis, as discussed in this article. Some of the recent findings have relevance for the sports physician. Exercise hyperpnea can cause an increased release of the cytokine interleukin-8, thus delaying infiltration of the respiratory epithelium by neutrophils and increasing vulnerability to upper respiratory infections.[3,4] There may also be a reduced secretion of the protective prostaglandin E2, exacerbating the tendency to bronchospasm,[5] plus a disruption of normal mucus clearance mechanisms. Recovery is generally rapid with a return to warm moist air, but concerns remain about the potential long-term consequences of the repair processes that are initiated, particularly an increased bronchial hyperresponsiveness.[6] Further study is needed, both on the likelihood of causing permanent injury and on methods of preventing long-term epithelial damage in athletes, whether from exposure to cold air or from the high concentrations of chlorine they encounter in some swimming pools.

R. J. Shephard, MD (Lond), PhD, DPE

References

1. Schaefer O, Eaton RD, Timmermans FJ, Hildes JA. Respiratory function impairment and cardiopulmonary consequences in long-time residents of the Canadian Arctic. *Can Med Assoc J.* 1980;123:997-1004.
2. Shephard RJ, Rode A. Cold, fitness and the exercise electrocardiogram. A 20 year longitudinal study of Canadian Inuit. *Int J Sports Med.* 1992;13:S176-S178.
3. Lloyd ELL. Environmental cold may be a major factor in some respiratory disorders. In: Fortuine R, ed. *Circumpolar Health' 84*. Seattle, WA: University of Washington Press; 1984:66-69.
4. Hashimoto S, Matsumoto K, Gon Y, Nakayama T, Takeshita I, Horie T. Hyperosmolarity-induced interleukin-8 expression in human bronchial epithelial cells through p38 mitogen-activated protein kinase. *Am J Respir Crit Care Med.* 1999;159:634-640.
5. Furuichi S, Hashimoto S, Gon Y, Matsumoto K, Horie T. p38 mitogen-activated protein kinase and c-Jun-NH2-terminal kinase regulate interleukin-8 and RANTES production in hyperosmolarity stimulated human bronchial epithelial cells. *Respirology.* 2002;7:193-200.
6. Hallstrand TS, Moody MW, Wurfel MM, Schwartz LB, Henderson WR Jr, Aitken ML. Inflammatory basis of exercise-induced bronchoconstriction. *Am J Respir Crit Care Med.* 2005;172:679-686.

Optimizing the 6-Min Walk Test as a Measure of Exercise Capacity in COPD

Chandra D, on behalf of the NETT Research Group (Univ of Pittsburgh, PA; et al)
Chest 142:1545-1552, 2012

Background.—It is uncertain whether the effort and expense of performing a second walk for the 6-min walk test improves test performance. Hence, we attempted to quantify the improvement in 6-min walk distance if an additional walk were to be performed.

Methods.—We studied patients consecutively enrolled into the National Emphysema Treatment Trial who prior to randomization and after 6 to 10 weeks of pulmonary rehabilitation performed two 6-min walks on consecutive days (N = 396). Patients also performed two 6-min walks at 6-month follow-up after randomization to lung volume reduction surgery (n = 74) or optimal medical therapy (n = 64). We compared change in the first walk distance to change in the second, average-of-two, and best-of-two walk distances.

Results.—Compared with the change in the first walk distance, change in the average-of-two and best-of-two walk distances had better validity and precision. Specifically, 6 months after randomization to lung volume reduction surgery, changes in the average-of-two ($r = 0.66$ vs $r = 0.58$, $P = .01$) and best-of-two walk distances ($r = 0.67$ vs $r = 0.58$, $P = .04$) better correlated with the change in maximal exercise capacity (ie, better validity). Additionally, the variance of change was 14% to 25% less for the average-of-two

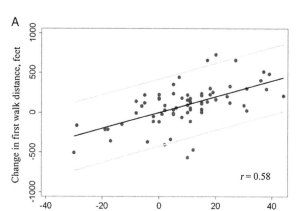

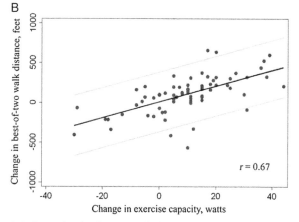

FIGURE 2.—A, B, Scatterplots for change in walk distance vs change in exercise capacity measured on cardiopulmonary exercise testing in patients undergoing lung volume reduction surgery ($n = 74$). Each plot has a fitted regression line with 95% confidence bands. The scatter was closer to the line, the 95% confidence bands were narrower, and the correlation (r) was stronger for best-of-two walk distances compared with change in the first walk distance. The increase in the correlation was significant for the best-of-two-walk distances vs that for the first walk distance ($r = 0.58$ vs $r = 0.67$, respectively, $P = .04$). (Reprinted from Chandra D, on behalf of the NETT Research Group. Optimizing the 6-min walk test as a measure of exercise capacity in COPD. *Chest.* 2012;142:1545-1552, © 2012, American College of Chest Physicians.)

walk distances and 14% to 33% less for the best-of-two walk distances than the variance of change in the single walk distance, indicating better precision.

Conclusions.—Adding a second walk to the 6-min walk test significantly improves its performance in measuring response to a therapeutic intervention, improves the validity of COPD clinical trials, and would result in a 14% to 33% reduction in sample size requirements. Hence, it should be strongly considered by clinicians and researchers as an outcome measure for therapeutic interventions in patients with COPD (Fig 2).

▶ The 6-minute walk is widely used in clinical practice, but, unlike many objective clinical tests, most observers make only a single assessment without any opportunity for practice of the test. The American Thoracic Society states somewhat equivocally: "A practice walk is not needed in most clinical settings but should be considered,"[1] although early users of the test suggested that results only became stable after several practice attempts.[2-4] The answer to this question probably depends in part on the use that is being made of the test. Some observers have used the measurement in an attempt to predict an individual's maximal oxygen intake, but like many alternative prediction procedures the standard deviation of the calculation is so large that such numbers provide little useful information about an individual's aerobic function. Changes in a patient's 6-minute walking distance may provide an indication of a change in the clinical condition of a given individual, and here it will probably be useful to make multiple measurements to reduce learning effects and reduce random error; this is particularly important if some provision must be made to provide the patient with oxygen during the test. The third potential use of walking test data is to examine the response of a large group of individuals to some form of treatment, as in the study of Chandra et al. Here again, the authors claim greater precision for duplicate measurements in terms of the ability to predict the change in exercise capacity in watts (Fig 2). The variance of the change in performance was reduced by 14% to 33% if the best of 2 estimates was considered. However, another alternative that the authors do not consider would be to make a single measurement but to double the number of patients in a study; this tactic would also reduce random errors by more than 30% and might improve other aspects of the study.

R. J. Shephard, MD (Lond), PhD, DPE

References

1. ATS Committee on Proficiency Standards for Clinical Pulmonary Function Laboratories. ATS statement: guidelines for the six-minute walk test. *Am J Respir Crit Care Med.* 2002;166:111-117.
2. Butland RJ, Pang J, Gross ER, Woodcock AA, Geddes DM. Two-, six-, and 12-minute walking tests in respiratory disease. *Br Med J (Clin Res Ed).* 1982;284:1607-1608.
3. McGavin CR, Gupta SP, McHardy GJ. Twelve-minute walking test for assessing disability in chronic bronchitis. *BMJ.* 1976;1:822-823.
4. Jenkins S, Cecins NM. Six-minute walk test in pulmonary rehabilitation: do all patients need a practice test? *Respirology.* 2010;15:1192-1196.

Effectiveness of exercise training in patients with COPD: the role of muscle fatigue

Burtin C, Saey D, Saglam M, et al (Katholieke Universiteit Leuven, Belgium; Université Laval, Quebec, Canada; Univ Hosps KULeuven, Leuven, Belgium)
Eur Respir J 40:338-344, 2012

The improvement in exercise performance in response to exercise training varies greatly from one patient with chronic obstructive pulmonary disease to another. It is possible that in a portion of patients the muscle stimulus applied during exercise training is insufficient to elicit training effects. We investigated whether patients presenting quadriceps contractile fatigue after training have more favourable effects of a rehabilitation programme.

46 patients followed a 3-month high-intensity exercise training programme. Exercise capacity, quadriceps force and quality of life were measured before and after the programme. Exercise training-induced quadriceps contractile fatigue was assessed after 1 month of rehabilitation with magnetic stimulation. A fall in quadriceps force of $\geq 15\%$, 15 min after training was considered as significant fatigue.

29 (63%) out of 46 patients developed significant fatigue. Patients with fatigue had a higher increase in 6-min walk distance (median (interquartile

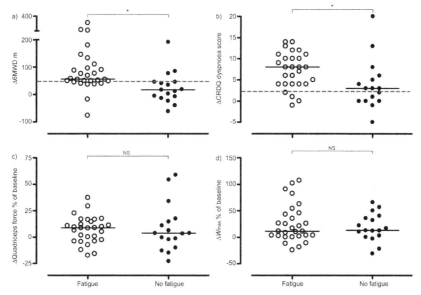

FIGURE 3.—Individual change (Δ) in a) 6-min walk distance (6MWD), b) Chronic Respiratory Disease Questionnaire (CRDQ) dyspnoea score, c) quadriceps force, and d) maximal workload (Wmax) during incremental exercise testing after the training programme in patients with and without quadriceps contractile fatigue. ————: median score of each group; - - - -: estimated clinical important difference for this variable. NS: nonsignificant.*: $p < 0.05$ between groups. (Reprinted from Burtin C, Saey D, Saglam M, et al. Effectiveness of exercise training in patients with COPD: the role of muscle fatigue. *Eur Respir J.* 2012;40:338-344, with permission from the European Respiratory Society.)

range) 57 (47–103) m *versus* 17 (−7–46) m; $p = 0.0023$) and Chronic Respiratory Disease Questionnaire score (mean ± SD 22 ± 12 points *versus* 14 ± 12 points; $p = 0.028$) after the training programme compared with patients without fatigue. Improvements in quadriceps force and maximal exercise capacity were similar in both subgroups.

Patients who develop quadriceps contractile fatigue during exercise training show greater training effects in terms of functional exercise capacity and health-related quality of life (Fig 3).

▶ Those who have worked in rehabilitation programs will know that it is much more difficult to motivate chronic obstructive pulmonary disease (COPD) patients to an adequate volume of exercise than it is for those who have sustained a myocardial infarction. This may be partly a reflection of inherent differences of personality between the 2 types of patients: a "type A" coronary patient is eager to succeed. But a further factor is that COPD is associated with muscular weakness that leads to both breathlessness and peripheral muscular fatigue. Breathlessness is the main factor that limits exercise for many patients,[1-3] and respiratory muscle training and adjustment of breathing patterns will often help such individuals. However, in other patients, it is the limb muscles that need strengthening. A corollary of this is that if their physical condition and quality of life are to be improved, the rehabilitation program must be of sufficient intensity to present an adequate training stimulus to the muscles.

This study used a combination of endurance training and resisted exercise on a leg press apparatus, and the benefit observed from rehabilitation was greatest in those who were exercising sufficiently to induce a decrease of quadriceps force 15 minutes after a training session (Fig 3). It is less clear why some patients did not train with adequate intensity; the authors claim to have eliminated breathlessness as a possible cause. Two other questions arise. Is there a method simpler than electrical stimulation to determine whether the skeletal muscles have been sufficiently fatigued, and are there potential techniques such as exercising 1 leg at a time that can increase the stimulus to the muscles?

R. J. Shephard, MD (Lond), PhD, DPE

References

1. Troosters T, Gosselink R, Decramer M. Exercise training in COPD: how to distinguish responders from nonresponders. *J Cardiopulm Rehabil.* 2001;21:10-17.
2. Zu Wallack RL, Patel K, Reardon JZ, Clark BA 3rd, Normandin EA. Predictors of improvement in the 12-minute walking distance following a six-week outpatient pulmonary rehabilitation program. *Chest.* 1991;99:805-808.
3. Plankeel JF, McMullen B, MacIntyre NR. Exercise outcomes after pulmonary rehabilitation depend on the initial mechanism of exercise limitation among non-oxygen-dependent COPD patients. *Chest.* 2005;127:110-116.

Exercise Training After Lung Transplantation Improves Participation in Daily Activity: A Randomized Controlled Trial

Langer D, Burtin C, Schepers L, et al (Faculty of Kinesiology and Rehabilitation Sciences, Heverlee, Belgium; et al)
Am J Transplant 12:1584-1592, 2012

The effects of exercise training after lung transplantation have not been studied in a randomized controlled trial so far. We investigated whether 3 months of supervised training, initiated immediately after hospital discharge, improve functional recovery and cardiovascular morbidity of patients up to 1 year after lung transplantation. Patients older than 40 years, who experienced an uncomplicated postoperative period, were eligible for this single blind, parallel group study. Sealed envelopes were used to randomly allocate patients to 3 months of exercise training (n = 21) or a control intervention (n = 19). Minutes of daily walking time (primary outcome), physical fitness, quality of life and cardiovascular morbidity were compared between groups adjusting for baseline assessments in a mixed models analysis. After 1 year daily walking time in the treated patients (n = 18) was 85 ± 27 min and in the control group (n = 16) 54 ± 30 min (adjusted difference 26 min [95%CI 8-45 min, $p = 0.006$]). Quadriceps force ($p = 0.001$), 6-minute walking distance ($p = 0.002$) and self-reported physical functioning ($p = 0.039$) were significantly higher in the intervention group. Average 24 h ambulatory blood pressures were significantly lower in the treated patients ($p \leq 0.01$). Based on these results patients should be strongly encouraged to participate in an exercise training intervention after lung transplantation (Fig 2).

▶ The most interesting points about this article seem to be that the substantial difference in outcome that was achieved after lung transplantation in the patients who received 3 months of supervised training (Fig 2) and that gains were well-maintained 9 months after the intensive outpatient rehabilitation had ended. The rehabilitation regimen was by no means nominal. Sessions were of 90 minutes' duration, 3 times per week, and activities included cycling, walking, stair climbing,

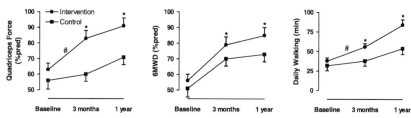

FIGURE 2.—Progression of quadriceps force, 6-minute walking distance (6MWD) and daily walking time during the intervention period (Baseline to 3 months) and during the follow-up period (3 months to 1 year). *, significant difference between groups; #, significant difference in slopes between groups. (Reprinted from Langer D, Burtin C, Schepers L, et al. Exercise training after lung transplantation improves participation in daily activity: a randomized controlled trial. *Am J Transplant*. 2012;12:1584-1592, with permission from The American Society of Transplantation and the American Society of Transplant Surgeons.)

and resistance exercise at an intensity reaching at least 60% of current maximal effort. One disappointing feature is that 40% of eligible patients refused to participate. It is unclear whether this was because of the need for subject randomization or because lengthy travel was sometimes required to reach the rehabilitation clinic. The latter problem can be a major disincentive to exercise participation, as others have noted.[1,2] The solution may be to have at least some of the training sessions performed at home, an approach that has proved very successful with cardiac patients at the Toronto Rehabilitation Center.[3] The other important question not answered by the present study is the impact of the exercise program upon complications of lung transplantation, including rejection. A much larger sample size would be needed to resolve this issue.

R. J. Shephard, MD (Lond), PhD, DPE

References

1. Wickerson L, Mathur S, Brooks D. Exercise training after lung transplantation: a systematic review. *J Heart Lung Transpl.* 2010;29:497-503.
2. Rochester CL. Pulmonary rehabilitation for patients who undergo lung-volume-reduction surgery or lung transplantation. *Respir Care.* 2008;53:1196-1202.
3. Vivodtzev I, Pison C, Guerrero K, et al. Benefits of home-based endurance training in lung transplant recipients. *Respir Physiol Neurobiol.* 2011;177:189-198.

7 Other Medical Conditions

Cancer

Insights Into the Reluctance of Patients With Late-Stage Cancer to Adopt Exercise as a Means to Reduce Their Symptoms and Improve Their Function
Cheville AL, Dose AM, Basford JR, et al (Mayo Clinic, Rochester, MN)
J Pain Symptom Manage 44:84-94, 2012

Context.—Exercise reduces cancer-related disablement and adverse symptoms, yet patients' attitudes toward exercise remain largely unexamined.

Objectives.—This qualitative study sought to characterize the beliefs of patients with late-stage disease regarding exercise, its relationship to their symptoms, and their clinicians' roles in providing related counseling.

Methods.—Semistructured interviews with 20 adults (half male and half aged 65 years or older) with Stage IIIB or IV nonsmall cell lung cancer were qualitatively analyzed. Participants were questioned about their levels of activity, the influence of their symptoms on their activities, perceived barriers and facilitators for exercise, and exercise-related instructions received from their professional caregivers.

Results.—Participants overwhelmingly cited usual daily activities as their source of "exercise." Symptoms, particularly treatment-related, discouraged participation, with fear of harm being a significant concern only among younger women. Exercise was recognized as important for physical and mental well-being but seldom as a means to mitigate symptoms. Weather, recalled levels of premorbid fitness, and exercise participation modulated current exercise behaviors. Although respondents preferred to receive guidance from their oncologist, none reported receiving more than general encouragement to "stay active." A lack of direction was typically accepted as a sanction of their current activity levels. Participants appeared less receptive to guidance from ancillary health professionals.

Conclusion.—Effective use of exercise and activity modification to ameliorate cancer-related symptoms appears to require a linkage to a patient's usual and past activities, proactive negotiation of potential barriers, education regarding symptoms and exercise, and the positive support of their oncologist.

▶ There is growing evidence that it is beneficial for patients to exercise following the treatment of a variety of types of carcinoma, but in practice the proportion of patients who follow such a plan is disappointingly low. Cheville and associates explore the reasons for this problem, using the technique of semistructured interviews. This is a relatively time-consuming approach, and perhaps for this reason they have accumulated information on only 20 individuals, treated for just 1 form of cancer. However, on the basis of 45 minutes per interview, they could usefully have looked at a larger sample. I also did not find any clear statement of how soon after treatment of the cancer the reactions of the individual were being analyzed. Symptoms were said to be the main factors precluding greater activity, with complaints of fatigue, nausea, malaise, and cold intolerance (the study was conducted in Minnesota). One disturbing feature of the interviews was that few oncologists had discussed appropriate patterns of exercise with their patients.

R. J. Shephard, MD (Lond), PhD, DPE

Physical Activity, Biomarkers, and Disease Outcomes in Cancer Survivors: A Systematic Review
Ballard-Barbash R, Friedenreich CM, Courneya KS, et al (Natl Insts of Health, Bethesda, MD; Univ of Alberta, Edmonton, Canada; et al)
J Natl Cancer Inst 104:815-840, 2012

Background.—Cancer survivors often seek information about how lifestyle factors, such as physical activity, may influence their prognosis. We systematically reviewed studies that examined relationships between physical activity and mortality (cancer-specific and all-cause) and/or cancer biomarkers.

Methods.—We identified 45 articles published from January 1950 to August 2011 through MEDLINE database searches that were related to physical activity, cancer survival, and biomarkers potentially relevant to cancer survival. We used the Preferred Reporting Items for Systematic Reviews and Meta-Analyses Statement to guide this review. Study characteristics, mortality outcomes, and biomarker-relevant and subgroup results were abstracted for each article that met the inclusion criteria (ie, research articles that included participants with a cancer diagnosis, mortality outcomes, and an assessment of physical activity).

Results.—There was consistent evidence from 27 observational studies that physical activity is associated with reduced all-cause, breast cancer—specific, and colon cancer—specific mortality. There is currently insufficient evidence regarding the association between physical activity and mortality for survivors of other cancers. Randomized controlled trials of exercise that included biomarker endpoints suggest that exercise may result in beneficial changes in the circulating level of insulin, insulin-related pathways,

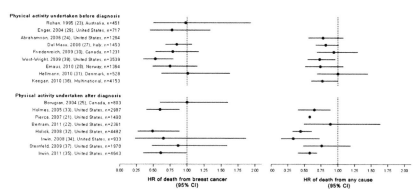

FIGURE 2.—Forest plot of risk estimates from observational studies of physical activity and mortality outcomes in breast cancer survivors. **Black circles** indicate hazard ratios (HRs), and **solid horizontal lines** represent 95% confidence intervals (CIs). The **vertical dotted line** indicates point of unity. (Reprinted from Ballard-Barbash R, Friedenreich CM, Courneya KS, et al. Physical activity, biomarkers, and disease outcomes in cancer survivors: a systematic review. *J Natl Cancer Inst*. 2012;104:815-840, by permission of Oxford University Press.)

inflammation, and, possibly, immunity; however, the evidence is still preliminary.

Conclusions.—Future research directions identified include the need for more observational studies on additional types of cancer with larger sample sizes; the need to examine whether the association between physical activity and mortality varies by tumor, clinical, or risk factor characteristics; and the need for research on the biological mechanisms involved in the association between physical activity and survival after a cancer diagnosis. Future randomized controlled trials of exercise with biomarker and cancer-specific disease endpoints, such as recurrence, new primary cancers, and cancer-specific mortality in cancer survivors, are warranted (Fig 2).

▶ There is good evidence that regular physical activity can reduce the risk of a number of cancers, particularly in the colon and the breast. Exercise programs are also recognized as generally safe and able to improve the quality of life following diagnosis and treatment of most cancers,[1] although there remains a need to evaluate whether cancer treatments such as anthracyclines or irradiation of the left side of the chest increase the risk of heart attacks. However, the effects of physical activity on long-term prognosis have received much less attention.[2,3] The present systematic review found 45 relevant articles looking at survival and/or cancer biomarkers, mostly published in the past 4 years. There was consistent evidence in 27 observational trials of a lower mortality among exercising patients with all-cause, colorectal, and particularly breast cancers (Fig 2), but data were as yet inconclusive for other types of cancer. There was also a suggestion from 11 randomized controlled trials of beneficial effects on cancer biomarkers, including circulating insulin level, insulin pathways, inflammation, and possibly immune function, although there is still scope for further investigations using objective biomarkers of risk of cancer recurrence. There is also a need for trials in which the amount of physical activity that has been undertaken is quantitated accurately using devices such as accelerometers. In the observational trials, it could be argued that the cancer survivors who were able to exercise were detected at an earlier stage or had more successful treatment, and that this explained their better prognosis. A randomized controlled trial of exercise for colon cancer survivors is currently in progress,[4] and the results of this investigation will be awaited with interest.

R. J. Shephard, MD (Lond), PhD, DPE

References

1. Schmitz KH, Courneya KS, Matthews C, et al. American College of Sports Medicine roundtable on exercise guidelines for cancer survivors. *Med Sci Sports Exerc.* 2010;42:1409-1426.
2. Cancer survivors: living longer, and now, better. *Lancet.* 2004;364:2153-2154.
3. *Physical Activity Guidelines Advisory Committee. Physical Activity Guidelines 2008.* Washington, DC: U.S. Department of Advisory Committee Report, Health and Human Services; 2008.
4. Courneya KS, Booth CM, Gill S, et al. The Colon Health and Life-Long Exercise Change trial: a randomized trial of the National Cancer Institute of Canada Clinical Trials Group. *Curr Oncol.* 2008;15:279-285.

Other Diseases

Physically active men show better semen parameters and hormone values than sedentary men

Vaamonde D, Da Silva-Grigoletto ME, García-Manso JM, et al (Univ of Córdoba, Spain; Andalusian Ctr of Sports Medicine and Scientific Sport Association, Córdoba, Spain; Univ of Las Palmas de Gran Canaria, Spain; et al)
Eur J Appl Physiol 112:3267-3273, 2012

Physical exercise promotes many health benefits. The present study was undertaken to assess possible semen and hormone differences among physically active (PA) subjects and sedentary subjects (SE). The analyzed qualitative sperm parameters were: volume, sperm count, motility, and morphology; where needed, additional testing was performed. The measured hormones were: follicle-stimulating hormone (FSH), luteinizing hormone (LH), testosterone (T), cortisol (C), and the ratio between T and C (T/C). Maximum oxygen consumption was also assessed to check for differences in fitness level. Statistically significant differences were found for several semen parameters such as total progressive motility (PA: 60.94 ± 5.03; SE: 56.07 ± 4.55) and morphology (PA: 15.54 ± 1.38, SE: 14.40 ± 1.15). The seminological values observed were supported by differences in hormones, with FSH, LH, and T being higher in PA than in SE (5.68 ± 2.51 vs. 3.14 ± 1.84; 5.95 ± 1.11 vs. 5.08 ± 0.98; 7.68 ± 0.77 vs. 6.49 ± 0.80, respectively). Likewise, the T/C ratio, index of anabolic versus catabolic status, was also higher in PA (0.46 ± 0.11 vs. 0.32 ± 0.07), which further supports the possibility of an improved hormonal environment. The present study shows that there are differences in semen and

TABLE 2.—Semen and Hormone Values of Physically Active Men and Sedentary Men. Values are Expressed as Mean ± SD

	Mean (±SD)		Mean dif		Sig	95% CI	
	Physically Active (N = 16)	Sedentary (N = 15)	PA-SE	$T^{\#}$	P	Lower	Upper
Concentration (*10^6/ml)	66.50 (±16.27)	58.38 (±16.19)	8.12	1.39	0.175	−3.81	20.05
Volume (ml)	3.24 (±0.81)	3.19 (±0.74)	0.05	0.178	0.783	−0.318	0.418
Vel a (%)	33.60 (±6.18)	32.27 (±8.75)	1.33	0.49	0.627	−4.20	6.87
Vel b (%)	27.35 (±7.18)	21.81 (±6.79)	5.54*	2.20	0.036	0.40	10.68
Vel a + b (%)	60.94 (±5.03)	56.07 (±4.55)	4.87*	2.82	0.009	1.34	8.40
Vel c (%)	8.54 (±4.00)	11.19 (±3.89)	−2.65	−1.87	0.072	−5.55	0.25
Vel d (%)	30.58 (±4.86)	34.78 (±5.69)	−4.20*	−2.22	0.035	−8.08	−0.32
Normal forms (%)	15.54 (±1.38)	14.40 (±1.15)	1.14*	2.49	0.019	0.20	2.08
T (μg/l)	7.68 (±0.77)	6.49 (±0.80)	1.19*	4.22	0.001	0.61	1.76
C (μg/dl)	19.25 (±4.15)	21.24 (±4.30)	−1.99	1.31	0.200	±5.09	1.11
T/C	0.46 (±0.11)	0.32 (±0.07)	0.14*	4.20	0.001	0.07	0.21
FSH (U/l)	5.68 (±2.51)	3.14 (±1.84)	2.54	3.20	0.003	0.91	4.17
LH (U/l)	5.95 (±1.11)	5.08 (±0.98)	0.87	2.31	0.028	0.09	1.64

*Significant difference between groups (P < 0.05).
$^{\#}$t Student's test.

hormone values of physically active subjects and sedentary subjects. Physically active subjects seem to have a more anabolic hormonal environment and a healthier semen production (Table 2).

▶ Some 40 years ago, I noticed that men who were heavily engaged in distance running had low scores on paper and pencil "masculinity" scales. My observations were greeted by shrieks of horrified disbelief! However, more recent research has vindicated these observations; investigators have shown low concentrations of testosterone and, probably consequently, a poor semen quality in ultraendurance athletes.[1,2] Although this trend is reversible with a period of detraining, it has become of increasing concern to many people, since various factors in the modern environment (including xenoestrogens, pesticides, and increasing ambient temperatures) have also been associated with a secular trend toward a progressive decrease in average sperm quality.[3-5] It is unclear if the impact on semen quality has any adverse effect on athletic motivation in the general public. However, for those health promoters who may have such concerns, the finding of normal or slightly better than normal semen characteristics in young men who were moderately active 3 days per week (a maximal oxygen intake of 51 mL/kg/min vs. 37 mL/kg/min in those classed as sedentary) (Table 2) is an encouraging finding; it would be interesting to see if their semen values reverted to the sedentary level with a period of abstinence from exercise. The authors are inclined to explain benefits in terms of a modulation of reactive oxygen species, but in my view it is more probable that moderate exercise promotes an overall anabolic environment.

R. J. Shephard, MD (Lond), PhD, DPE

References

1. Vaamonde D, Da Silva-Grigoletto ME, García-Manso JM, et al. Sperm morphology normalcy is inversely correlated to cycling kilometers in elite triathletes. *Rev Andal Med Deporte*. 2009;2:43-46.
2. Vaamonde D, Da Silva-Grigoletto ME, García-Manso JM, Vaamonde-Lemos R, Swanson RJ, Oehninger SC. Response of semen parameters to three training modalities. *Fertil Steril*. 2009;92:1941-1946.
3. Carlsen E, Giwercman A, Keiding N, Skakkebaek NE. Evidence for decreasing quality of semen during past 50 years. *BMJ*. 1992;305:609-613.
4. De Mouzon J, Thonneau P, Spira A, Multigner L. Declining sperm count. Semen quality has declined among men born in France since 1950. *BMJ*. 1996;313:43.
5. Merzenich H, Zeeb H, Blettner M. Decreasing sperm quality: a global problem? *BMC Public Health*. 2010;10:24.

Correlation Between Seminal Oxidative Stress Biomarkers and Antioxidants with Sperm DNA Damage in Elite Athletes and Recreationally Active Men

Tartibian B, Maleki BH (Urmia Univ, Iran)
Clin J Sport Med 22:132-139, 2012

Objective.—To evaluate the seminal plasma 8-isoprostane, reactive oxygen species (ROS), malondialdehyde (MDA), superoxide dismutase (SOD), catalase, total antioxidant capacity (TAC), and levels of sperm DNA fragmentation in elite athletes and recreationally active men.

Design.—Prospective design was used for this study.

Setting.—The study was performed in the Exercise Physiology Laboratory of the Urmia University.

Participants.—Fifty-six elite athletes and 52 recreationally active men (18–28 years) participated in this study.

Intervention.—All subjects had a semen sampling at baseline.

Main Outcome Measures.—Total antioxidant capacity and SOD activity were measured by colorimetric assay. Levels of ROS were measured by a chemiluminescence assay. Malondialdehyde levels were measured by thiobarbituric acid reactive substance assay. Catalase activity was measured by monitoring the initial rate of disappearance of hydrogen peroxide. Concentration of free 8-isoprostane was measured by enzyme immunoassay method. Sperm DNA fragmentation was evaluated with the terminal deoxynucleotidyl transferase—mediated fluorescein dUTP nick end-labeling assay.

Results.—Recreationally active men have significantly higher levels of body fat, seminal SOD, TAC, and catalase and lower levels of $\dot{V}o_2$max, seminal ROS, MDA, and 8-isoprostane and subsequently lower rate of sperm DNA fragmentation when compared with elite athletes ($P < 0.001$). Significantly negative correlation was observed between sperm DNA fragmentation with body fat, seminal SOD, catalase, and TAC levels ($P < 0.001$). Significantly positive correlation was observed between sperm DNA fragmentation with $\dot{V}o_2$max, seminal 8-isoprostane, ROS, and MDA levels ($P < 0.001$).

TABLE 2.—Comparison of Semen Parameters, Seminal Antioxidants, and Oxidative Stress Biomarkers in Different Groups of the Study

Variables	Elite Athletes	Groups Recreationally Active Men	Significance*
No. spermatozoa ($\times 10^6$)	46.9 ± 15.5	89.2 ± 27.5	<0.001*
Volume, mL	2.5 ± 0.8	4.7 ± 0.7	<0.001*
Motility, first hour	24.3 ± 11.6	67.6 ± 14.9	<0.001*
Morphology, %	18.3 ± 5.8	33.5 ± 5	<0.001*
Concentration, $\times 10^6$/mL	64.4 ± 6.9	38.6 ± 6.6	<0.001*
8-Isoprostane, ng/mL	11.1 ± 5.4	2.4 ± 1.4	<0.001*
ROS, RLU	731 ± 204	172 ± 136	<0.001*
MDA, nmol/mL	0.8 ± 0.3	0.2 ± 0.1	<0.001*
SOD, U/mL	4.1 ± 1.7	8.9 ± 2.6	<0.001*
Catalase, U/mL	24 ± 12.1	44.7 ± 9.6	<0.001*
TAC, mM	1.3 ± 0.8	2.9 ± 1.3	<0.001*
Sperm TUNEL positive, %	7.2 ± 3.6	2.3 ± 1.3	<0.001*

Sperm TUNEL positive (%): the number of TUNEL-positive cells.
RLU, relative light unit; TUNEL, terminal deoxynucleotidyl transferase—mediated fluorescein dUTP nick end-labeling.
*$P < 0.001$, significant difference among the groups.

Conclusion.—Spermatozoa from recreationally active men may be less susceptible to oxidative stress—induced DNA damage and hence infertility (Table 2).

▶ There have been previous reports of temporary infertility in high-performance athletes, with low sperm counts, poor motility, and limited semen volumes, but the data of these authors are particularly striking in this regard (Table 2); they also include data showing an increase in DNA fragmentation. The athletes concerned were all engaged in sports such as wrestling, boxing, judo, and tae kwon do, and it is possible that some aspect of this type of sport (whether physical injury to the scrotum or the wearing of compression shorts and jockstraps) may have contributed to these adverse findings. Other potential causes of male infertility include an inadequate intake of food energy and an increase of intrascrotal temperatures. The athlete participants in this study were performing at least 2 hours of high-intensity exercise 4 to 5 days per week, whereas the comparison group was engaged in only moderate activity (heart rate around 130 beats per minute, 2 to 3 days per week), with corresponding differences in maximal oxygen intake (62.3 vs 50.1 mL/[kg/min]) and body fat content (6.4% vs 9.2%, method not specified). Spermatozoa can themselves generate reactive oxygen species, and in modest amounts this seems to play an enabling role,[1,2] but if reactive oxygen species are present in greater amounts, this may affect the integrity of the DNA[3] or render the sperm infertile.[4] Most previous studies have shown reversal of the changes in sperm counts with a relaxation of training; it seems important to check in future studies that the DNA fragmentation is also reversed.

R. J. Shephard, MD (Lond), PhD, DPE

References

1. Thundathil J, de Lamirande E, Gagnon C. Nitric oxide regulates the phosphorylation of the threonine-glutamine-tyrosine motif in proteins of human spermatozoa during capacitation. *Biol Reprod.* 2003;68:1291-1298.
2. Rivlin J, Mendel J, Rubinstein S, Etkovitz N, Breitbart H. Role of hydrogen peroxide in sperm capacitation and acrosome reaction. *Biol Reprod.* 2004;70: 518-522.
3. Aitken RJ, Krausz C. Oxidative stress, DNA damage and the Y chromosome. *Reproduction.* 2001;122:497-506.
4. Sikka S. Role of oxidative stress and antioxidants in andrology and assisted reproductive technology. *J Androl.* 2004;25:5-18.

Physical fitness, but not muscle strength, is a risk factor for death in amyotrophic lateral sclerosis at an early age
Mattsson P, Lönnstedt I, Nygren I, et al (Uppsala Univ, Sweden; Statisticon AB, Uppsala, Sweden)
J Neurol Neurosurg Psychiatry 83:390-394, 2012

Background.—Amyotrophic lateral sclerosis (ALS) is a rare neurodegenerative disorder mainly characterised by motor symptoms. Extensive physical activity has been implicated in the aetiology of ALS. Differences in anthropometrics, physical fitness and isometric strength measured at 18−19 years were assessed to determine if they are associated with subsequent death in ALS.

Method.—Data on body weight and height, physical fitness, resting heart rate and isometric strength measured at conscription were linked with data on death certificates in men born in 1951−1965 in Sweden (n = 809 789). Physical fitness was assessed as a maximal test on an electrically braked bicycle ergometer. Muscle strength was measured as the maximal isometric strength in handgrip, elbow flexion and knee extension in standardised positions, using a dynamometer. Analyses were based on 684 459 (84.5%) men because of missing data. A matched case control study within this sample was performed. The population was followed until 31 December 2006, and 85 men died from ALS during this period.

Results.—Weight adjusted physical fitness (W/kg), but not physical fitness per se, was a risk factor for ALS (OR 1.98, 95% CI 1.32 to 2.97), whereas resting pulse rate, muscle strength and other variables were not.

Conclusions.—Physical fitness, but not muscle strength, is a risk factor for death at early age in ALS. This may indicate that a common factor underlies both fitness (W/kg) and risk of ALS (Table 1).

▶ Exercise scientists are accustomed to hearing uniformly good news about the preventive value of regular physical activity, and it is important to remember that there are a few medical conditions in which the outcome is less favorable. Amyotrophic lateral sclerosis (ALS) seems one such example. The impact of physical activity on the risk of developing this condition remains controversial,[1,2] but 1 recent report suggested that there was a 10-fold increase of risk in Italian

TABLE 1.—Measures of Anthropometrics, Physical Fitness and Isometric Strength in Amyotrophic Lateral Sclerosis (ALS) Cases and Controls

	Cases (n = 85) (Mean (SD))	Controls* (n = 2531) (Mean (SD))	OR	95% CI	*p* Value
Anthropometrics					
Weight (kg)	66.3 (8.6)	68.5 (10.8)	0.98	0.96 to 1.00	0.06
Height (cm)	177.6 (6.0)	178.5 (6.4)	0.98	0.94 to 1.01	0.18
Physical fitness					
WMAX[†] (W)	246.7 (38.6)	240.2 (36.5)	1.01	1.00 to 1.01	0.09
WMAX[†‡] (W/kg)	3.75 (0.55)	3.55 (0.55)	1.98	1.32 to 2.97	0.001
Resting heart rate (bpm)	77.0 (13.7)	74.6 (12.9)	1.02	1.00 to 1.03	0.09
Isometric strength					
Handgrip[‡] (N)	595.7 (98.5)	612.8 (98.8)	1.00	1.00 to 1.00	0.10
Handgrip[‡] (N/kg)	9.0 (1.3)	9.1 (1.5)	0.98	0.85 to 1.14	0.84
Elbow flexion (N)	378.3 (87.2)	378.5 (81.4)	1.00	1.00 to 1.00	0.99
Elbow flexion[‡] (N/kg)	5.7 (1.2)	5.6 (1.1)	1.14	0.94 to 1.39	0.19
Knee extension (N)	542.6 (99.1)	535.7 (108.9)	1.00	1.00 to 1.00	0.57
Knee extension[‡] (N/kg)	8.2 (1.3)	7.9 (1.5)	1.15	1.00 to 1.33	0.05

OR expresses the risk of developing amyotrophic lateral sclerosis.
WMAX, maximum physical working capacity.
*Number of controls varied between 2504 and 2531.
[†]Physical fitness from ergometer test.
[‡]Isometric muscle strength per kg body weight.

professional football players.[3] The present study was based on a population sample of Swedes born between 1951 and 1965. A total of 85 subsequently fatal late-onset cases of ALS with strength and fitness measurements were identified, and 2531 matched case control subjects were assigned, with a follow-up as long as 25 years. The cases with ALS initially had a higher peak weight-adjusted work output on the cycle ergometer, but no difference in strength measurements (Table 1). The authors of this report thus suggest that there is an underlying phenotype with a high proportion of type I muscle fibers that is vulnerable to ALS; type I fibers are known to be affected earlier and more severely in ALS.[4,5] If the findings are indeed a reflection of phenotype, then there is no reason to curtail normal physical activity in this group of individuals.

R. J. Shephard, MD (Lond), PhD, DPE

References

1. Armon C. An evidence-based medicine approach to the evaluation of the role of exogenous risk factors in sporadic amyotrophic lateral sclerosis. *Neuroepidemiology.* 2003;22:217-228.
2. Armon C. Sports and trauma in amyotrophic lateral sclerosis revisited. *J Neurol Sci.* 2007;262:45-53.
3. Chiò A, Benzi G, Dossena M, Mutani R, Mora G. Severely increased risk of amyotrophic lateral sclerosis among Italian professional football players. *Brain.* 2005; 128:472-476.
4. Patten BM, Zito G, Harati Y. Histologic findings in motor neuron disease. Relation to clinically determined activity, duration, and severity of disease. *Arch Neurol.* 1979; 36:560-564.
5. Iwasaki Y, Sugimoto H, Ikeda K, et al. Muscle morphometry in amyotrophic lateral sclerosis. *Int J Neurosci.* 1991;58:165-170.

Clinical features of brain motor control and influence in upper motor neuron dysfunction

Brown JM, Tansey KE (Univ of California at San Diego School of Medicine; Emory Univ School of Medicine, Atlanta, GA)
Clin Neurol Neurosurg 114:441-446, 2012

Background.—The upper motor neuron (UMN) syndrome results when neurons or their axons are disrupted or with loss of conduction through these axons involving the central nervous system (CNS) motor pathways. The problem may be caused by trauma; vascular issues; or inflammatory, metabolic, neoplastic, inherited, developmental, or degenerative disorders. The resulting motor control impairment varies widely. The residual capacity of the nervous system to respond to interventions remains unknown. The ability to detect subtle changes that may result from such interventions is also compromised. Neurologic tests that can be performed in clinical settings and how these assessment protocols provide evidence of subclinical motor control were outlined.

Tests.—The postural consequences of CNS injury can manifest as inabilities to maintain a standing posture, rise to a standing position, sit upright, or roll from supine to lateral positions. Posture (sitting or standing) is tested with outstretched upper limbs. It is important to assess the whole body with neck and limb posture, adding volitional motor tasks for the contralateral limb, rostral, or caudal body segments when postural alteration must be enhanced.

Tone is increased with the UMN syndrome. Passive muscle stretch is examined to document increased tone severity. After controlling for environmental conditions (noise and distractions), which can alter test results, the patient's relaxed limb is moved through its normal range at a predetermined rate of speed (very slow, moderate, and then very fast), with the response at each velocity noted. The pendulum test can also be used, where the thigh is supported horizontally and the leg is held straight out by the examiner and then dropped to swing freely from the knee. Amplitude, rate, and number of oscillations are noted. The arm can be tested as well. Vibration can also be applied if the patient has fixed shortenings or contractures that do not permit other tone tests.

Assessing phasic stretch response uses the patellar knee-jerk or percussion of the tendons of the biceps or triceps and Achilles' tendon. Other muscles may also be tested.

The plantar withdrawal reflex is assessed to elicit muscle hypertonia. A nociceptive cutaneous stimulus is delivered to the plantar surface of the foot, eliciting either a brisk or a prolonged withdrawal movement. Other cutaneomuscular reflexes can be tested, noting the threshold at which a response is elicited, amplitude of the primary response, and radiation of the response to ipsilateral and contralateral muscles.

Volitional motor activity is no longer smoothly integrated with UMN injury. Muscles are directly palpated while the subject performs motor tasks at various speeds.

Subclinical motor control is assessed in patients who exhibit no overt movement at individual joints. Additional sensory input and increased effort are applied and any changes observed. Once this assessment is completed, the examiner returns to test the tone, phasic reflex, and withdrawal reflexes to determine subclinical motor control. Reinforcement maneuvers help to assess residual supraspinal modulation of segmental excitability. These maneuvers include forcefully closing the eyes, clenching the jaw, and making a fist. The patient is then asked to attempt to first assist, then resist, movements by the examiner. Similar retests are done for phasic stretch and withdrawal reflexes.

Conclusions.—Once the clinical diagnosis of UMN control impairment has been made, it is necessary to determine the degree of impairment and the type and extent of residual motor control present. This information helps in predicting spontaneous recovery, response to interventions, and spastic features as well as residual motor control.

▶ Clinicians commonly recognize motor control impairment from disruption of cortical motor neuronal function as upper motor neuron (UMN) syndrome. Disruption of function may be caused by vascular issues such as stroke, traumatic issues such as spinal cord injury, or acquired brain injury, or they may manifest because of degenerative or developmental disease, among other causes. The dysfunction observed in these patient populations is heterogeneous, and, therefore, establishing what is or is not dysfunctional is often a challenge. This article provides an excellent discussion of a range of clinically based neurological testing procedures that if performed correctly will provide evidence of subclinical motor control, thereby potentially uncovering functional capabilities in the client heretofore absent with traditional assessments alone. The authors provide the most up-to-date information on assessment of posture, tone, phasic stretch reflexes, withdrawal reflexes, and volitional activity. It is the latter component that is of most interest and the 1 that may be lacking or inadequately performed in systematic assessments of motor function. Intentional (volitional) movement is what we do in our everyday lives, and without an intact integration of both descending and ascending control, the performance of even the most simple volitional task becomes problematic or even impossible, such as one would observe in a complete lesion of the spinal cord at high cervical spinal segment levels. Although muscle tone would be high and resistance to passive stretch considerable, volitional movement would be absent because of the spastic paralysis usually consequent to such a lesion of the spinal cord. However, one may be able to observe multijoint patterned movement in the absence of control of discrete movements. When assessing for subclinical motor control, the authors make the very important point of the need to provide additional sensory (mechanosensory or proprioceptive) input and come up with ways to facilitate the movement with increased effort. Furthermore, the volitional facilitation or suppression of reflex activity provides another way of uncovering heretofore silent, supraspinal responses. Only detailed assessments of UMN function will provide a true picture of the capacity for motor control in clients with dysfunctional central nervous systems, thereby giving the rehabilitation clinician insight into targeted interventions.

V. Galea, PhD

Effects of Motor Cortex Modulation and Descending Inhibitory Systems on Pain Thresholds in Healthy Subjects

Reidler JS, Mendonca ME, Santana MB, et al (Harvard Med School, Boston, MA; et al)
J Pain 13:450-458, 2012

Pain modulation can be achieved using neuromodulatory tools that influence various levels of the nervous system. Transcranial direct current stimulation (tDCS), for instance, has been shown to reduce chronic pain when applied to the primary motor cortex. In contrast to this central neuromodulatory technique, diffuse noxious inhibitory controls (DNIC) refers to endogenous analgesic mechanisms that decrease pain following the introduction of heterotopic noxious stimuli. We examined whether combining top-down motor cortex modulation using anodal tDCS with a bottom-up DNIC induction paradigm synergistically increases the threshold at which pain is perceived. The pain thresholds of 15 healthy subjects were assessed before and after administration of active tDCS, sham tDCS, cold-water-induced DNIC, and combined tDCS and DNIC. We found that both tDCS and the DNIC paradigm significantly increased pain thresholds and that these approaches appeared to have additive effects. Increase in pain threshold following active tDCS was positively correlated with baseline N-acetylaspartate in the cingulate cortex and negatively correlated with baseline glutamine levels in the thalamus as measured by magnetic resonance spectroscopy. These results suggest that motor cortex modulation may have a greater analgesic effect when combined with bottom-up neuromodulatory mechanisms, presenting new avenues for modulation of pain using noninvasive neuromodulatory approaches.

Perspective.—This article demonstrates that both noninvasive motor cortex modulation and a descending noxious inhibitory controls paradigm significantly increase pain thresholds in healthy subjects and appear to have an additive effect when combined. These results suggest that existing pain therapies involving DNIC may be enhanced through combination with noninvasive brain stimulation.

▶ The experience of pain is a result of modulatory neural network activity that arises in both the central and peripheral nervous systems. It can manifest as a necessary response to a nociceptive stimulus, such as touching a hot stove, or as a persistent tingling or burning sensation in those who experience chronic central pain such as amputees who develop a painful phantom limb. The effective treatment of pain remains an area of intensive investigation, particularly in the management of chronic pain. While pharmaceutical interventions are commonplace, clients often experience habituation to the dosage, necessitating ever-increasing dosages or possibly moving to narcotic medications placing them at higher risk of addiction. The search for noninvasive, nonpharmaceutical pain management strategies continues. In this publication, Reidler and co-workers address the use of neuromodulation with a top-down approach using transcranial direct current stimulation (tDCS)[1] and a bottom-up approach using diffuse noxious inhibitory controls (DNIC). Using these tools, they showed an additive effect in healthy volunteers by increasing the pressure-pain thresholds as measured by a pain algometer. An increase in pain threshold is desirable for the simple reason that greater stimulation is then required to trigger pain pathways. One very interesting aspect of this study (and there are many) is the fact that tDCS applied to the primary motor cortex is an effective pain control. This type of cortical stimulation is pain free and possibly modulates pain through direct cortical effects on thalamic nuclei and more downstream effects on the anterior cingulate and brain stem all via connections to neurons in primary motor cortex.[2] DNIC is also known as conditioned pain modulation and is effective in modulating pain by the introduction of a conditioning stimulus, which triggers descending inhibitory control from areas of the caudal medulla.[3] In the authors' words, this is essentially a situation in which pain inhibits pain. To investigate the relationship between brain metabolites and changes in pain threshold, Reidler and colleagues used magnetic resonance spectroscopy to measure baseline levels of glutamate, glutamine, creatine-phosphocreatine, and other metabolites. While the results of the MRS were in line with expectations, the small number of participants necessitates cautious interpretation. Overall, the encouraging results of this study allow for use of these neuromodulatory tools in patients with chronic pain of both central and peripheral origin.

V. Galea, PhD

References

1. Lang N, Siebner HR, Ward NS, et al. How does transcranial DC stimulation of the primary motor cortex alter regional neural activity in the human brain? *Eur J Neurosci*. 2005;22:495-504.
2. Garcia-Larrea L, Peyron R, Mertens P, et al. Electrical stimulation of motor cortex for pain control: a combined PET-scan and electrophysiological study. *Pain*. 1999; 83:259-273.
3. Le Bars D, Dickenson AH, Besson JM. Diffuse noxious inhibitory controls (DNIC). I. Effects on dorsal horn convergent neurones in the rat. *Pain*. 1979;6:283-304.

Active Video Game Play in Children With Cerebral Palsy: Potential for Physical Activity Promotion and Rehabilitation Therapies
Howcroft J, Klejman S, Fehlings D, et al (Holland Bloorview Kids Rehabilitation Hosp, Toronto, Ontario, Canada)
Arch Phys Med Rehabil 93:1448-1456, 2012

Objective.—To evaluate the potential of active video game (AVG) play for physical activity promotion and rehabilitation therapies in children

TABLE 4.—Summary of AVG Characteristics With Respect to Intensity of Physical Activity, Nature of Movements, Most Active Muscle Groups, Frequency of Movements, and Suitability for Potential Therapeutic Goals

Game	Intensity of Physical Activity	Nature of Movements	Most Active Muscles (Upper Limb)	Movement Frequency	Therapeutic Goals
Boxing	Moderate	Bilateral	WE	High	- Wrist extension/flexion - Wrist medial/lateral deviation - High velocity movements - Hand-eye coordination
DDR	Moderate	Quadrilateral	WE	Low* to medium	- Primarily lower body (balance, strength) - Whole body coordination
Tennis	Light	Unilateral	WE	Medium	- Shoulder abduction/adduction - Wrist extension/flexion - Wrist medial/lateral deviation - Hand-eye coordination
Bowling	Light	Unilateral	WE	Low	- Shoulder flexion/extension - Elbow flexion/extension

*Low frequency is associated with beginner levels similar to those tested in this study.

with cerebral palsy (CP) through a quantitative exploration of energy expenditure, muscle activation, and quality of movement.

Design.—Single-group, experimental study.

Setting.—Human movement laboratory in an urban rehabilitation hospital.

Participants.—Children (N = 17; mean age ± SD, 9.43 ± 1.51y) with CP.

Intervention.—Participants played 4 AVGs (bowling, tennis, boxing, and a dance game).

Main Outcome Measures.—Energy expenditure via a portable cardio-pulmonary testing unit; upper limb muscle activations via single differential surface electrodes; upper limb kinematics via an optical motion capture system; and self-reported enjoyment via the Physical Activity Enjoyment Scale (PACES).

Results.—Moderate levels of physical activity were achieved during the dance (metabolic equivalent for task [MET] = 3.20 ± 1.04) and boxing (MET = 3.36 ± 1.50) games. Muscle activations did not exceed maximum voluntary exertions and were greatest for the boxing AVG and for the wrist extensor bundle. Angular velocities and accelerations were significantly larger in the dominant arm than in the hemiplegic arm during bilateral play. A high level of enjoyment was reported on the PACES (4.5 ± 0.3 out of 5).

Conclusions.—AVG play via a low-cost, commercially available system can offer an enjoyable opportunity for light to moderate physical activity in children with CP. While all games may encourage motor learning to some extent, AVGs can be strategically selected to address specific therapeutic goals (eg, targeted joints, bilateral limb use). Future research is needed to address the challenge of individual variability in movement patterns/play styles. Likewise, further study exploring home use of AVGs for physical activity promotion and rehabilitation therapies, and its functional outcomes, is warranted (Table 4).

▶ There has been a lot of discussion about the value of active videogames in increasing the physical activity of children.[1] Such a concept probably has little merit for those in normal health. The activity is commonly arm swinging or stepping, and the intensity of effort is usually rather low. The healthy child would be better employed enjoying a vigorous game in the sunshine with some friends and learning some skills that could be carried forward into adult life. However, there may be value in active video gaming in conditions such as cerebral palsy, because such children are generally much less active than their peers,[2-4] and the games can potentially be adapted to provide specifically desired forms of exercise and attain certain therapeutic goals (Table 4); for instance, a boxing game can encourage the development of faster wrist movements. Even in cerebral palsy, the level of activity obtained by active gaming is relatively low (typically, 2—3 metabolic equivalents),[5] and this is unlikely to do much to correct obesity or improve poor overall physical condition. Moreover, commercially available equipment was used by the authors, and the children then tended to use the non-spastic limb when playing; there is a need for games that force use of the spastic limb. However, that they enjoyed the games may encourage regularity with this form of exercise.

R. J. Shephard, MD (Lond), PhD, DPE

References

1. Mears D, Hansen L. Active gaming: definitions, options, and implementation. *Strateg J Phys Sport Educ.* 2009;23:1-40.
2. Bandini LG, Curtin C, Hamad C, Tybor DJ, Must A. Prevalence of overweight in children with developmental disorders in the continuous national health and nutrition examination survey (NHANES) 1999-2002. *J Pediatr.* 2005;146:738-743.
3. Hurvitz EA, Green LB, Hornyak JE, Khurana SR, Koch LG. Body mass index measures in children with cerebral palsy related to gross motor function classification: a clinic-based study. *Am J Phys Med Rehabil.* 2008;87:395-403.
4. Rimmer JH. Physical fitness levels of persons with cerebral palsy. *Dev Med Child Neurol.* 2001;43:208-212.
5. Biddiss E, Irwin J. Active video games to promote physical activity in children and youth: a systematic review. *Arch Pediatr Adolesc Med.* 2010;164:664-672.

Exercise and non-alcoholic fatty liver disease: A systematic review and meta-analysis
Keating SE, Hackett DA, George J, et al (Univ of Sydney, Australia)
J Hepatol 57:157-166, 2012

Background & Aims.—Exercise is an integral component of lifestyle intervention aimed at weight loss, but an independent benefit of exercise in NAFLD has also been suggested.

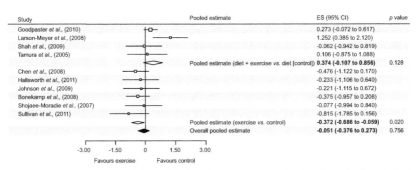

FIGURE 2.—Meta-analysis of the pooled effect of exercise *vs.* control on liver fat with sub-analysis of: the effect of combined exercise and diet *vs.* diet and exercise *vs.* non-exercise control. (Reprinted from Keating SE, Hackett DA, George J, et al. Exercise and non-alcoholic fatty liver disease: a systematic review and meta-analysis. *J Hepatol.* 2012;57:157-166, with permission from European Association for the Study of the Liver.)

Methods.—We aimed to evaluate the efficacy of aerobic exercise and/or progressive resistance training for the modulation of liver fat and alanine aminotransferase (ALT) levels in adults. Relevant databases were searched up to August 2011 for controlled trials, which compared regular exercise *vs.* a non-exercise control on change in liver fat and/or ALT.

Results.—Of the 16,822 studies from the initial search, 12 were included. There was a significant pooled effect size (ES) for the comparison between exercise therapy *vs.* control (ES = −0.37, 95% CI: −0.06 to −0.69; $p = 0.02$), but only when interventions which compared combined exercise and diet *vs.* diet-alone and achieved substantial weight loss, were omitted. The benefit of exercise on liver fat occurred with minimal or no weight loss. There was no effect of exercise alone *vs.* control on ALT (ES = −0.15, 95% CI: 0.14 to −0.45; $p = 0.32$).

Conclusions.—Individual reports of exercise interventions often have low sample sizes and insufficient power to detect clinically meaningful hepatic benefits. By pooling current research, we show clear evidence for a benefit of exercise therapy on liver fat but not ALT levels. This benefit is apparent with minimal or no weight loss and at exercise levels below current exercise recommendations for obesity management. Given the paucity of current treatment options, exercise provides a valid, low-cost therapy for disorders characterised by fatty liver (Fig 2).

▶ Nonalcoholic fatty liver is surprisingly prevalent in developed societies, affecting up to a third of the adult population,[1] mainly those who are obese.[2] Although in general the prognosis is good, the condition can progress to cirrhosis and hepatic carcinoma; it is also a risk factor for insulin resistance and cardiovascular disease. Pharmaceutical options are few. Although thiazolidine-diones reduce liver fat, there are concerns about their safety.[3,4] There is thus growing interest in the potential of exercise to address this condition, given inverse correlations between disease prevalence and activity[5] or physical fitness.[6,7] The present authors carried out a meta-analysis of 12 prospective trials. Data were pooled, despite differences in exercise programs between trials. Some evidence of benefit was found from exercise programs with no added dietary intervention (Fig 2), but there were no parallel changes in serum alanine transferase (ALT) activity. It seems a little surprising that benefit was observed despite little or no weight loss. Further trials are warranted to discover the type and dose of exercise that is most effective and to see if there are still no effects on ALT if patients have higher initial values for this enzyme.

R. J. Shephard, MD (Lond), PhD, DPE

References

1. Szczepaniak LS, Nurenberg P, Leonard D, et al. Magnetic resonance spectroscopy to measure hepatic triglyceride content: prevalence of hepatic steatosis in the general population. *Am J Physiol Endocrinol Metab.* 2005;288:E462-E468.
2. Bellentani S, Saccoccio G, Masutti F, et al. Prevalence of and risk factors for hepatic steatosis in Northern Italy. *Ann Intern Med.* 2000;132:112-117.
3. Sanyal A, Chalasani N, Kowdley K, et al. Pioglitazone, vitamin E, or placebo for nonalcoholic steatohepatitis. *N Engl J Med.* 2010;362:1675-1685.
4. Musso G, Gambino R, Cassader M, et al. A meta-analysis of randomized trials for the treatment of nonalcoholic fatty liver disease. *Hepatology.* 2010;52:79-104.
5. Perseghin G, Lattuada G, De Cobelli F, et al. Habitual physical activity is associated with intrahepatic fat content in humans. *Diabetes Care.* 2007;30:683-688.
6. Nguyen-Duy T-B, Nichaman MZ, Church TS, et al. Visceral fat and liver fat are independent predictors of metabolic risk factors in men. *Am J Physiol Endocrinol Metab.* 2003;284:E1065-E1071.
7. Kantartzis K, Thamer C, Peter A, et al. High cardiorespiratory fitness is an independent predictor of the reduction in liver fat during a lifestyle intervention in non-alcoholic fatty liver disease. *Gut.* 2009;58:1281-1288.

Physical Activity as a Protective Factor in Relapse Following Smoking Cessation in Participants with a Depressive Disorder

Bernard P, Ninot G, Guillaume S, et al (Univ of Montpellier, France; Inserm U1061, Montpellier, France)
Am J Addict 21:348-355, 2012

The factors predicting smoking abstinence in depressive smokers, and the role of physical activity in precessation, were investigated. One hundred thirty-three smokers with current major depressive disorders (score ≥ 10 on the Depression subscale of Hospital Anxiety and Depression Scale) were recruited from a large prospective cohort of smokers ($n = 1,119$). Over a maximum period of 3 years, regression modeling, adjusted for potential confounders, showed that physical activity was associated with relapse (relapse rate $= 0.54$, 95% confidence interval $= 0.34-0.85, p = .008$). Also, antidepressants, anxiolytics, level of education, and number of attempts to quit were associated with relapse. The protective role of physical activity on relapse rate could be a modifiable factor in smoking cessation for smokers with depressive disorders.

▶ The prevention of relapse in former smokers must be one of the most discouraging tasks facing a physician. The problem is even more difficult if there is an associated depression. The prevalence of smoking among French psychiatric patients was as high as 59% in 2002.[1] Smokers with depressive disorders also smoke more and are more likely to be dependent.[2] Moreover, those with depression are more likely to show recidivism.[3,4] There is some evidence that physical activity increases the likelihood of successful smoking cessation in healthy individuals.[5,6] These authors tested, over a 3-year period, the value of exercise in helping smoking cessation in a relatively small cross-sectional study of individuals with severe depression. The initial cessation program was a standard combination of counseling and pharmacotherapy. The assessment of continued abstinence from smoking is a little suspect, since it was based on telephone reports rather than carbon monoxide or cotinine determinations. Although relapses were apparently less frequent in those who were physically active, no exercise program was instituted, and this seems a major weakness in the study, since it could be that a lower level of depression in some individuals allowed both physical activity and successful smoking cessation.

R. J. Shephard, MD (Lond), PhD, DPE

References

1. Poirier MF, Canceil O, Baylé F, et al. Prevalence of smoking in psychiatric patients. *Prog Neuropsychopharmacol Biol Psychiatr.* 2002;26:529-537.
2. Trosclair A, Dube SR. Smoking among adults reporting lifetime depression, anxiety, anxiety with depression, and major depressive episode, United States, 2005–2006. *Addict Behav.* 2010;35:438-443.
3. Cinciripini PM, Wetter DW, Fouladi RT, et al. The effects of depressed mood on smoking cessation: mediation by postcessation self-efficacy. *J Consult Clin Psychol.* 2003;71:292-301.
4. Niaura R, Britt DM, Shadel WG, Goldstein M, Abrams D, Brown R. Symptoms of depression and survival experience among three samples of smokers trying to quit. *Psychol Addict Behav.* 2001;15:13-17.
5. Paavola M, Vartiainen E, Puska P. Smoking cessation between teenage years and adulthood. *Health Educ Res.* 2001;16:49-57.
6. Ussher M, Taylor A, Faulkner G. Exercise interventions for smoking cessation. *Cochrane Database Syst Rev.* 2008;(4):CD002295.

Effect of exercise on depression severity in older people: systematic review and meta-analysis of randomised controlled trials
Bridle C, Spanjers K, Patel S, et al (Univ of Warwick, Coventry, UK)
Br J Psychiatry 201:180-185, 2012

Background.—The prevelance of depression in older people is high, treatment is inadequate, it creates a substantial burden and is a public health priority for which exercise has been proposed as a therapeutic strategy.

Aims.—To estimate the effect of exercise on depressive symptoms among older people, and assess whether treatment effect varies depending on the depression criteria used to determine participant eligibility.

Method.—Systematic review and meta-analysis of randomised controlled trials of exercise for depression in older people.

| Study or subgroup | Excercise | | | Control | | | SMD | SMD |
	Mean	s.d.	Total	Mean	s.d.	Total	IV, Random, 95% CI	IV, Random, 95% CI
Chou (2004)[23]	15.3	9.8	7	39.1	9.7	7	−2.29 (−3.73 to −0.84)	
Tsang (2006)[24]	3.4	2.5	48	5.7	1.5	34	−1.06 (−1.53 to −0.59)	
Singh (2001)[18]	9.2	2.8	15	11	2.36	14	−0.67 (−1.43 to 0.08)	
Mather (2002)[20]	11.5	3.3	42	13.7	3.3	43	−0.66 (−1.10 to −0.22)	
Brenes (2007)[16]	4.5	2.9	14	6.3	3.5	12	−0.55 (−1.33 to 0.24)	
Clechanowski (2004)[17]	0.82	0.62	72	1.01	0.46	66	−0.34 (−0.68 to −0.01)	
Williams (2008)[19]	9.7	6.6	16	11.8	8.1	12	−0.28 (−1.03 to 0.47)	
Kerse (2010)[22]	2.4	2.2	94	2.8	2.2	87	−0.18 (−0.47 to 0.11)	
Sims (2006)[21]	11.5	6.7	14	11.9	4.9	18	−0.07 (−0.77 to 0.63)	

-2 -1 0 1 2
Favours excercise   Favours control

FIGURE 2.—Trial-level data, effect estimates and forest plots for depression severity. SMD, standard mean difference. (Reprinted from Bridle C, Spanjers K, Patel S, et al. Effect of exercise on depression severity in older people: systematic review and meta-analysis of randomised controlled trials. *Br J Psychiatry*. 2012;201:180-185, with permission from the Royal College of Psychiatrists.)

Results.—Nine trials met the inclusion criteria and seven were meta-analysed. Exercise was associated with significantly lower depression severity (standardised mean difference (SMD) = −0.34, 95% CI −0.52 to −0.17), irrespective of whether participant eligibility was determined by clinical diagnosis (SMD = −0.38, 95% CI −0.67 to −0.10) or symptom checklist (SMD = −0.34, 95% CI −0.62 to −0.06). Results remained significant in sensitivity analyses.

Conclusions.—Our findings suggest that, for older people who present with clinically meaningful symptoms of depression, prescribing structured exercise tailored to individual ability will reduce depression severity (Fig 2).

▶ There have been many reports suggesting that exercise programs are helpful for people with depression, but often the evidence has been cross-sectional in type; mood-state may then influence exercise participation, rather than the converse. The study of Bridle et al is a meta-analysis that is restricted to 7 randomized controlled trials in patients > 60 years, and significant benefit is found from individually prescribed exercise programs over a follow-up > 3 months (Fig 2). The standardized mean difference (SMD) of 0.34 is equivalent to 63% of exercisers having a lower depression score than controls at the end of the study, and 13% of the exercisers doing better than expected. This is roughly equivalent to what might be expected from psychotherapy[1] or use of antidepressant medication.[2] The basis of exercise was quite varied; endurance or strength training, or even tai chi, usually three to five 30- to 45-minute sessions per week. There are at least 3 qualifications to these findings. One possibility is that participation in the exercise group provided additional social contacts, and only some of the studies included in the meta-analysis attempted to provide equal social contacts for the control group. A second potential source of bias is that the more severely depressed patients tend to drop out of the exercise program, and not all of the trials based their analyses on "intention to treat." Finally, there may have been a publication bias favoring positive outcomes. Nevertheless, an average benefit matching that obtained from drugs or psychotherapy merits serious consideration.

R. J. Shephard, MD (Lond), PhD, DPE

References

1. Cuijpers P, van Straten A, Bohlmeijer E, Hollon SD, Andersson G. The effects of psychotherapy for adult depression are overestimated: a meta-analysis of study quality and effect size. *Psychol Med.* 2010;40:211-223.
2. Taylor D, Meader N, Bird V, Pilling S, Creed F, Goldberg D. Pharmacological interventions for people with depression and chronic physical health problems: systematic review and meta-analyses of safety and efficacy. *Br J Psychiatry.* 2011;198:179-188.

Relationship between Physical Activity and Brain Atrophy Progression

Yuki A, Lee S, Kim H, et al (Natl Ctr for Geriatrics and Gerontology, Obu city, Aichi prefecture, Japan; Tokaigakuen Univ, Miyoshi, Aichi Prefecture, Japan; et al)
Med Sci Sports Exerc 44:2362-2368, 2012

Introduction.—Brain atrophy is associated with impairment in cognitive function and learning function. The aim of this study was to determine whether daily physical activity prevents age-related brain atrophy progression.

Methods.—The participants were 381 men and 393 women who had participated in both the baseline and the follow-up surveys (mean duration = 8.2 yr). Magnetic resonance imaging of the frontal and temporal lobes was performed at the time of the baseline and follow-up surveys. The daily physical activities and total energy expenditures of the participants were recorded at baseline with uniaxial accelerometry sensors. Multiple logistic regression models were fit to determine the association between activity energy expenditure, number of steps, and total energy expenditure variables and frontal and temporal lobe atrophy progression while controlling for possible confounders.

Results.—In male participants, the odds ratio of frontal lobe atrophy progression for the fifth quintile compared with the first quintile in activity energy expenditure was 3.408 (95% confidence interval = 1.205−9.643) and for the number of steps was 3.651 (95% confidence interval = 1.304−10.219). Men and women with low total energy expenditure were at risk for frontal lobe atrophy progression. There were no significant differences between temporal lobe atrophy progression and physical activity or total energy expenditure.

Conclusion.—The results indicate that physical activity and total energy expenditure are significant predictors of frontal lobe atrophy progression during an 8-yr period. Promoting participation in activities may be beneficial for attenuating age-related frontal lobe atrophy and for preventing dementia (Table 4).

▶ The volume of gray matter in the brain decreases by about 15% from young adult life through to the 70s,[1] and the cumulative loss of brain tissue seems particularly marked in those with Alzheimer's disease.[2] Thus, magnetic resonance imaging (MRI) of the brain may offer a noninvasive quantitative method of

TABLE 4.—Adjusted Odds Ratios of Frontal and Temporal Lobe Atrophy Progression in Male Participants Distributed into Quintiles of Physical Activity and Total Energy Expenditure Data

	Quintile 1	Quintile 2	Odds Ratio, 95% CI Quintile 3	Quintile 4	Quintile 5
Frontal lobe (*n*)	76	76	76	76	77
Activity energy expenditure (kcal·d^{-1})	3.408, 1.205–9.643 (<143.2)	1.054, 0.321–3.462 (143.2 to <184.4)	1.623, 0.523–5.035 (184.4 to <226.2)	2.054, 0.691–6.904 (226.2 to <284.4)	1.00, referent (≥284.4)
No. of step per day	3.651, 1.304–10.219 (<5736.0)	1.216, 0.383–3.863 (5736.0 to <6955.0)	1.487, 0.471–4.689 (6955.0 to <8261.4)	2.403, 0.819–7.052 (8261.4 to <10,407.4)	1.00, referent (≥10,407.4)
Total energy expenditure (kcal·d^{-1})	4.816, 1.037–22.376 (<1771.4)	2.758, 0.652–11.672 (1771.4 to <1897.4)	4.639, 1.191–18.067 (1897.4 to <1983.4)	2.275, 0.553–9.358 (1983.4 to <2091.2)	1.00, referent (≥2091.2)
Temporal lobe (*n*)	76	76	76	76	77
Activity energy expenditure (kcal·d^{-1})	1.015, 0.473–2.178 (<143.2)	1.293, 0.617–2.708 (143.2 to <184.4)	0.800, 0.364–1.756 (184.4 to <226.2)	0.845, 0.390–1.833 (226.2 to <284.4)	1.00, referent (≥284.4)
No. of step per day	0.938, 0.435–2.024 (<5736.0)	1.100, 0.519–2.330 (5736.0 to <6955.0)	1.142, 0.538–2.425 (6955.0 to <8261.4)	1.123, 0.528–2.389 (8261.4 to <10,407.4)	1.00, referent (≥10,407.4)
Total energy expenditure (kcal·d^{-1})	1.045, 0.388–2.816 (<1771.4)	1.303, 0.554–3.065 (1771.4 to <1897.4)	1.229, 0.537–2.810 (1897.4 to <1983.4)	1.006, 0.439–2.307 (1983.4 to <2091.2)	1.00, referent (≥2091.2)

Odds ratios were controlled for age, BMI, education history, medical history (stroke, ischemic heart disease, hypertension, hyperlipidemia, and diabetes), current smoking, and alcohol intake in a multinomial logistic regression model.

assessing lifestyle factors that are reputed to slow the deterioration of mental function with aging, including a regular exercise program.[3,4] Yuki et al tested the benefits of physical activity over an 8-year follow-up of a substantial sample of 381 men and 393 women, with a 4-grade assessment of the degree of atrophy as seen in the frontal and temporal lobes.[5,6] Habitual physical activity patterns were assessed by uniaxial accelerometer over a 7-day period (which is rather short for obtaining representative data in the elderly). Whether activity was expressed as the number of steps taken per day, the total active energy expenditure, or the total energy expenditure per day, active individuals had substantial protection against frontal (but not temporal) lobe atrophy over the 8 years, even when data were standardized for body mass index (Table 4). Further studies are needed to examine the influence of differences in habitual physical activity on the amyloid content of the brain lobes as seen at postmortem examination. However, the data of Yuki et al certainly support the value of regular exercise as a means of conserving brain function in the elderly.

R. J. Shephard, MD (Lond), PhD, DPE

References

1. Taki Y, Kinomura S, Sato K, Goto R, Kawashima R, Fukuda H. A longitudinal study of gray matter volume decline with age and modifying factors. *Neurobiol Aging.* 2011;32:907-915.
2. Killiany RJ, Gomez-Isla T, Moss M, et al. Use of structural magnetic resonance imaging to predict who will get Alzheimer's disease. *Ann Neurol.* 2000;47: 430-439.
3. Boyke J, Driemeyer J, Gaser C, Büchel C, May A. Training-induced brain structure changes in the elderly. *J Neurosci.* 2008;28:7031-7035.
4. Draganski B, May A. Training-induced structural changes in the adult human brain. *Behav Brain Res.* 2008;192:137-142.
5. Manolio TA, Kronmal RA, Burke GL, et al. Magnetic resonance abnormalities and cardiovascular disease in older adults. The Cardiovascular Health Study. *Stroke.* 1994;25:318-327.
6. Middleton LE, Manini TM, Simonsick EM, et al. Activity energy expenditure and incident cognitive impairment in older adults. *Arch Intern Med.* 2011;171: 1251-1257.

Exercise and Mental Illness: Results From the National Epidemiologic Survey on Alcohol and Related Conditions (NESARC)
Dakwar E, Blanco C, Lin K-H, et al (Columbia Univ, NY; et al)
J Clin Psychiatry 73:960-966, 2012

Background.—Regular exercise is thought to be associated with low rates of mental illness, but this association has been inadequately studied. The purpose of this study was to test the hypotheses that the recommended amount of self-reported vigorous exercise would be cross-sectionally associated with reduced prevalence and incidence of various *DSM-IV* psychiatric disorders, as well as increased rates of remission.

Method.—Data were collected from 2001 to 2005 as part of the National Epidemiologic Survey on Alcohol and Related Conditions (NESARC),

TABLE 2.—Prevalence of Psychiatric Disorders in the 3 Exercise Groups at Wave 2 (N = 23,505) and Comparisons[a,b]

Disorder	Public Health Dose (n = 8,871; % = 37.74)		Some Exercise (n = 7,683; % = 32.69)		No Exercise (n = 6,951; % = 29.57)		Public Health Dose vs No Exercise (ref)			Some Exercise vs No Exercise (ref)		
	%	SEM	%	SEM	%	SEM	AOR[b]	CI		AOR[b]	CI	
Any Axis I disorder	37.57	0.83	36.21	0.76	31.68	0.95	1.22	1.12	1.34	1.24	1.13	1.35
Any substance use disorder	25.68	0.77	23.69	0.68	18.95	0.80	1.16	1.08	1.33	1.26	1.14	1.42
Alcohol abuse	7.52	0.36	6.82	0.37	4.25	0.33	1.17	0.99	1.38	1.16	1.01	1.42
Alcohol dependence	6.12	0.33	5.23	0.32	3.45	0.26	1.35	1.12	1.66	1.38	1.12	1.69
Drug abuse	2.19	0.19	2.02	0.19	1.46	0.23	0.99	0.68	1.44	1.14	0.78	1.66
Drug dependence	1.01	0.16	0.84	0.13	0.58	0.12	1.51	0.89	2.56	1.58	0.93	2.70
Nicotine dependence	15.34	0.64	14.63	0.59	12.99	0.66	1.13	1.00	1.29	1.23	1.08	1.37
Any depressive disorder	5.27	0.32	5.84	0.32	6.21	0.37	0.96	0.81	1.15	1.01	0.84	1.18
Major depressive disorder	5.04	0.29	5.71	0.32	5.87	0.36	0.96	0.82	1.15	1.03	0.86	1.24
Dysthymia	0.69	0.13	0.36	0.07	0.89	0.13	0.94	0.61	1.49	0.49	0.29	0.83
Any bipolar disorder	4.13	0.28	3.53	0.25	3.08	0.27	1.48	1.18	1.86	1.33	1.05	1.69
Bipolar I	2.88	0.22	2.63	0.23	2.48	0.25	1.27	0.97	1.65	1.23	0.92	1.65
Bipolar II	1.25	0.15	0.86	0.13	0.58	0.09	2.29	1.39	3.76	1.74	1.06	2.72
Any anxiety disorder	12.23	0.48	12.81	0.48	12.04	0.53	1.13	0.99	1.29	1.14	1.00	1.33
Panic disorder	2.35	0.21	2.51	0.21	2.28	0.21	1.14	0.86	1.51	1.19	0.93	1.53
Social phobia	2.21	0.19	2.83	0.25	2.31	0.22	0.98	0.76	1.27	1.29	0.98	1.69
Specific phobia	7.22	0.39	7.89	0.41	7.45	0.43	1.11	0.94	1.29	1.15	0.98	1.35
Generalized anxiety disorder	3.4	0.28	3.57	0.28	3.42	0.31	1.16	0.91	1.51	1.15	0.87	1.51

Abbreviation: AOR = adjusted odds ratio, ref = reference.
[a]Shaded areas represent associations in which the CI does not cross 1.
[b]Adjusted for significant sociodemographic variables: sex, race, nativity, age, education, individual income, employment status, and marital status.

a 2-wave face-to-face survey conducted by the National Institute on Alcohol Abuse and Alcoholism. For this study, the sample consisted of 23,505 nondisabled adults aged between 18 and 65 years.

Results.—Individuals who engaged in vigorous exercise at Wave 2 were significantly more likely than were nonexercisers to be diagnosed with a current psychiatric disorder (adjusted odds ratio [AOR] = 1.22, 95% CI, 1.12−1.34 for the nationally recommended amount vs no exercise), significantly less likely to attain remission from a psychiatric disorder between waves (AOR = 0.77, 95% CI, 0.65−0.91), and significantly more likely to relapse or be newly diagnosed with a psychiatric disorder between waves (AOR = 1.15, 95% CI, 1.02−1.30). Alcohol dependence and bipolar II disorder were the disorders most strongly associated with exercise.

Conclusions.—This investigation suggests that the pursuit of vigorous exercise is associated with a vulnerability to mental illness. This surprising finding may be due to reward-related factors that influence both exercise engagement and the expression of certain psychiatric disorders. Prospective trials will be helpful in further clarifying the associations between exercise and mental illness, as the relationships between the 2 are more complex than previously believed (Table 2).

▶ The positive association between engagement in vigorous exercise and psychiatric disorder reported here is, at first inspection, quite surprising, particularly because several previous reports have suggested negative associations between exercise and conditions such as anxiety and depression.[1] However, there has been at least 1 previous cross-sectional report that exercise had little positive influence on the prevalence of substance abuse disorders.[2] A simple questionnaire was used in the present study, and it focused specifically on vigorous activity sufficient to cause heavy sweating or large increases in heart rate or breathing. It was this criterion, rather than moderate physical activity, that was used to determine if people were meeting current public health recommendations for exercise. Although there was a small positive association between such vigorous exercise and the prevalence of depression and bipolar disorders, there was a much larger association between vigorous exercise and substance abuse (Table 2). One possible factor may be the partying that follows participation in some team sports. It is also possible that vigorous activity, by producing opioids,[3,4] stimulates the same reward centers that are activated by drugs, or it could even be that the psychiatric disorder modifies the individual's response to the questionnaire. It is certainly surprising that 38% of the sample claimed to be taking the US recommendation for vigorous exercise. Before too much significance is attached to this report, there is a need for more longitudinal observations looking at the impact of exercise on substance abuse.

R. J. Shephard, MD (Lond), PhD, DPE

References

1. Carek PJ, Laibstein SE, Carek SM. Exercise for the treatment of depression and anxiety. *Int J Psychiatr Med.* 2011;41:15-28.
2. Goodwin RD. Association between physical activity and mental disorders among adults in the United States. *Prev Med.* 2003;36:698-703.
3. Boecker H, Sprenger T, Spilker ME, et al. The runner's high: opiodergic mechanisms in the human brain. *Cereb Cortex.* 2008;18:2523-2531.
4. Dietrich A, McDaniel WF. Endocannaboids and exercise. *Br J Sports Med.* 2004; 38:536-541.

The Association Between Physical Activity and the Risk of Incident Psoriasis
Frankel HC, Han J, Li T, et al (Brigham and Women's Hosp and Harvard Med School, Boston, MA)
Arch Dermatol 148:918-924, 2012

Objective.—To examine the association between total physical activity, walking, and vigorous exercise and the incidence of psoriasis in women.

Design.—Cohort study.

Setting.—The Nurses' Health Study II, a cohort of 116 430 women aged 27 to 44 years in 1991.

Participants.—The study population included 86 655 US female nurses who reported whether they had ever been diagnosed as having psoriasis and who completed detailed physical activity questionnaires in 1991, 1997, and 2001. We excluded participants with a history of psoriasis prior to 1991.

Main Outcome Measures.—Risk of psoriasis by quintile of physical activity as measured by a metabolic equivalent task score.

Results.—We documented 1026 incident psoriasis cases during 1 195 703 person-years of follow-up (14 years, 1991-2005). After adjusting for age, smoking, and alcohol use, increasing physical activity was

TABLE 3.—Age-Adjusted and Multivariate RRs for Confirmed Incident Psoriasis by Amount and Type of Physical Activity[a]

Variable	No. of Incident Cases of Psoriasis	Age Adjusted RR (95% CI)	Age Adjusted P Value for Trend	Multivariate[b] RR (95% CI)	Multivariate[b] P Value for Trend	Multivariate[b,c] RR (95% CI)	Multivariate[b,c] P Value for Trend
Physical activity, MET-hours/wk[d]							
0.2-3.8	118	1 [Reference]		1 [Reference]		1 [Reference]	
3.9-9.0	125	1.06 (0.82-1.36)		1.07 (0.83-1.38)		1.14 (0.88-1.46)	
9.1-16.9	131	1.10 (0.86-1.42)	<.001	1.12 (0.87-1.44)	.001	1.25 (0.97-1.61)	.08
17.0-31.8	104	0.87 (0.67-1.14)		0.89 (0.68-1.16)		1.02 (0.78-1.33)	
≥31.9	72	0.62 (0.46-0.83)		0.62 (0.46-0.84)		0.75 (0.56-1.02)	
Vigorous activity, MET-hours/wk[d,e]							
None	167	1 [Reference]		1 [Reference]		1 [Reference]	
0.1-4.5	72	0.72 (0.54-0.95)		0.73 (0.55-0.96)		0.75 (0.57-1.00)	
4.6-9.7	122	0.89 (0.70-1.13)	<.001	0.88 (0.69-1.11)	.002	0.91 (0.72-1.16)	.03
9.8-20.8	115	0.84 (0.66-1.07)		0.84 (0.66-1.08)		0.91 (0.71-1.16)	
≥20.9	74	0.56 (0.42-0.73)		0.57 (0.43-0.76)		0.64 (0.48-0.86)	

Abbreviations: MET, metabolic equivalent task; RR, relative risk.
[a]Incident psoriasis was confirmed using the Psoriasis Screening Tool.
[b]Adjusted for age, smoking (never, past, or current, including 1-14, 15-34, or ≥35 cigarettes per day), and alcohol intake in quintiles of drinks per week (none, 0.1-0.3, 0.4-0.7, 0.8-1.1, 1.2-2.3, and ≥2.4).
[c]Adjusted for body mass index (calculated as weight in kilograms divided by height in meters squared) (<21.0, 21.0-22.9, 23.0-24.9, 25.0-27.4, 27.5-29.9, 30.0-34.9, and ≥35.0).
[d]Calculated by multiplying the MET score by the participant's reported activity in hours per week.
[e]Defined as at least 6 METs per hour.

inversely associated with the risk of psoriasis. The most physically active quintile of women had a lower multivariate relative risk (RR) of psoriasis (0.72 [95% CI, 0.59-0.89; $P < .001$ for trend]) compared with the least active quintile. Vigorous physical activity (≥ 6 metabolic equivalents) was associated with a reduced risk of psoriasis (multivariate RR for the highest quintile, 0.66 [95% CI, 0.54-0.81; $P < .001$ for trend]); this association remained significant after adjusting for body mass index (RR, 0.73 [95% CI, 0.60-0.90; $P = .009$ for trend]). Walking was not associated with psoriasis risk. In a subset of 550 confirmed psoriasis cases, we observed a similarly reduced risk of psoriasis associated with vigorous physical activity (multivariate RR for the highest quintile, 0.64 [95% CI, 0.48-0.86; $P = .03$ for trend]).

Conclusion.—In this study of US women, vigorous physical activity is independently associated with a reduced risk of incident psoriasis (Table 3).

▶ Psoriasis is a troublesome condition. The fairly strong negative association with vigorous activity (but not with walking) seen in a large-scale prospective trial is a new finding, and it points to a potential suggestion the physician can offer patients who are affected with this condition. The main weakness in this study is reliance on self-reports of psoriasis. The amount of exercise linked to a 30% reduction in risk is not impossible to achieve: 21 metabolic equivalents hours per week, equivalent to 105 minutes of running or 180 minutes of swimming, and this would confer many other health benefits in addition to a possible reduction in the risk of psoriasis. It is less clear whether the relation to vigorous exercise is a causal one. Although psoriasis is associated with a high body mass index,[1] it is also positively associated with smoking[2] and alcohol intake,[3] which are harbingers of an overall poor lifestyle. However, the association with vigorous activity does not seem to be weakened by statistical adjustment for smoking and alcohol intake (Table 3). One possible mechanism of benefit might be a modulation of chronic inflammatory processes by vigorous exercise (ie, a lowering of concentrations of proinflammatory cytokines such as tumor necrosis factor).[4] Alternatively, exercise might act through an elevation of mood state.

R. J. Shephard, MD (Lond), PhD, DPE

References

1. Setty AR, Curhan G, Choi HK. Obesity, waist circumference, weight change, and the risk of psoriasis in women: Nurses' Health Study II. *Arch Intern Med.* 2007; 167:1670-1675.
2. Setty AR, Curhan G, Choi HK. Smoking and the risk of psoriasis in women: Nurses' Health Study II. *Am J Med.* 2007;120:953-959.
3. Qureshi AA, Dominguez PL, Choi HK, Han J, Curhan G. Alcohol intake and risk of incident psoriasis in US women: a prospective study. *Arch Dermatol.* 2010;146: 1364-1369.
4. Kondo T, Kobayashi I, Murakami M. Effect of exercise on circulating adipokine levels in obese young women. *Endocr J.* 2006;53:189-195.

The Association Between Physical Activity and the Risk of Incident Psoriasis
Frankel HC, Han J, Li T, et al (Brigham and Women's Hosp and Harvard Med School, Boston, MA)
Arch Dermatol 148:918-924, 2012

Objective.—To examine the association between total physical activity, walking, and vigorous exercise and the incidence of psoriasis in women.

Design.—Cohort study.

Setting.—The Nurses' Health Study II, a cohort of 116 430 women aged 27 to 44 years in 1991.

Participants.—The study population included 86 655 US female nurses who reported whether they had ever been diagnosed as having psoriasis and who completed detailed physical activity questionnaires in 1991, 1997, and 2001. We excluded participants with a history of psoriasis prior to 1991.

Main Outcome Measures.—Risk of psoriasis by quintile of physical activity as measured by a metabolic equivalent task score.

Results.—We documented 1026 incident psoriasis cases during 1 195 703 person-years of follow-up (14 years, 1991-2005). After adjusting for age, smoking, and alcohol use, increasing physical activity was inversely associated with the risk of psoriasis. The most physically active quintile of women had a lower multivariate relative risk (RR) of psoriasis (0.72 [95% CI, 0.59-0.89; $P < .001$ for trend]) compared with the least active quintile. Vigorous physical activity (≥ 6 metabolic equivalents) was associated with a reduced risk of psoriasis (multivariate RR for the highest quintile, 0.66 [95% CI, 0.54-0.81; $P < .001$ for trend]); this association remained significant after adjusting for body mass index (RR, 0.73 [95% CI, 0.60-0.90; $P = .009$ for trend]). Walking was not associated with psoriasis risk. In a subset of 550 confirmed psoriasis cases, we observed a similarly reduced risk of psoriasis associated with vigorous physical activity (multivariate RR for the highest quintile, 0.64 [95% CI, 0.48-0.86; $P = .03$ for trend]).

Conclusion.—In this study of US women, vigorous physical activity is independently associated with a reduced risk of incident psoriasis.

▶ Psoriasis is a common skin condition that causes skin redness, irritation, and thick skin with flaky, silver-white patches. Psoriasis is considered an immunologic disorder with systemic inflammation. Risk factors for psoriasis include higher body mass index (BMI), adult weight gain, high alcohol intake, and smoking.[1] Previous studies have been unclear regarding the role of physical activity in psoriasis prevention. In this study of US women, participation in at least 20.9 MET-hours per week of vigorous exercise (equivalent to 105 minutes of running) was associated with a 25% to 30% reduced risk of psoriasis. The association between vigorous activity and psoriasis risk remained significant after adjustment for BMI. This amount of vigorous activity is roughly equivalent to the current US Department of Health and Human Services recommendation for greater health benefits. The authors speculated that systemic inflammation is related to psoriasis and is best reduced through vigorous exercise. Stressful life events are associated with new-onset psoriasis and may trigger psoriasis. Psychological stress may affect psoriasis via immune system modulation. Correspondingly, the authors surmised that the protective benefits of physical activity on psoriasis could be mediated through its effect on mood. Exercise decreases anxiety, stress, and depression, and improves emotional well-being.

D. C. Nieman, DrPH

Reference

1. Menter A, Griffiths CE, Tebbey PW, Horn EJ, Sterry W; International Psoriasis Council. Exploring the association between cardiovascular and other disease-related risk factors in the psoriasis population: the need for increased understanding across the medical community. *J Eur Acad Dermatol Venereol.* 2010;24:1371-1377.

Lack of Endogenous Pain Inhibition During Exercise in People With Chronic Whiplash Associated Disorders: An Experimental Study

Van Oosterwijck J, Nijs J, Meeus M, et al (Vrije Universiteit Brussel, Belgium; et al)
J Pain 13:242-254, 2012

A controlled experimental study was performed to examine the efficacy of the endogenous pain inhibitory systems and whether this (mal)functioning is associated with symptom increases following exercise in patients with chronic whiplash-associated disorders (WAD). In addition, 2 types of exercise were compared. Twenty-two women with chronic WAD and 22 healthy controls performed a submaximal and a self-paced, physiologically limited exercise test on a cycle ergometer with cardiorespiratory monitoring on 2 separate occasions. Pain pressure thresholds (PPT), health status, and activity levels were assessed in response to the 2 exercise bouts. In chronic WAD, PPT decreased following submaximal exercise, whereas they increased in healthy subjects. The same effect was established in response to the self-paced, physiologically limited exercise, with exception of the PPT at the calf which increased. A worsening of the chronic WAD symptom complex was reported post-exercise. Fewer symptoms were reported in response to the self-paced, physiologically limited exercise. These observations suggest abnormal central pain processing during exercise in patients with chronic WAD. Submaximal exercise triggers post-exertional malaise, while a self-paced and physiologically limited exercise will trigger less severe symptoms, and therefore seems more appropriate for chronic WAD patients.

Perspective.—The results from this exercise study suggest impaired endogenous pain inhibition during exercise in people with chronic WAD. This finding highlights the fact that one should be cautious when evaluating

TABLE 1.—Changes in Health Status in Response to Submaximal Exercise in Patients With Chronic WAD (n = 22) and Healthy Sedentary Control Subjects (n = 22)

	Chronic WAD Patients (Mean ± Standard Deviation)	Control Subjects (Mean ± Standard Deviation)	Between-Groups Comparison (F-Value; P Value)
Pain (mm)			
Pre-exercise	50.7 ± 26.7	18.4 ± 22.7* ●	
Post-exercise	62.2 ± 28.6	15.4 ± 20.5* ●	6.8; .013[‡]
24 hours post-exercise	54.9 ± 31.2	9.0 ± 10.7* ●	3.4; .038[‡]
Headache (mm)			
Pre-exercise	25.0 ± 31.2	5.7 ± 14.3	
Post-exercise	34.7 ± 33.9	6.5 ± 11.6	5.6; .023[‡]
24 hours post-exercise	35.2 ± 32.7	4.6 ± 13.8	3.0; .057
Sore throat (mm)			
Pre-exercise	13.2 ± 22.2	6.6 ± 15.1	
Post-exercise	15.6 ± 24.2	4.3 ± 8.1	2.8; .100
24 hours post-exercise	14.3 ± 25.6	2.8 ± 5.0	2.4; .095
Fatigue (mm)			
Pre-exercise	54.2 ± 25.3	27.2 ± 24.2	
Post-exercise	61.6 ± 30.6	16.9 ± 17.0	13.5; .001[‡]
24 hours post-exercise	54.9 ± 35.0	15.8 ± 17.6	4.3; .016[‡]
Fatigue after physical activity (mm)			
Pre-exercise	57.9 ± 30.8	27.1 ± 21.3	
Post-exercise	65.2 ± 31.4	13.8 ± 13.1	7.9; .008[‡]
24 hours post-exercise	62.0 ± 32.3	15.9 ± 20.5	4.0; .022[‡]
Symptom severity total score (mm)			
Pre-exercise	42.0 ± 20.5	14.5 ± 9.7	
Post-exercise	44.8 ± 22.9	10.9 ± 8.2	11.5; .002[‡]
24 hours post-exercise	41.7 ± 23.8	8.9 ± 8.4	4.8; .011[‡]
SF-36[†] bodily pain			
Pre-exercise	44.2 ± 21.6	81.6 ± 21.2	
Post-exercise	40.6 ± 21.6	89.8 ± 27.0	5.5; .024[‡]
24 hours post-exercise	40.1 ± 22.9	83.1 ± 19.3	3.3; .042[‡]
SF-36 general health			
Pre-exercise	32.8 ± 19.7	54.8 ± 16.2	
Post-exercise	33.4 ± 22.2	54.1 ± 16.6	.268; .607
24 hours post-exercise	28.9 ± 21.0	53.4 ± 18.7	1.6; .218

*Time × group interaction effects were examined using 2-factor repeated measures ANOVA with group (chronic WAD and controls) and time (pre- and post-exercise) as factors.
● Time × group interaction effects were examined using 2-factor repeated measures ANOVA with group (chronic WAD and controls) and time (pre-exercise, post-exercise, 24 hours post-exercise) as factors.
[†] Medical Outcomes Short Form 36 Health Status Survey.
[‡] Statistically significant results.

and recommending exercise in people with chronic WAD, and that the use of more individual, targeted exercise therapies is recommended (Table 1).

▶ The treatment of chronic pain is a dilemma for many physicians. Whiplash is one of the more common causes with up to 50% of patients showing long-lasting symptoms,[1,2] with major economic implications.[3] When the pain becomes chronic, the problem often reflects abnormal central processing of information rather than persisting anatomic abnormalities of the spine.[4,5] All too often, however, the prescription of pain-relieving medications such as oxytocin leads to an addiction that is difficult to resolve. The potential to profit from an exercise-induced secretion of endorphins is thus an interesting possibility. In normal individuals, vigorous exercise (at least 75% of maximal oxygen intake) increases pain thresholds, probably through an opioid-linked descending inhibition of symptoms.[6] Unfortunately, as the study of Oosterwijk and colleagues demonstrates, this does not seem to happen following a whiplash injury; instead, a prescribed submaximal bout of exercise leads to worsening rather than an improvement of perceptions of a standard pain signal (Table 1). There is a danger that this hypersensibility will in turn lead to exercise avoidance by such patients.[7] Decreased pain thresholds are less marked with self-paced exercise, and this thus seems the best recommendation to offer such individuals.

R. J. Shephard, MD (Lond), PhD, DPE

References

1. Carroll LJ, Holm LW, Hogg-Johnson S, et al. Course and prognostic factors for neck pain in whiplash-associated disorders (WAD): results of the Bone and Joint Decade 2000-2010 Task Force on Neck Pain and Its Associated Disorders. *Spine (Phila Pa 1976)*. 2008;33:S83-S92.
2. Kamper SJ, Rebbeck TJ, Maher CG, McAuley JH, Sterling M. Course and prognostic factors of whiplash: a systematic review and meta-analysis. *Pain*. 2008; 138:617-629.
3. Barnseley L, Lord S, Bogduk N. Whiplash injury. *Pain*. 1994;58:283-307.
4. Kasch H, Qerama E, Bach FW, Jensen TS. Reduced cold pressor pain tolerance in non-recovered whiplash patients: a 1-year prospective study. *Eur J Pain*. 2005;9: 561-569.
5. Sterling M, Jull G, Vicenzino B, Kenardy J. Sensory hypersensitivity occurs soon after whiplash injury and is associated with poor recovery. *Pain*. 2003;104: 509-517.
6. Hoffman MD, Shepanski MA, Ruble SB, Valic Z, Buckwalter JB, Clifford PS. Intensity and duration threshold for aerobic exercise-induced analgesia to pressure pain. *Arch Phys Med Rehabil*. 2004;85:1183-1187.
7. Vlaeyen JW, Linton SJ. Fear-avoidance and its consequences in chronic musculoskeletal pain: a state of the art. *Pain*. 2000;85:317-332.

8 Environmental Factors

Air Pollutants

Small Things Make a Big Difference: Particulate Matter and Exercise
Cutrufello PT, Smoliga JM, Rundell KW (Univ of Scranton, PA; High Point Univ, NC; Pharmaxis Inc, Exton, PA)
Sports Med 42:1041-1058, 2012

The increased risk of morbidity and mortality among adults and children with pre-existing cardiovascular or respiratory illness from emission-derived particulate matter (PM) is well documented. However, the detrimental effects of PM inhalation on the exercising, healthy population is still in question. This review will focus on the acute and chronic responses to PM inhalation during exercise and how PM exposure influences exercise performance. The smaller ultrafine PM (<0.01 μm aerodynamic diameter) appears to have the most severe health consequences compared with the larger coarse PM ($2.5 < PM < 10$ μm aerodynamic diameter). While the response to PM inhalation may affect those with a pre-existing condition, the healthy population is not immune to the effects of PM inhalation, especially during exercise. This population, including the competitive athlete, is susceptible to pulmonary inflammation, decreased lung function (both acute and chronic in nature), the increased risk of asthma, vascular endothelial dysfunction, mild elevations in pulmonary artery pressure and diminished exercise performance. PM exposure is usually associated with vehicular traffic, but other sources of PM, including small engines from lawn and garden equipment, cigarette smoke, wood smoke and cooking, may also impair health and performance. The physiological effects of PM are dependent on the source of PM, various environmental factors, physical attributes and nature of exercise. There are a number of measures an athlete can take to reduce exposure to PM, as well as the deleterious effects that result from the inevitable exposure to PM. Considering the acute and chronic physiological responses to PM inhalation, individuals living and exercising in urban areas in close proximity to major roadways should consider ambient air pollution levels (in particular, PM and ozone) prior to engaging in vigorous exercise, and those exposed to PM through other sources may need to make

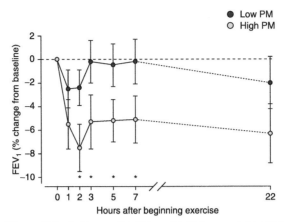

FIGURE 3.—Effect on FEV_1 of a 2-hour walk in high-particle/high-ozone air (high PM) vs a 2-hour walk in low-particle/low-ozone air (low PM) in subjects with asthmatic airways (data from McCreanor et al.[70]). Bars represent means and standard errors. FEV_1 = forced expiratory volume in the first second; PM = particulate matter; *indicates significant differences between high PM and low PM at the $p < 0.05$ level. *Editor's Note*: Please refer to original journal article for full references. (Reprinted from from Cutrufello PT, Smoliga JM, Rundell KW. Small things make a big difference: particulate matter and exercise. *Sports Med.* 2012;42:1041-1058, with permission from Springer International Publishing AG.)

lifestyle alterations to avoid the deleterious effects of PM inhalation. Although it is clear that PM exposure is detrimental to healthy individuals engaging in exercise, further research is necessary to better understand the role of PM on athlete health and performance, as well as measures that can attenuate the harmful effects of PM (Fig 3).

▶ The adverse effects of smog on human health were recognized by the dramatic increases of death rates among the frail elderly in London over 2 prolonged foggy spells in London during the 1950s. The main culprit was found to be the coal smoke that was emitted at a low level by millions of domestic fireplaces, a combination of sulfur dioxide and large-sized particulate matter. The health problem arising from this type of pollution was apparently solved by banning the burning of coal in domestic fireplaces. However, more recently, attention has focused on the hazards arising from fine particulate matter (< 2.5 microns in diameter) and the finest particles (< 0.1 microns), with vehicle exhaust as the principal source of both pollutants. The fine particulate matter does not cause the thick yellow, sulfurous mist typical of the old London fogs, but it does leave a pronounced haze over busy highways, and because a high proportion of the very fine particulate matter is retained within the lungs, it can have an adverse effect on pulmonary function. This is particularly likely in those who exercise and thus increase their dosage of pollutants 10- to 20-fold. Concerns were expressed about pollutants at both the Los Angeles and the Barcelona Games. A study in Athens concluded that nitrogen dioxide, ozone, and particulate matter (all coming mainly from vehicle exhaust, not forgetting the ice-rink Zamboni) were the main atmospheric hazards faced by competitors.[1] Although the effects of particulate matter on forced expiratory volume are quite dramatic (Fig 3), they are also temporary, and no conclusive evidence of a long-term effect on athlete health has yet been demonstrated. Prudent measures are to avoid exercising at rush hours and to situate exercise venues away from busy highways. Vegetation around a playing field may also help to trap some of the particulate matter.[2] Other possible measures are to treat competitors with leukotriene receptor antagonists and antioxidants.

R. J. Shephard, MD (Lond), PhD, DPE

References

1. Florida-James G, Donaldson K, Stone V. Athens 2004: the pollution climate and athletic performance. *J Sports Sci.* 2004;22:967-980.
2. Rundell KW, Caviston R, Hollenbach AM, Murphy K. Vehicular air pollution, playgrounds, and youth athletic fields. *Inhal Toxicol.* 2006;18:541-547.

Circadian Rhythms

Effect of a phase advance and phase delay of the 24-h cycle on energy metabolism, appetite, and related hormones

Gonnissen HKJ, Rutters F, Mazuy C, et al (Maastricht Univ, Netherlands)
Am J Clin Nutr 96:689-697, 2012

Background.—The disruption of the circadian system has been associated with the development of obesity.

Objective.—We examined the effects of circadian misalignment on sleep, energy expenditure, substrate oxidation, appetite, and related hormones.

Design.—Thirteen subjects [aged 24.3 ± 2.5 (mean ± SD) y; BMI (in kg/m^2): 23.6 ± 1.7 (mean ± SD)] completed a randomized crossover study. For each condition, subjects stayed time blinded in the respiration chamber during 3 light-entrained circadian cycles that resulted in a phase advance (3 × 21 h) and a phase delay (3 × 27 h) compared with during a 24-h cycle. Sleep, energy expenditure, substrate oxidation, and appetite were quantified. Blood and saliva samples were taken to determine melatonin, glucose, insulin, ghrelin, leptin, glucagon-like peptide 1 (GLP-1), and cortisol concentrations.

Results.—Circadian misalignment, either phase advanced or phase delayed, did not result in any changes in appetite or energy expenditure, whereas meal-related blood variables (glucose, insulin, ghrelin, leptin, and GLP-1) followed the new meal patterns. However, phase-advanced misalignment caused flattening of the cortisol-secretion pattern ($P < 0.001$), increased insulin concentrations ($P = 0.04$), and increased carbohydrate oxidation ($P = 0.03$) and decreased protein oxidation ($P = 0.001$). Phase-delayed misalignment increased rapid eye movement sleep ($P < 0.001$) and the sleeping metabolic rate ($P = 0.02$), increased glucose ($P = 0.02$) and decreased GLP-1 ($P = 0.02$) concentrations, and increased carbohydrate oxidation ($P = 0.01$) and decreased protein oxidation ($P = 0.003$).

Conclusions.—The main effect of circadian misalignment, either phase advanced or phase delayed, is a concomitant disturbance of the glucose-insulin metabolism and substrate oxidation, whereas the energy balance

TABLE 2.—Outcome Variables of Energy Expenditure, EI, EB, and Substrate Oxidation During the Third Day of the 21- and 27-h Cycles Compared With During the 24-h Cycle[1]

Outcome Variable	24 h	21-h, Day 3	27-h, Day 3
TEE (kJ/min)	6.19 ± 0.16	6.14 ± 0.18	6.21 ± 0.18
SMR (kJ/min)	4.41 ± 0.13	4.47 ± 0.13	4.51 ± 0.13*
RMR (kJ/min)	5.04 ± 0.17	5.04 ± 0.17	5.08 ± 0.15
AEE (kJ/min)	1.15 ± 0.05	1.10 ± 0.07	1.12 ± 0.06
DIT (kJ/min)	0.63 ± 0.06	0.57 ± 0.04	0.57 ± 0.05
RQ	0.91 ± 0.02	0.92 ± 0.01*	0.92 ± 0.01
EI (kJ/min)	6.49 ± 0.22	6.49 ± 0.22	6.49 ± 0.22
EB (kJ/min)	0.29 ± 0.11	0.35 ± 0.12	0.28 ± 0.10
Pox (kJ/min)	0.86 ± 0.05	0.60 ± 0.04*	0.66 ± 0.03*
Fox (kJ/min)	1.22 ± 0.12	1.24 ± 0.11	1.21 ± 0.07
CHOox (kJ/min)	3.88 ± 0.14	4.07 ± 0.11*	4.08 ± 0.12*

[1]All values are means ± SEMs, except RQ values, which are means ± SDs. ANOVA repeated measures with Bonferroni correction was performed ($n = 13$).

*Significantly different from the 24-h cycle. AEE, activity-induced energy expenditure; CHOox, carbohydrate oxidation; DIT, diet-induced energy expenditure; EB, energy balance; EI, energy intake; Fox, fat oxidation; Pox, protein oxidation; RMR, resting metabolic rate; RQ, respiratory quotient; SMR, sleeping metabolic rate; TEE, total energy expenditure.

or sleep is not largely affected. Chronically eating and sleeping at unusual circadian times may create a health risk through a metabolic disturbance. This trial was registered at the International Clinical Trials Registry Platform (http://apps.who.int/trialsearch/) as NTR2926 (Table 2).

▶ This study was conducted with a view to examining the possible impact of displacement of the circadian rhythm upon the genesis of obesity. There was in fact little change in overall energy balance. However, the findings may possibly have relevance for endurance athletes who compete in foreign time zones. Whether the body clock was advanced or retarded, a 3-hour shift was sufficient to increase glucose metabolism substantially at the expense of protein metabolism (Table 2). There seems scope for further studies looking at the effects of 5- to 6-hour changes, as with transcontinental or trans-Atlantic journeys. Investigators should also test whether a similar increase of glucose metabolism occurs in those who are exercising vigorously, when the circadian rhythm has been disrupted.

R. J. Shephard, MD (Lond), PhD, DPE

Jet Lag and Travel Fatigue: A Comprehensive Management Plan for Sport Medicine Physicians and High-Performance Support Teams
Samuels CH (Centre for Sleep and Human Performance, Calgary, Alberta, Canada)
Clin J Sport Med 22:268-273, 2012

The impact of transcontinental travel and high-volume travel on athletes can result in physiologic disturbances and a complicated set of physical symptoms. Jet lag and travel fatigue have been identified by athletes, athletic

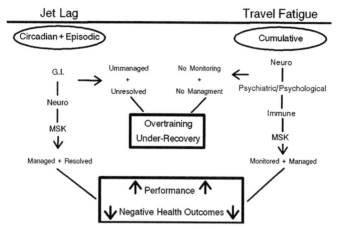

FIGURE 1.—Jet lag and travel fatigue symptoms and management algorithm. The symptoms of jet lag are a function of circadian desynchronization and largely episodic, whereas the symptoms of travel fatigue are cumulative and chronic. The goal is to minimize jet lag symptoms by effectively addressing circadian resynchronization while monitoring the athlete for cumulative fatigue, managing the impact of travel, and preventing the health consequences associated with travel. (Reprinted from Samuels CH. Jet lag and travel fatigue: a comprehensive management plan for sport medicine physicians and high-performance support teams. *Clin J Sport Med.* 2012;22:268-273, with permission from Lippincott Williams & Wilkins.)

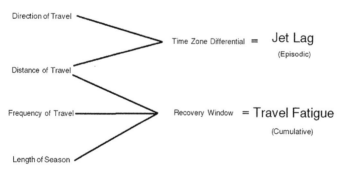

FIGURE 2.—A conceptual model of jet lag and travel fatigue. Several factors influence the time zone differential and the recovery window associated with jet lag and travel fatigue. Time zone differential is a circadian phenomenon that accounts for time of day factors and circadian resynchronization that affects performance. The recovery window refers to time available for athletes and teams to recover from competition and travel in preparation for upcoming competition throughout a season. (Reprinted from Samuels CH. Jet lag and travel fatigue: a comprehensive management plan for sport medicine physicians and high-performance support teams. *Clin J Sport Med.* 2012;22:268-273, with permission from Lippincott Williams & Wilkins.)

trainers, coaches, and physicians as important but challenging problems that could benefit from practical solutions. Currently, there is a culture of disregard and lack of knowledge regarding the negative effects of jet lag and travel fatigue on the athlete's well-being and performance. In addition, the key physiologic metric (determination of the human circadian phase) that guides jet lag treatment interventions is elusive and thus limits

TABLE.—Jet Lag and Fatigue Management Intervention Strategies

	East		West	
		Direction of Travel		
Interventions	< 3 Time Zones	≥ 3 Time Zones	< 4 Time Zones	≥ 4 Time Zones
Jet lag				
Pharmacologic	Postflight: medium-acting and medium half-life hypnotic*[5]	3-mg to 5-mg melatonin, 30 minutes before bed[17,18] In-flight: ultra short-acting and short half-life hypnotic*[5] Postflight: medium-acting and medium half-life hypnotic*[5]	Postflight: medium-acting and medium half-life hypnotic*[5]	3-mg to 5-mg melatonin, 30 minutes before bed[17,18] In-flight: ultra short-acting and short half-life hypnotic*[5] Postflight: medium-acting and medium half-life hypnotic*[5]
Circadian phase shifting	Meals and bedtime 1-2 h earlier, 2 d before departure (optional)[5,12]	Meals and bedtime 1-2 h earlier, 2 d before departure (optional)[5,12] Seek/avoid light according to jet lag calculator†	Meals and bedtime 1-2 h later, 2 d before departure (optional)[12]	Meals and bedtime 1-2 h later, 2 d before departure (optional)[5,12] Seek/avoid light according to jet lag calculator†
Jet lag symptom management				
GI irregularities	Antacids, bismuth subsalicylate, etc	→		
Headache	Analgesics and antiinflammatory	→		
Decreased mental performance	Strategic use of caffeine (see Fatigue Countermeasures: Caffeine)	→		
Decreased physical performance	Modified training routines (see Fatigue countermeasures: training)	→		
Sleep disturbance	Sedatives and sleep hygiene (see Pharmacologic interventions)	→		

Travel fatigue			
Pharmacologic	No intervention required. Use clinical judgment.	3-5 mg melatonin, 30 min before bed[17,18] In-flight: ultra short-acting and short half-life hypnotic*§ Postflight: medium-acting and medium half-life hypnotic*§	No intervention required. Use clinical judgment.	3-5 mg melatonin, 30 min before bed[17,18] In-flight: ultra short-acting and short half-life hypnotic*§ Postflight: medium-acting and medium half-life hypnotic*§
Fatigue countermeasures			
Feeding	No changes	Smaller, more frequent, recovery content meals on destination schedule	No changes	Smaller, more frequent, recovery content meals on destination schedule
Hydration	Maintain extra hydration	Maintain extra hydration	Maintain extra hydration	Maintain extra hydration
Training	No intervention required	Reduced for 2-4 d postflight	No intervention required	Reduced for 2-4 d postflight
Sleep hygiene	Maximize rest and sleep during travel	Maximize rest and sleep during travel	Maximize rest and sleep during travel	Maximize rest and sleep during travel
Naps	20-30 min at the circadian nadir	20-30 min at the circadian nadir	20-30 min at the circadian nadir	20-30 min at the circadian nadir
Light	As required: Mid AM light exposure (30-60 min) Mid afternoon light avoidance	Initial 2 days of arrival: Mid AM light exposure (30-60 min) Mid afternoon light avoidance	As required: Late afternoon light exposure (30-60 min) Late PM light avoidance	Initial 2 days of arrival: Late afternoon light exposure (30-60 min) Late PM light avoidance
Caffeine	50-200 mg as required	50-200 mg, mornings on waking and in the minutes before a nap	50-200 mg as required	50-200 mg, late afternoons and in the minutes before a nap

Therapeutic interventions are based on the direction of travel and the number of time zones or distance traveled from the origin of departure. Travel < 3 time zones eastward and < 4 time zones westward involves time of day influences and should focus on a specific set of interventions to manage the effects of jet lag and travel fatigue on performance. Longer flights extending ≥ 3 time zones eastward and ≥ 4 time zones westward require similar time of day interventions but also involve additional interventions and in-flight/postflight considerations to manage more complex circadian adjustment.

Editor's Note: Please refer to original journal article for full references.

*The physician's clinical judgment should determine the need for a hypnotic based on whether or not the athlete suffers from insomnia with travel.

†Available at: http://www.fleerstreetclinic.com/calc.php.

evidence-based therapeutic advice. A better understanding of preflight, inflight, and postflight management options, such as use of melatonin or the judicious application of sedatives, is important for the sports clinician to help athletes limit fatigue symptoms and maintain optimal performance. The purpose of this article was to provide a practical applied method of implementing a travel management program for athletic teams (Figs 1 and 2, Table).

▶ High-level athletic competition and international travel bring with them the inevitable evils of jet lag and travel fatigue, both of which can be extremely detrimental to optimal performance. Given the incredible investment of time, energy, and resources (including financial) in preparation for major events such as world championships or the Olympic Games, it is somewhat surprising that more attention is not paid to a management plan for these common conditions. Despite the lack of generalizable research, there are some concrete measures that can be taken to help offset the impact of transcontinental and high-volume travel on athletes. This article offers an algorithm (Fig 1) for symptoms and management and a conceptual model of how they interact (Fig 2). A comprehensive and helpful outline of pharmacologic and physical intervention strategies is included (Table).

C. Lebrun, MDCM, MPE, CCFP, Dip Sport Med, FACSM

Heat and Cold

Partial heat acclimation of athletes with spinal cord lesion

Castle PC, Kularatne BP, Brewer J, et al (Univ of Bedfordshire, UK; Disability Target Shooting Great Britain, Buckinghamshire, UK; et al)
Eur J Appl Physiol 113:109-115, 2013

Heat acclimation (HA) can improve thermoregulatory stability in able-bodied athletes in part by an enhanced sweat response. Athletes with spinal cord lesion are unable to sweat below the lesion and it is unknown if they can HA. Five paralympic shooting athletes with spinal cord lesion completed seven consecutive days HA in hot conditions (33.4 ± 0.6 °C, 64.8 ± 3.7 %rh). Each HA session consisted of 20 min arm crank exercise at 50 % $\dot{V}O_{2peak}$ followed by 40 min rest, or simulated shooting. Aural temperature (T_{aur}) was recorded throughout. Body mass was assessed before and after each session and a sweat collection swab was fixed to T12 of the spine. Fingertip whole blood was sampled at rest on days 1 and 7 for estimation of the change in plasma volume. Resting T_{aur} declined from 36.3 ± 0.2 °C on day 1 to 36.0 ± 0.2 °C by day 6 ($P < 0.05$). During the HA sessions mean, T_{aur} declined from 37.2 ± 0.2 °C on day 1, to 36.7 ± 0.3 °C on day 7 ($P < 0.05$). Plasma volume increased from day 1 by 1.5 ± 0.6 % on day 7 ($P < 0.05$). No sweat secretion was detected or changes in body mass observed from any participant. Repeated hyperthermia combined with limited evaporative heat loss was sufficient to increase plasma volume, probably by alterations in fluid regulatory hormones. In conclusion,

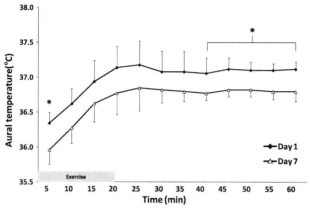

FIGURE 2.—Mean ± SD aural temperature (°C) at 5 min intervals during the 60 min heat acclimation session on day 1 and day 7. *Asterisk* indicates a significant difference compared to day 1 ($P < 0.05$). (With kind permission from Springer Science+Business Media: Castle PC, Kularatne BP, Brewer J, et al. Partial heat acclimation of athletes with spinal cord lesion. *Eur J Appl Physiol.* 2013;113:109-115, with permission from Springer-Verlag.)

we found that although no sweat response was observed, athletes with spinal cord lesion could partially HA (Fig 2).

▶ One of the hazards faced by athletes with spinal injury is a poor tolerance of hot environmental conditions.[1,2] They are thus at a correspondingly increased risk of heat illness during competitions. Not only do they face a loss of vasoregulation, but there is also a total absence of sweat secretion below the level of the spinal cord lesion.[1] Attempts to precool such athletes by devices such as an ice vest[3] are hampered by hypersensitivity to extremely cold temperatures. This study is the first to examine the possibility of inducing a more long-term heat acclimation in individuals with paraplegia and quadriplegia. Despite the inability to sweat over most of the body, some adaptation was observed over 7 one-hour exposures to hot and humid conditions in terms of both core temperatures (Fig 2) and heart rates. This was attributed to a 1.5% increase of plasma volume, presumably mediated by changes in the secretion of fluid regulatory hormones.[4,5] After acclimation, subjects apparently began the heat exposure with the advantage of a substantially lower core temperature, although, because of the absence of sweating below the lesion, the rate of increase of auricular temperature during the heat exposure remained unchanged. One weakness in this study was that no tests were made of a possible increase in sweating above the level of the lesion; one investigator has suggested that this may increase as much as 6-fold with heat acclimation.[6] There were also no controls to allow for possible changes in the external environment. Nevertheless, this small-scale study does suggest that there may be value in heat acclimation programs for some categories of athletes with spinal injuries who are proposing to compete in a hot climate. There is plainly a need for controlled studies to examine whether benefit is observed not only in target shooters but also in those who are more vulnerable to heat stress, particularly those involved in endurance sports.

R. J. Shephard, MD (Lond), PhD, DPE

References

1. Totel GL. Physiological responses to heat of resting man with impaired sweating capacity. *J Appl Physiol.* 1974;37:346-352.
2. Webborn ADJ. Heat-related problems for the Paralympic Games, Atlanta 1996. *Int J Ther Rehabil.* 1996;3:429-436.
3. Webborn N, Price MJ, Castle PC, Goosey-Tolfrey VL. Effects of two cooling strategies on the thermoregulatory responses of tetraplegic athletes during repeated intermittent exercise in the heat. *J Appl Physiol.* 2005;98:2101-2107.
4. Francesconi RP, Sawka MN, Pandolf KB. Hypohydration and heat acclimation: plasma renin and aldosterone during exercise. *J Appl Physiol.* 1983;55:1790-1794.
5. Garrett AT, Goosens NG, Rehrer NG, Patterson MJ, Cotter JD. Induction and decay of short-term heat acclimation. *Eur J Appl Physiol.* 2009;107:659-670.
6. Petrofsky JS. Thermoreugulatory stress during rest and exercise in heat in patients with spinal cord injury. *Eur J Appl Physiol.* 1992;64:503-507.

Pre-Cooling and Sports Performance: A Meta-Analytical Review
Wegmann M, Faude O, Poppendieck W, et al (Saarland Univ, Saarbrücken, Germany)
Sports Med 42:545-564, 2012

Pre-cooling is used by many athletes for the purpose of reducing body temperature prior to exercise and, consequently, decreasing heat stress and improving performance. Although there are a considerable number of studies showing beneficial effects of pre-cooling, definite conclusions on the effectiveness of pre-cooling on performance cannot yet be drawn. Moreover, detailed analyses of the specific conditions under which pre-cooling may be most promising are, so far, missing. Therefore, we conducted a literature search and located 27 peer-reviewed randomized controlled trials, which addressed the effects of pre-cooling on performance. These studies were analysed with regard to performance effects and several test circumstances (environmental temperature, test protocol, cooling method, aerobic capacity of the subjects).

Eighteen studies were performed in a hot (> 26°C) environment and eight in a moderate. The cooling protocols were water application (n = 12), cooling packs (n = 3), cold drinks (n = 2), cooling vest (n = 6) and a cooled room (n = 4). The following different performance tests were used: short-term, high-intensity sprints (n = 2), intermittent sprints (n = 6), time trials (n = 10), open-end tests (n = 7) and graded exercise tests (n = 2). If possible, subjects were grouped into different aerobic capacity levels according to their maximal oxygen consumption ($\dot{V}O_{2max}$): medium 55−65 mL/kg/min (n = 11) and high > 65 mL/kg/min (n = 6). For all studies the relative changes of performance due to pre-cooling compared with a control condition, as well as effect sizes (Hedges' g) were calculated.

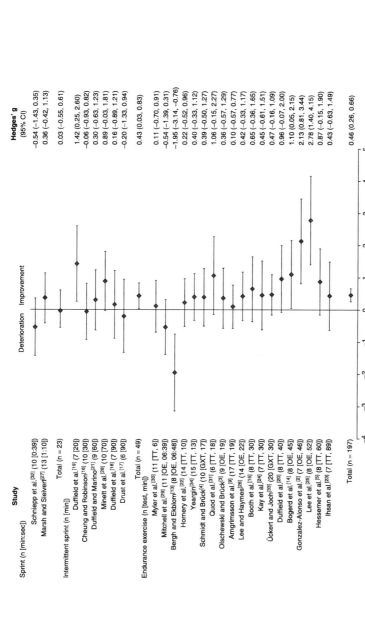

FIGURE 4.—Effects of pre-cooling on performance related to exercise type and duration. The magnitude of the effect size indicates: 0–0.19 = negligible effect, 0.20–0.49 = small effect, 0.50–0.79 = moderate effect, ≥ 0.80 = large effect. CI = confidence interval; GXT = graded exercise test; n = number of subjects; OE = open-end test; TT = time trials. *Editor's Note:* Please refer to original journal article for full references. (Reprinted from Wegmann M, Faude O, Poppendieck W, et al. Pre-Cooling and sports performance: a meta-analytical review. *Sports Med.* 2012;42:545-564, with permission from Springer International Publishing AG.)

Mean values were weighted according to the number of subjects in each study.

Pre-cooling had a larger effect on performance in hot (+6.6%, g = 0.62) than in moderate temperatures (+1.4%, g = 0.004). The largest performance enhancements were found for endurance tests like open-end tests (+8.6%, g = 0.52), graded exercise tests (+6.0%, g = 0.44) and time trials (+4.2%, g = 0.44). A similar effect was observed for intermittent sprints (+3.3%, g = 0.43), whereas performance changes were smaller during short-term, high-intensity sprints (−0.5%, g = 0.03). The most promising cooling methods were cold drinks (+15.0%, g = 1.68), cooling packs (+5.6%, g = 0.70) and a cooled room (+10.7%, g = 0.49), whereas a cooling vest (+4.8%, g = 0.31) and water application (+1.2%, g = 0.21) showed only small effects. With respect to aerobic capacity, the best results were found in the subjects with the highest. $\dot{V}O_{2max}$ (high +7.7%, g = 0.65; medium +3.8%, g = 0.27). There were four studies analysing endurance-trained athletes under time-trial conditions, which, in a practical sense, seem to be most relevant. Those studies found an average effect on performance of 3.7% (g = 0.48).

In summary, pre-cooling can effectively enhance endurance performance, particularly in hot environments, whereas sprint exercise is barely affected. In particular, well trained athletes may benefit in a typical competition setting with practical and relevant effects. With respect to feasibility, cold drinks, cooling packs and cooling vests can be regarded as best-practice methods (Fig 4).

▶ This seems a careful meta-analysis of peer-reviewed studies of the effects of precooling on athletic performance, as seen in randomized crossover trials on male athletes with a maximal oxygen intake > 55 mL/kg/min. Funnel plots have been used to check data for publication bias. Not surprisingly, cooling offered the greatest benefit in endurance events, and it had a slight negative effect in some sprint trials (Fig 4). Under hot conditions, cooling could boost endurance performance by 5% to 10%. The authors suggest that the most effective methods of cooling were cold drinks, cooling packs, and a cold room. However, they did not separate out the effects of a desert climate from hot and humid heat, and this should be done in a future analysis. Under hot and dry conditions, wetting of the clothing seems likely to be a simple and very effective aid to endurance performance. I certainly found this to be the case when I climbed Masada on a very hot day. All other members of a fitness symposium thought I was courting heat stress and waited for the lift to start operating, but I finished the climb cool and refreshed! The present authors found only one published trial of precooling in female athletes, and this is another obvious area for future enquiry.

R. J. Shephard, MD (Lond), PhD, DPE

High and Low Ambient Pressures

Effectiveness of Preacclimatization Strategies for High-Altitude Exposure

Fulco CS, Beidleman BA, Muza SR (United States Army Res Inst of Environmental Medicine, Natick, MA)
Exerc Sport Sci Rev 41:55-63, 2013

Acute mountain sickness (AMS) and large decrements in endurance exercise performance occur when unacclimatized individuals rapidly ascend to high altitudes. Six altitude and hypoxia preacclimatization strategies were evaluated to determine their effectiveness for minimizing AMS and improving performance during altitude exposures. Strategies using hypobaric chambers or true altitude were much more effective overall than those using normobaric hypoxia (breathing, <20.9% oxygen) (Table 3).

▶ Athletes who must compete at high altitudes, or patients who are planning events such as a Himalayan trek, may well inquire what is the most effective method of preparation for such activity. Fulco and associates review the outcomes of several potential tactics, including living at an actual altitude of 2200 m for a week or longer or spending time in a hypobaric chamber or breathing hypoxic mixtures for varying parts of the day or night over 1-2 weeks. The target altitude after acclimatization was arbitrarily set at 4300 m. All of the suggested treatments reduced the risk of acute mountain sickness (Table 3), but use of the hypobaric chamber (intermittent altitude exposure [IAE] 7 or IAE 15) and/or staging at Pike's Peak (2200 m) was more effective than exposure to normobaric hypoxia. The degree of ventilatory adaptation achieved by the optimal tactic was the equivalent of living 4 days at 4300 m. The greater benefit from exposure to the actual altitude (acclimatization) rather than conditions simulated by hypoxic gas mixtures (acclimation) is in keeping with studies in other adverse environments such as very hot climates, and it is supported by some direct comparisons of the two approaches to high altitude adaptation.[1]

R. J. Shephard, MD (Lond), PhD, DPE

Reference

1. Miller GP, Faiss R, Pialoux VP, et al. Counterpoint. Hypobaric hypoxia induces/does not induce different responses than normobaric hypoxia. *J Appl Physiol.* 2012;112:1781-1796.

TABLE 3.—Strategy Effectiveness When Assessed at the Target Altitude of 4300 m

Reference	Short Title	PetCO$_2$	SaO$_2$	AMS Prevalence	Exercise Performance
(8,12,13,20,21,24)	Benchmark (24 h)	35 mm Hg	80%–81%	80%–100%	−60% to −70%
	Benchmark (After prolonged exposure)	Lower +++++	Higher +++++	Zero	Improved +++
(2,3)	IAE 15	Lower +++++	Higher +++	Zero	Improved +++++
(4)	IAE 7	n/a	Higher +++	n/a	Improved +++
(1,10)	Staging	Lower +++	Higher +++	45%	Improved +++
(14)	MAR	Lower +++++	Higher +++++	Zero	No reduction in exercise intensity from 2200 m +++++
(9)	NH (Sleep)	No effect	No effect	64%	No effect
(5,19)	NH (Awake)	Lower +	No effect	50%	No effect

+++++, ≥4 mm Hg reduction in PetCO$_2$, an increase of ≥5% in SaO$_2$, or >20% endurance exercise performance improvement.
+++, 3 or 4 mm Hg reduction in PetCO$_2$, a 3% to 5% increase in SaO$_2$, or a 10% to 20% Endurance exercise performance improvement.
+, 1 or 2 mm Hg reduction in PetCO$_2$, or a 1% or 2% increase in SaO$_2$. No effect, no difference from Sham.
Editor's Note: Please refer to original journal article for full references.

Influence of rest and exercise at a simulated altitude of 4,000 m on appetite, energy intake, and plasma concentrations of acylated ghrelin and peptide YY

Wasse LK, Sunderland C, King JA, et al (Loughborough Univ, Nottingham, UK; Nottingham Trent Univ, UK; et al)
J Appl Physiol 112:552-559, 2012

The reason for high altitude anorexia is unclear but could involve alterations in the appetite hormones ghrelin and peptide YY (PYY). This study examined the effect of resting and exercising in hypoxia (12.7% O_2; ~4,000 m) on appetite, energy intake, and plasma concentrations of acylated ghrelin and PYY. Ten healthy males completed four, 7-h trials in an environmental chamber in a random order. The four trials were control-normoxia, control-hypoxia, exercise-normoxia, and exercise-hypoxia. During exercise trials, participants ran for 60 min at 70% of altitude-specific maximal oxygen consumption ($\dot{V}o_{2max}$) and then rested. Participants rested throughout control trials. A standardized meal was consumed at 2 h and an ad libitum buffet meal at 5.5 h. Area under the curve values for hunger (assessed using visual analog scales) tended to be lower during hypoxic trials than normoxic trials (repeated-measures ANOVA, $P = 0.07$). Ad libitum energy intake was lower ($P = 0.001$) in hypoxia (5,291 ± 2,189 kJ) than

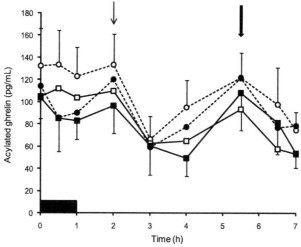

FIGURE 2.—Plasma acylated ghrelin concentrations during the normoxic control trial (OE), normoxic exercise trial (●), hypoxic control trial (□), and hypoxic exercise trial (■). Values are means ± SE; $n = 10$. Some error bars have been omitted for clarity (trial means ± SE values for omitted trials are as follows: normoxic exercise: 92 ± 18 pg/ml and hypoxic control: 85 ± 19 pg/ml). Black rectangle indicates treadmill running, thin downward arrow indicates standardized meal consumption, and bold downward arrow indicates buffet meal consumption. Repeated-measures ANOVA revealed a main effect of altitude ($P = 0.005$), exercise ($P = 0.001$), and time ($P < 0.001$) and an exercise × time interaction ($P < 0.05$). (Reprinted from Wasse LK, Sunderland C, King JA, et al. Influence of rest and exercise at a simulated altitude of 4,000 m on appetite, energy intake, and plasma concentrations of acylated ghrelin and peptide YY. *J Appl Physiol.* 2012;112:552-559, with permission from the American Physiological Society.)

normoxia (7,718 ± 2,356 kJ; means ± SD). Mean plasma acylated ghrelin concentrations were lower in hypoxia than normoxia (82 ± 66 vs. 100 ± 69 pg/ml; $P = 0.005$) while PYY concentrations tended to be higher in normoxia (32 ± 4 vs. 30 ± 3 pmol/l; $P = 0.059$). Exercise suppressed hunger and acylated ghrelin and increased PYY but did not influence ad libitum energy intake. These findings confirm that hypoxia suppresses hunger and food intake. Further research is required to determine if decreased concentrations of acylated ghrelin orchestrate this suppression (Fig 2).

▶ There are probably many components to the progressive deterioration of physical condition that besets mountaineers. However, one important issue is high-altitude anorexia,[1] with an associated decrease in lean body mass.[2] Possible reasons for a poor appetite and loss of body mass include a limited availability of food, a lack of palatability in the meals that are improvised,[3] and an extremely high daily energy expenditure. Acute mountain sickness has also been suggested as a possible contributing factor, although the poor appetite and weight loss often persists after mountain sickness has subsided.[4] Problems of poor appetite are also observed during decompression chamber simulations of Everest ascents, despite the provision of appetizing food and the elimination of most extraneous environmental stressors,[3,5] thus raising the possibility that one cause of anorexia may be a direct action of hypoxia on hormonal appetite regulating mechanisms. At least 1 previous report has noted a short-term decrease in total ghrelin at high altitude.[6] In the present study, Wasse et al looked at the effects of simulated altitude upon concentrations of the biologically active component of ghrelin (acylated ghrelin) and on the anorectic gut hormone peptide PPY. They observed a substantial 31% decrease of ad libitum energy intake in response to just 7 hours' exposure to a simulated altitude of 4000 m, with a parallel decrease in serum ghrelin (Fig 2); there were also statistically nonsignificant trends to a decrease in appetite and an increase of PPY. No remedies are suggested in this article, but isolation of the causal role of acylated ghrelin may be a first step in countering high-altitude anorexia.

R. J. Shephard, MD (Lond), PhD, DPE

References

1. Barry PW, Pollard AJ. Altitude illness. *BMJ.* 2003;326:915-919.
2. Kayser B. Nutrition and energetics of exercise at altitude. Theory and possible practical implications. *Sports Med.* 1994;17:309-323.
3. Westerterp-Plantenga MS, Westerterp KR, Rubbens M, Verwegen CR, Richelet JP, Gardette B. Appetite at "high altitude" [Operation Everest III (Comex-'97)]: a simulated ascent of Mount Everest. *J Appl Physiol.* 1999;87:391-399.
4. Tschöp M, Morrison KM. Weight loss at high altitude. *Adv Exp Med Biol.* 2001; 502:237-247.
5. Rose MS, Houston CS, Fulco CS, et al. Operation Everest. II: nutrition and body composition. *J Appl Physiol.* 1988;65:2545-2551.
6. Quintero P, Milagro FI, Campón J, Martinez JA. Impact of oxygen availability on body weight management. *Med Hypotheses.* 2010;74:901-907.

Effects of experience and commercialisation on survival in Himalayan mountaineering: retrospective cohort study

Westhoff JL, Koepsell TD, Littell CT (Madigan Healthcare System, Tacoma, WA; Univ of Washington, Seattle)
BMJ 344:e3782, 2012

Objectives.—To determine whether previous Himalayan experience is associated with a decreased risk of climbing death, and whether mountaineers participating in commercial expeditions differ in their risk of death relative to those participating in traditional climbs.

Design.—Retrospective cohort study.

Setting.—Expeditions in the Nepalese Himalayan peaks, from 1 January 1970 to the spring climbing season in 2010.

Participants.—23 995 non-porters venturing above base camp on 39 038 climbs, 23 295 on 8000 m peaks.

Outcome.—Death.

Results.—After controlling for use of standard route, peak, age, season, sex, summit success, and year of expedition, increased Himalayan experience was not associated with a change in the odds of death (odds ratio 1.00, 95% confidence interval 0.96 to 1.05, $P = 0.904$). Participation in a commercial climb was associated with a 37% lower odds of death relative to a traditional venture, although not significantly (0.63, 0.37 to 1.09, $P = 0.100$). Choice of peak was clearly associated with altered odds of death (omnibus $P < 0.001$); year of expedition was associated with a significant trend toward reduced odds of death (0.98, 0.96 to 0.99, $P = 0.011$).

Conclusions.—No net survival benefit is associated with increased Himalayan experience or participation in a traditional (versus commercial) venture. The incremental decrease in risk associated with calendar year suggests that cumulative, collective knowledge and general innovation are more important than individual experience in improving the odds of survival (Table 2).

▶ Few would argue against the fact that mountain climbing is a dangerous sport, particularly when tackling higher elevations such as Mount Everest.[1,2] Nevertheless, about 100 million people explore high peaks every year, and the number participating in commercial expeditions is rising continuously[3]; indeed, the number of trekkers in Nepal has increased 450% between 1994 and 2000.[4] A recent estimate of risk for climbing the Nepalese peaks (based on 30 days' exposure per climb of peaks higher than 8000 m) set the frequency of deaths at 544 per million days of exposure; this may be compared with only 1.1 death per million days of downhill skiing in the Alps.[4]

This article examined the relative importance of experience to risk and the possible differences between amateur and commercial expeditions. They were able to amass data on more than 39 000 ascents between 1970 and 2010. They found no differences in risk with commercial operations versus amateur or with the level of experience of the climbers, but there was a welcome trend toward

TABLE 2.—Characteristics of Traditional Versus Commercial Climbs by Climbers on Constituent Himalayan Peaks, 1970-2010. Data are No (%)

Variable	Traditional	Commercial	Total
Sex of climber			
Male	28 457 (91.6)	6993 (87.9)	35 450 (90.8)
Female	2625 (8.5)	962 (12.1)	3587 (9.2)
Unknown	1	0	1
Age of climber (years)			
≤19	156 (0.5)	34 (0.4)	190 (0.5)
20-29	8710 (28.0)	1035 (13.0)	9745 (25.0)
30-39	12 280 (39.5)	2833 (35.6)	15 113 (38.7)
40-49	6355 (20.5)	2472 (31.1)	8827 (22.6)
50-59	2136 (6.9)	1183 (14.9)	3319 (8.5)
≥60	578 (1.9)	334 (4.2)	912 (2.3)
Unknown	868 (2.8)	64 (0.8)	932 (2.4)
Expedition number			
1	18 796 (60.5)	4624 (58.1)	23 420 (60.0)
2-4	9033 (29.1)	2330 (29.3)	11 363 (29.1)
5-9	2356 (7.6)	642 (8.1)	2998 (7.7)
≥10	872 (2.8)	353 (4.4)	1225 (3.1)
Unknown	26 (0.1)	6 (0.1)	32 (0.1)
Route			
Non-standard	15 793 (50.8)	1563 (19.7)	17 356 (44.5)
Standard	15 290 (49.2)	6392 (80.4)	21 682 (55.5)
Season			
Spring	14 139 (45.5)	3688 (46.4)	17 827 (45.7)
Summer	354 (1.1)	24 (0.3)	378 (1.0)
Autumn	15 160 (48.8)	4131 (51.9)	19 291 (49.4)
Winter	1430 (4.6)	112 (1.4)	1542 (4.0)
Altitude of peak (m)			
≤7000	5641 (18.2)	1731 (21.8)	7372 (18.9)
7000-7999	7210 (23.2)	1161 (14.6)	8371 (21.4)
≥8000	18 232 (58.7)	5063 (63.7)	23 295 (59.7)
8000 m peaks*			
Annapurna I	1144 (6.3)	55 (1.1)	1199 (5.2)
Cho Oyu	3632 (19.9)	2055 (40.6)	5687 (24.4)
Dhaulagiri I	1503 (8.2)	164 (3.2)	1667 (7.2)
Everest	7004 (38.4)	2331 (46.0)	9335 (40.1)
Kangchenjunga	1005 (5.5)	28 (0.6)	1033 (4.4)
Lhotse	1191 (6.5)	132 (2.6)	1323 (5.7)
Makalu	1368 (7.5)	58 (1.2)	1426 (6.1)
Manaslu	1385 (7.6)	240 (4.7)	1625 (7.0)
Success	8712 (28.0)	3534 (44.4)	12 246 (31.4)
Death	524 (1.7)	55 (0.7)	579 (1.5)
Mechanism of death†			
Acute mountain sickness	28 (5.3)	5 (9.1)	33 (5.7)
Exposure	49 (9.4)	8 (14.5)	57 (9.8)
Fall	216 (41.2)	29 (52.7)	245 (42.3)
Crevasse	13 (2.5)	1 (1.8)	14 (2.4)
Avalanche	162 (30.9)	3 (5.5)	165 (28.5)
Falling debris	11 (2.1)	1 (1.8)	12 (2.1)
Other	20 (3.8)	6 (10.9)	26 (4.5)
Unknown	25 (4.8)	2 (3.6)	27 (4.7)

*Percentages of 8000 m peak climbs only.
†Percentages of total deaths for traditional or commercial expeditions.

decreased mortality over the 40 years of observation. The main causes of death were falls and avalanches (Table 2).

R. J. Shephard, MD (Lond), PhD, DPE

References

1. Huey RB, Eguskitza X. Supplemental oxygen and mountaineer death rates on Everest and K2. *JAMA*. 2000;284:181.
2. Firth PG, Zheng H, Windsor JS, et al. Mortality on Mount Everest, 1921-2006: descriptive study. *BMJ*. 2008;337:a2654.
3. Weinbruch S, Nordby KC. Fatal accidents among elite mountaineers: a historical perspective from the European Alps. *High Alt Med Biol*. 2010;11:147-151.
4. Burtscher M. Climbing the Himalayas more safely. *BMJ*. 2012;344:e3778.

Ibuprofen Prevents Altitude Illness: A Randomized Controlled Trial for Prevention of Altitude Illness With Nonsteroidal Anti-inflammatories
Lipman GS, Kanaan NC, Holck PS, et al (Stanford Univ School of Medicine, Palo Alto, CA; Univ of Hawaii, Honolulu; et al)
Ann Emerg Med 59:484-490, 2012

Study Objective.—Acute mountain sickness occurs in more than 25% of the tens of millions of people who travel to high altitude each year. Previous studies on chemoprophylaxis with nonsteroidal anti-inflammatory drugs are limited in their ability to determine efficacy. We compare ibuprofen versus placebo in the prevention of acute mountain sickness incidence and severity on ascent from low to high altitude.

Methods.—Healthy adult volunteers living at low altitude were randomized to ibuprofen 600 mg or placebo 3 times daily, starting 6 hours before ascent from 1,240 m (4,100 ft) to 3,810 m (12,570 ft) during July and August 2010 in the White Mountains of California. The main outcome measures were acute mountain sickness incidence and severity, measured by the Lake Louise Questionnaire acute mountain sickness score with a diagnosis of ≥3 with headache and 1 other symptom.

Results.—Eighty-six participants completed the study; 44 (51%) received ibuprofen and 42 (49%) placebo. There were no differences in demographic characteristics between the 2 groups. Fewer participants in the ibuprofen group (43%) developed acute mountain sickness compared with those receiving placebo (69%) (odds ratio 0.3, 95% confidence interval 0.1 to 0.8; number needed to treat 3.9, 95% confidence interval 2 to 33). The acute mountain sickness severity was higher in the placebo group (4.4 [SD 2.6]) than individuals receiving ibuprofen (3.2 [SD 2.4]) (mean difference 0.9%; 95% confidence interval 0.3% to 3.0%).

Conclusion.—Compared with placebo, ibuprofen was effective in reducing the incidence of acute mountain sickness.

▶ This is a randomized clinical trial of substantial size showing that ibuprofen taken 6 hours before ascent to altitude reduces the likelihood of mountain sickness relative to control subjects (2 of 42 vs 6 of 44); however, the difference in Lake Louise score of 1 point was less than the investigators had hoped for. It is reasonable to anticipate some benefit from nonsteroidal anti-inflammatory drugs (NSAIDs), since they inhibit the inflammatory cyclo-oxygenase cascade and subsequent vasodilatation and increase of vascular permeability due to the release of prostaglandins and thromboxanes.[1] Previous studies have shown some benefit against headaches,[2,3] but it has not been clearly established that NSAIDs protect against other manifestations of mountain sickness.[4,5] In this article, a convenience sample of low-altitude residents received 4 doses of ibuprofen. The first was taken at an altitude of 1240 m and the remaining 3 over the following day, after driving to an altitude of 3545 m and then hiking to 3810 m. The clinical benefit seems of a similar order to what would have been expected with acetazolamide,[6,7] although this conclusion would have been stronger if a fraction of the subjects had received acetazolamide as an alternative treatment. The big advantage of ibuprofen is, of course, that it is widely available as an over-the-counter medication, and for most people the side effects may be less than the nausea, dizziness, and fatigue sometimes associated with acetazolamide use.

R. J. Shephard, MD (Lond), PhD, DPE

References

1. Ray CJ, Abbas MR, Coney AM, Marshall JM. Interactions of adenosine, prostaglandins and nitric oxide in hypoxia-induced vasodilatation: in vivo and in vitro studies. *J Physiol*. 2002;544:195-209.
2. Burtscher M, Likar R, Nachbauer W, Schaffert W, Philadelphy M. Ibuprofen versus sumatriptan for high-altitude headache. *Lancet*. 1995;346:254-255.
3. Gertsch JH, Lipman GS, Holck PS, et al. Prospective, double-blind, randomized, placebo-controlled comparison of acetazolamide versus ibuprofen for prophylaxis against high altitude headache: the Headache Evaluation at Altitude Trial (HEAT). *Wilderness Environ Med*. 2010;21:236-243.
4. Meehan RT, Cymerman A, Rock P, et al. The effect of naproxen on acute mountain sickness and vascular responses to hypoxia. *Am J Med Sci*. 1986;292:15-20.
5. Kayser B, Hulsebosch R, Bosch F. Low-dose acetylsalicylic acid analog and acetazolamide for prevention of acute mountain sickness. *High Alt Med Biol*. 2008; 9:15-23.
6. van Patot MC, Leadbetter G 3rd, Keyes LE, Maakestad KM, Olson S, Hackett PH. Prophylactic low-dose acetazolamide reduces the incidence and severity of acute mountain sickness. *High Alt Med Biol*. 2008;9:289-293.
7. Basnyat B, Murdoch DR. High-altitude illness. *Lancet*. 2003;361:1967-1974.

Increases in $\dot{V}O_{2max}$ with "live high–train low" altitude training: role of ventilatory acclimatization
Wilhite DP, Mickleborough TD, Laymon AS, et al (Indiana Univ, Bloomington)
Eur J Appl Physiol 113:419-426, 2013

The purpose of this study was to estimate the percentage of the increase in whole body maximal oxygen consumption ($\dot{V}O_{2max}$) that is accounted for by increased respiratory muscle oxygen uptake after altitude training. Six elite male distance runners ($\dot{V}O_{2max} = 70.6 \pm 4.5$ ml kg^{-1} min^{-1}) and

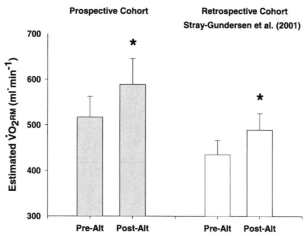

FIGURE 3.—Changes in the estimated respiratory muscle oxygen consumption ($\dot{V}O_{2RM}$) during maximal exercise from pre- to post-altitude training. *Pre-Alt* pre-altitude; *Post-Alt* post-altitude. Values are mean ± SE. *Significantly different from *Pre-Alt*, $p \leq 0.05$. (With kind permission from Springer Science+Business Media: Wilhite DP, Mickleborough TD, Laymon AS, et al. Increases in $\dot{V}O_{2max}$ with "live high—train low" altitude training: role of ventilatory acclimatization. *Eur J Appl Physiol.* 2013;113:419-426, with permission from Springer-Verlag.)

one elite female distance runner ($\dot{V}O_{2max} = 64.7\ \mathrm{ml\,kg^{-1}\,min^{-1}}$) completed a 28-day "live high—train low" training intervention (living elevation, 2,150 m). Before and after altitude training, subjects ran at three submaximal speeds, and during a separate session, performed a graded exercise test to exhaustion. A regression equation derived from published data was used to estimate respiratory muscle $\dot{V}O_2$ ($\dot{V}O_{2RM}$) using our ventilation ($\dot{V}_E$) values. $\dot{V}O_{2RM}$ was also estimated retrospectively from a larger group of distance runners ($n = 22$). $\dot{V}O_{2max}$ significantly ($p < 0.05$) increased from pre- to post-altitude ($196 \pm 59\ \mathrm{ml\,min^{-1}}$), while $\dot{V}_E$ at $\dot{V}O_{2max}$ also significantly ($p < 0.05$) increased ($13.3 \pm 5.3\ \mathrm{l\,min^{-1}}$). The estimated $\dot{V}O_{2RM}$ contributed 37% of $\Delta\dot{V}O_{2max}$. The retrospective group also saw a significant increase in $\dot{V}O_{2max}$ from pre- to post-altitude ($201 \pm 36\ \mathrm{ml\,min^{-1}}$), along with a $10.8 \pm 2.1\ \mathrm{l\,min^{-1}}$ increase in $\dot{V}_E$, thus requiring an estimated 27% of $\Delta\dot{V}O_{2max}$. Our data suggest that a substantial portion of the improvement in $\dot{V}O_{2max}$ with chronic altitude training goes to fuel the respiratory muscles as opposed to the musculature which directly contributes to locomotion. Consequently, the timecourse of decay in ventilatory acclimatization following return to sea-level may have an impact on competitive performance (Fig 3).

▶ Many endurance athletes have now embraced the "live high train low" regimen.[1] Such a pattern of training induces an increased secretion of erythropoietin, a resultant increase of hemoglobin level, and a larger maximal oxygen intake.[2,3] It is often assumed that there will be a proportional increase in endurance performance. However, in addition to stimulating erythropoietin production, life at high altitude leads to an adjustment of acid/base balance in an attempt to permit a compensatory hyperventilation. This acid/base shift has consequences when exercising at sea level, leading to a greater ventilation for a given power output.[2] One adverse result is that an increased fraction of the individual's maximal oxygen intake is directed to the chest muscles (Fig 3), rather than to the muscles of locomotion.[4] Any gain of performance is thus quite a bit smaller than might be inferred from the increase of oxygen transport. In the present study, a 28-day sojourn at Flagstaff, AZ (2150 m), increased the athlete's peak sea level ventilation by 13 L/min, and the respiratory muscles were estimated to have consumed 37% of the gain in oxygen transport. This problem may be compounded by a reflex diversion of blood flow from the limbs to the chest muscles[5] and by a viscosity-related decrease of peak cardiac output. The net impact of a living high, training low regimen on performance must therefore be assessed from trials on the track instead of making inferences based on the measurement of maximal oxygen intake.

R. J. Shephard, MD (Lond), PhD, DPE

References

1. Wilber RL. Application of altitude/hypoxic training by elite athletes. *Med Sci Sports Exerc.* 2007;39:1610-1624.
2. Levine BD, Stray-Gundersen J. "Living high-training low": effect of moderate-altitude acclimatization with low-altitude training on performance. *J Appl Physiol.* 1997;83:102-112.
3. Levine BD, Stray-Gundersen J. The effects of altitude training are mediated primarily by acclimatization, rather than by hypoxic exercise. *Adv Exp Med Biol.* 2001;502:75-88.
4. Shephard RJ. The oxygen cost of breathing during vigorous exercise. *Q J Exp Physiol Cogn Med Sci.* 1966;51:336-350.
5. Dempsey JA, Romer L, Rodman J, Miller J, Smith C. Consequences of exercise-induced respiratory muscle work. *Respir Physiol Neurobiol.* 2006;28:242-250.

Risks factors for recurrent neurological decompression sickness in recreational divers: a case-control study

Gempp E, Louge P, Blatteau J-E, et al (Sainte Anne's Military Hosp, Toulon, France; Inst of Biomedical Res of French Armed Forces Res Team in Operational Diving, Toulon, France)
J Sports Med Phys Fitness 52:530-536, 2012

Aim.—Individual or environmental factors that predispose to the recurrence of neurological decompression sickness (DCS) in scuba divers are not known and preventive measures designed to mitigate the risk of a subsequent episode remain empirical. The aim of this controlled study was to examine some potential risk factors predictive of recurrent DCS event that may lead to practical recommendations for divers who wish to continue diving after an initial episode.

Methods.—Age, gender, diving experience, presence of a large right-to-left shunt (RLS) and diving practice following post-DCS resumption were

TABLE 2.—Low and Average Levels for Diving Certifications Consisted of Divers with a Certificate of Open-Water Diver, Rescue Diver and Advanced Open-Water Diver or Equivalent While High Level Comprised Divemasters and Diving Instructors

Variables	Univariate Analysis			Multivariate Analysis		
	Recurrence	No Recurrence	P	OR (95% CI)	P	Adj OR (95% CI)
Age (yr)			0.44	1.6 (0.5-4.6)		
≥47	17	30				
<47	7	20				
Gender			0.74	1.5 (0.4-6.3)		
Male	21	41				
Female	3	9				
Diving experience after initial DCS (median nb of dives)			0.43	1.6 (0.6-4.3)		
≥210	14	35				
<210	10	15				
Diving certification			0.14	2.2 (0.8-6.3)	0.03	3.8 (1.1-14)
High level	17	26				
Low and average levels	7	24				
Large right-to-left shunt			0.006	4.9 (1.6-14.5)	0.006	5.4 (1.5-19.7)
Yes	18	19				
No	6	31				
Changes in diving practice			0.0001	9.7 (2.8-32.9)	0.001	8.4 (2.3-31.1)
No	20	17				
Yes	4	33				

evaluated as potential predictors of a further DCS in recreational divers admitted in our hyperbaric facility over a period of 12 years.

Results.—Twenty-four recurrent cases and 50 divers treated for a single DCS episode which continued diving were recruited after review of medical forms and follow-up interview by telephone. After controlling for potential confounding variables between groups, multivariate analysis revealed that experienced divers (OR, 3.8; 95% CI, 1.1-14; $P = 0.03$), the presence of large RLS (OR, 5.4; 95% CI, 1.5-19.7; $P = 0.006$) and the lack of changes in the way of diving after prior DCS (OR, 8.4; 95% CI, 2.3-31.1; $P = 0.001$) were independently associated with a repeated episode.

Conclusion.—The findings highlight the importance for divers to adopt conservative dives profiles or to use preferentially oxygen-enriched breathing mixtures after an initial DCS. Closure of a documented RLS through a large patent foramen ovale as a secondary preventive procedure for individuals that cannot adapt their diving practice remains debatable (Table 2).

▶ When I was testing test pilots for decompression sickness at the RAF Institute of Aviation Medicine, the onset of the neurologic form of decompression sickness was regarded as a major emergency, and it is disturbing to read that one coastal hospital in France was able to accumulate 24 recurrent cases of neurologic decompression sickness among recreational divers in less than 13 years. One report sets the official incidence of the syndrome at 0.02% to 0.03% per dive.[1] The observed incidence, of course, depends on the manifestations that are included when making the diagnosis. In this study, these were quite broad, including paresthesias, numbness, motor weakness, ataxia, visual disturbances, altered higher function or speech, and inner ear disorders occurring within 6 hours of surfacing. In addition to the depth and duration of the dive, the water temperature, and the ascent protocol, the risk of decompression sickness is increased by various personal factors, including age, a low level of fitness, obesity, and a patent foramen ovale. There is also some evidence that a person who has had one attack is at greater biological risk of a recurrence.[2] However, these authors argue that much of the risk of recurrence reflects the presence of a large septal defect and a failure of the individual concerned to modify diving patterns after an initial episode (Table 2). Certainly, one episode of neurologic decompression sickness brings an urgent warning to change diving behavior. My own preference with those who show the more severe manifestations would be to recommend an alternative form of recreation.

R. J. Shephard, MD (Lond), PhD, DPE

References

1. Vann RD, Butler FK, Mitchell SJ, et al. Decompression illness. *Lancet.* 2011;377: 153-164.
2. Mollerlokken A, Eftedal I. Individual risk of decompression sickness: possible effects of genomic or epigenomic variation altering gene expresson. In: Lang M, Brubakk A, eds. *The Future of Diving: 100 Years of Haldane and Beyond.* Washington, DC: Smithsonian Institute Scholarly Press; 2009:53-57.

Persistence of critical flicker fusion frequency impairment after a 33 mfw SCUBA dive: evidence of prolonged nitrogen narcosis
Balestra C, Lafère P, Germonpré P (DAN Europe Res Division, Brussels, Belgium)
Eur J Appl Physiol 112:4063-4068, 2012

One of the possible risks incurred while diving is inert gas narcosis (IGN), yet its mechanism of action remains a matter of controversy. Although providing insights in the basic mechanisms of IGN, research has been primarily limited to animal studies. A human study, in real diving conditions, was needed. Twenty volunteers within strict biometrical criteria (male, age 30–40 years, BMI 20–23, non smoker) were selected. They performed a nodecompression dive to a depth of 33 mfw for 20 min and were assessed by the means of critical flicker fusion frequency (CFFF) measurement before the dive, during the dive upon arriving at the bottom, 5 min before the ascent, and 30 min after surfacing. After this late measurement, divers breathed oxygen for 15 min and were assessed a final time. Compared to the pre-dive value the mean value of each measurement was significantly different ($p < 0.001$). An increase of CFFF to 104 ± 5.1 % upon arriving to the bottom is followed by a decrease to 93.5 ± 4.3 %. This impairment of CFFF persisted 30 min after surfacing, still decreased to $96.3 \pm 8.2\%$ compared to pre-dive CFFF. Post-dive measures made

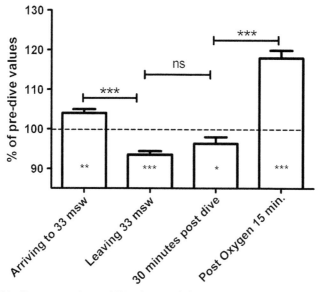

FIGURE 1.—Percentage variation of CFFF during and after a 20 min dive to 33 mfw/110 ffw. Pre-dive CFFF value is taken as 100%. Each subject is compared to his own pre-dive value. (***$p < 0.001$; **$p < 0.01$; *$p < 0.05$; *ns* not significant) ($n = 20$). (Reprinted from Balestra C, Lafère P, Germonpré P. Persistence of critical flicker fusion frequency impairment after a 33 mfw SCUBA dive: evidence of prolonged nitrogen narcosis. *Eur J Appl Physiol.* 2012;112:4063-4068, with permission from Springer-Verlag.)

after 15 min of oxygen were not different from control (without nitrogen supersaturation), 124.4 ± 10.8 versus 124.2 ± 3.9 %. This simple study suggests that IGN (at least partially) depends on gas-protein interactions and that the cerebral impairment persists for at least 30 min after surfacing. This could be an important consideration in situations where precise and accurate judgment or actions are essential (Fig 1).

▶ Inert gas narcosis is a well-recognized hazard for the SCUBA diver, with issues of temporal and spatial disorientation, loss of physical coordination, mood disorders, and memory disturbances.[1,2] It is thus important not to undertake a further dive until symptoms have ended. The critical flicker fusion test is finding increasing use in diving investigations as an objective measure of cerebral arousal; with responses that parallel electroencephalogram changes, it can often reveal subtle but persistent abnormalities of neural function that are not revealed by subjective questioning.[3] The results of Balestra and associates were obtained on 20 non-obese and experienced middle-aged divers after they had descended to 33 meters of fresh water for 20 minutes. Thirty minutes after returning to the surface, there was some recovery, but the flicker fusion score still showed significant impairment relative to the predive value; this deficit was corrected rapidly by administration of oxygen (Fig 1). The beneficial effects of oxygen may reflect a facilitation of nerve conduction[4] and/or a decreased production of GABA and thus an inhibition of inhibitory circuits in the brain.[5] Further study is needed to explore whether the oxygen is also facilitating the washout of nitrogen or whether it is acting competitively in a gas—protein interaction.

R. J. Shephard, MD (Lond), PhD, DPE

References

1. Lowry C. Inert gas narcosis. In: Edmons C, Lowry C, Pennefather J, et al., eds. *Diving and Subaquatic Medicine*. 4th ed. London, UK: Hodder Arnold; 2005:183-193.
2. Richardson D, Kinsella D, Schreeves K. Gas narcosis. In: Richardson D, Kinsella D, Schreeves K, eds. *The Encyclopedia of Recreational Diving*. Rancho Santa Margarita, CA: PADI; 2005:20-23.
3. Seki K, Hugon M. Critical flicker frequency (CFF) and subjective fatigue during an oxyhelium saturation dive at 62 ATA. *Undersea Biomed Res*. 1976;3:235-247.
4. Brerro-Saby C, Delliaux S, Steinberg JG, Jammes Y. The changes in neuromuscular excitability with normobaric hyperoxia in humans. *Exp Physiol*. 2010;95:153-159.
5. Banister EW, Singh AK. The central role of ammonia in OHD-inducted convulsions. In: Bachrach AJ, Matzen MM, eds. *Underwater Physiology VII*. Bethesda, MD: Undersea Med Soc Inc; 1981:37-44.

Should children dive with self-contained underwater breathing apparatus (SCUBA)?
Winkler BE, Muth C-M, Tetzlaff K (Univ of Ulm, Germany; Univ of Tuebingen, Germany)
Acta Paediatr 101:472-478, 2012

Diving with self-contained underwater breathing apparatus (SCUBA) has become a popular recreational activity in children and adolescents. This article provides an extensive review of the current literature.

Conclusions.—Medical contraindications to SCUBA diving for adults apply to children and adolescents, too, but must be adapted. Additional restrictions to the fitness to dive must apply to both, children and adolescents. Children should always be accompanied by a trained adult when diving (Fig 1).

▶ The authors of this report focus mainly on potential medical hazards that may increase risks for the young SCUBA diver, but the most alarming section of their article is that devoted to the epidemiology of SCUBA accidents in children and adolescents, particularly because these authors are suggesting that children as young as 8 years old can engage in this sport. This policy is apparently supported by commercial SCUBA diving associations such as the Professional Association of Diving Instructors and an ever-growing number of young children are being certified (Fig 1). Between 1989 and 2002, the Divers Alert Network documented 1248 fatal accidents among divers; 24 of these were in individuals younger than 18 years of age.[1] Over a 20-year period, the University of Hawaii alone treated 6 children with arterial gas embolism and 16 cases of decompression sickness, often arising from a defiance of basic diving rules. Another common source of difficulty was an emergency ascent associated with an underwater panic attack, in some cases linked to pre-existing asthma. Nine children also had to make an emergency

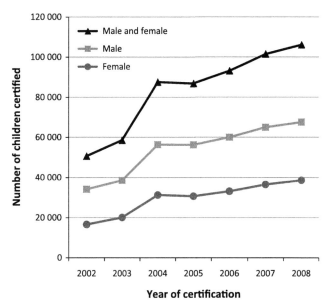

FIGURE 1.—Certifications in 8–14-year-old children by Professional Association of Diving Instructors (PADI). From 2002 till 2008, the numbers of male, female and total certifications per year are presented. (Reprinted from Winkler BE, Muth C-M, Tetzlaff K. Should children dive with self-contained underwater breathing apparatus (SCUBA)? *Acta Paediatr.* 2012;101:472-478, with permission from John Wiley and Sons.)

ascent because their gas tank was exhausted. As might perhaps be anticipated, the risk of a problem seems to be particularly high in children labeled as suffering from attention deficit disorder.[2]

R. J. Shephard, MD (Lond), PhD, DPE

References

1. Caruso JL, Uguccioni DM, Ellis JE, et al. Diving fatalities involving children and adolescents. *Undersea Hyperb Med.* 2004;31:329.
2. Smerz R. Epidemiology and treatment of decompression illness in children and adolescents in Hawaii, 1983–2003. *SPUMS J.* 2005;35:5-10.

Should Children Be SCUBA Diving?: Cerebral Arterial Gas Embolism in a Swimming Pool

Johnson V, Adkinson C, Bowen M, et al (Hennepin County Med Ctr, Minneapolis, MN; Children's Hosps and Clinics of Minnesota, Minneapolis)
Pediatr Emerg Care 28:361-362, 2012

Cerebral arterial gas embolism (CAGE) is a well-known serious complication of self-contained breathing apparatus (SCUBA) diving. Most serious complications of SCUBA diving occur in adults because most of SCUBA divers are adults. However, young age is an independent risk factor for injury in SCUBA diving and shallow-water SCUBA diving is the riskiest environment for CAGE. We present a case of a 10-year-old boy who developed CAGE while taking SCUBA diving lessons in a university swimming pool. This case illustrates the potential danger of SCUBA diving for children who lack understanding of the physics of diving as well as the often unappreciated risk of shallow-water SCUBA diving. Our intent is to educate providers of primary care to children, so that they may appropriately advise parents about SCUBA diving, and to educate providers of emergency care to children, so that they will recognize this uncommon but serious emergency condition.

▶ Cerebral artery embolism can occur during scuba diving if a person ascends without exhaling; a differential pressure between gas within the lungs and water on the outside of the chest wall allows overexpansion of the lungs, rupturing pulmonary vessels and allowing entry of gas bubbles into the pleura, the mediastinum, or the arterial circulation. The water does not need to be particularly deep— an ascent of as little as 1 m can be sufficient to cause such damage.[1,2] The only treatment currently recommended is immediate hyperbaric oxygen, which (as in this article) possibly increases the supply of oxygen to the affected area of the brain, reducing symptoms of cerebral injury.[3] The current lower age limit for scuba instruction in the United States is 12 years,[4] and the patient in this report was only aged 10 years. However, given the risks involved, it may be questioned whether all boys of 12 years have the maturity to use such equipment safely.

R. J. Shephard, MD (Lond), PhD, DPE

References

1. Cooperman EM, Hogg J, Thurlbeck WM. Mechanisms of death in shallow-water scuba diving. *Can Med Assoc J*. 1968;99:1128-1131.
2. Polak B, Adams H. Traumatic air embolism in submarine escape training. *U S Nav Med Bull*. 1932;30:165-177.
3. Muth CM, Shank ES. Gas embolism. *N Engl J Med*. 2000;342:476-482.
4. Dembert ML, Keith JF 3rd. Evaluating the potential pediatric scuba diver. *Am J Dis Child*. 1986;140:1135-1141.

Other Environmental Problems

Urban Sprawl, Physical Activity, and Body Mass Index: Nurses' Health Study and Nurses' Health Study II

James P, Troped PJ, Hart JE, et al (Harvard School of Public Health, Boston, MA; Purdue Univ, West Lafayette, IN; et al)
Am J Public Health 103:369-375, 2013

Objectives.—We evaluated the association between the county sprawl index, a measure of residential density and street accessibility, and physical activity and body mass index (BMI).

Methods.—We conducted a multilevel cross-sectional analysis in a sample of Nurses' Health Study participants living throughout the United States in 2000 to 2001 (n = 136 592).

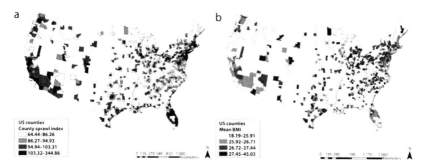

FIGURE 1.—County sprawl index and mean body mass index in participants and counties: United States, Nurses' Health Study, 2000, and Nurses' Health Study II, 2001. (Reprinted with permission from the American Public Health Association. James P, Troped PJ, Hart JE, et al. Urban sprawl, physical activity, and body mass index: Nurses' Health Study and Nurses' Health Study II. *Am J Public Health.* 2013;103:369-375 Copyright 2013.)

Results.—In analyses adjusted for age, smoking status, race, and husband's education, a 1-SD (25.7) increase in the county sprawl index (indicating a denser, more compact county) was associated with a 0.13 kilograms per meters squared (95% confidence interval [CI] = −0.18, −0.07) lower BMI and 0.41 (95% CI = 0.17, 0.65) more metabolic equivalent (MET) hours per week of total physical activity, 0.26 (95% CI = 0.19, 0.33) more MET hours per week of walking, and 0.47 (95% CI = 0.34, 0.59) more MET hours per week of walking, bicycling, jogging, and running. We detected potential effect modification for age, previous disease status, husband's education level (a proxy for socioeconomic status), and race.

Conclusions.—Our results suggest that living in a dense, compact county may be conducive to higher levels of physical activity and lower BMI in women (Fig 1).

▶ Physical activity and obesity are linked to the "built environment" or the land-use patterns, transportation systems, and design features that provide opportunities for travel and physical activity.[1] Important attributes of the built environment include density, street connectivity, and land-use mix, and enhance opportunities for walking and overall physical activity because homes, stores, and other destinations are closer. This large study of geographically diverse female nurses found an inverse relationship between the county sprawl index and body mass index (BMI), and positive associations between the county sprawl index and physical activity (Fig 1). In other words, women who lived in denser counties with more accessible street designs had lower BMIs and were more active.

D. C. Nieman, DrPH

Reference

1. Brownson RC, Hoehner CM, Day K, Forsyth A, Sallis JF. Measuring the built environment for physical activity: state of the science. *Am J Prev Med.* 2009;36: S99-S123.e12.

9 Special Considerations: Children, Women, the Elderly, and Special Populations

Children

Physical Therapy Reduces Bone Resorption and Increases Bone Formation in Preterm Infants

Vignochi CM, Silveira RC, Miura E, et al (Universidade Federal do Rio Grande do sul, Brazil; Fundação Federal de Ciências da Saúde, Porto Alegre, Brazil)

Am J Perinatol 29:573-578, 2012

Aim.—To evaluate bone metabolism in newborn preterm infants before and after a physical therapy protocol.

Method.—This randomized controlled clinical trial included 30 newborn preterm infants with gestational age <35 weeks and appropriate weight for gestational age, who were randomized into control group (CG) and physiotherapy group (PG). The PG protocol consisted of 15 minutes of daily passive movements with gentle joint compression 5 days a week. Daily data were obtained on feeding and body weight. Measurements of bone-specific alkaline phosphatase (BAP) and urinary deoxypyridinoline (DPD) were collected before and after intervention in both groups. The analysis of covariance test was performed to compare the means of both groups.

Results.—At baseline, gestational age and corrected gestational age, birth weight, and gender were similar between both groups. Nutrient supply, length of total parenteral nutrition, and mechanical ventilation were also similar. BAP level increase in PG was 22.44 ± 3.49 U/L, whereas in CG was 2.87 ± 3.99 U/L ($p = 0.003$). There was a reduction of DPD levels in PG of 28.21 ± 11.05 nmol/mmol, and an increase of 49.95 ± 11.05 nmol/mmol ($p < 0.001$) in GC.

Conclusion.—The benefits of prevention and treatment of metabolic bone disease of prematurity, in addition to an adequate diet, should include these passive exercises with gentle joint compressions to improve the quality of premature infant's bones.

▶ This is an interesting study regarding osteopenia in preterm infants. The prevalence of osteopenia has been found to be relatively high in this population and is related to gestational age; birth weight and corticosteroid use (to treat respiratory disorders) may further aggravate osteopenia and in severe cases the risk of fracture has been found to be high. There is emerging evidence regarding mobilizations, which will produce mechanical stimuli promoting bone formation and growth in preterm infants. This study adds to this body of knowledge. A simple physiotherapy protocol performed 5 days a week for 15 minutes, including passive mobilizations in flexion and extension with soft articular compression of upper and lower limbs, led to a significant and clinically important increase in bone formation markers. The conclusions of the authors are sound and the authors warrant longer follow-up studies to see the long-term effects of this type of intervention. These results are promising and this type of intervention could also be taught to parents.

F. Desmeules, PT, PhD

Moderate to Vigorous Physical Activity and Sedentary Time and Cardiometabolic Risk Factors in Children and Adolescents

Ekelund U, for the International Children's Accelerometry Database (ICAD) Collaborators (Inst of Metabolic Science, Cambridge, UK; et al)
JAMA 307:704-712, 2012

Context.—Sparse data exist on the combined associations between physical activity and sedentary time with cardiometabolic risk factors in healthy children.

Objective.—To examine the independent and combined associations between objectively measured time in moderate- to vigorous-intensity physical activity (MVPA) and sedentary time with cardiometabolic risk factors.

Design, Setting, and Participants.—Pooled data from 14 studies between 1998 and 2009 comprising 20 871 children (aged 4-18 years) from the International Children's Accelerometry Database. Time spent in MVPA and sedentary time were measured using accelerometry after reanalyzing raw data. The independent associations between time in MVPA and sedentary time, with outcomes, were examined using meta-analysis. Participants were stratified by tertiles of MVPA and sedentary time.

Main Outcome Measures.—Waist circumference, systolic blood pressure, fasting triglycerides, high-density lipoprotein cholesterol, and insulin.

Results.—Times (mean [SD] min/d) accumulated by children in MVPA and being sedentary were 30 (21) and 354 (96), respectively. Time in MVPA was significantly associated with all cardiometabolic outcomes independent of sex, age, monitor wear time, time spent sedentary, and waist circumference (when not the outcome). Sedentary time was not associated

TABLE 5.—Associations Between Total Physical Activity, Time Spent in MVPA, and Sedentary Time with Cardiometabolic Risk Factors in 20 871 Children

	β Coefficients (95% CI)[a]				
	Waist Circumference, cm (n = 20 871)	SBP, mm Hg[b] (n = 15 062)	Insulin, pmol/L[b] (n = 5261)	Triglycerides, mg/dL[b] (n = 5689)	HDL Cholesterol, mg/dL (n = 8360)
Total PA, cpm	−0.35 (−0.50 to −0.16)	−0.10 (−0.26 to 0.05)	−0.026 (−0.033 to −0.020)	−0.021 (−0.026 to −0.016)	0.19 (−0.11 to 0.48)
MVPA, min/d	−0.52 (−0.76 to −0.28)	−0.15 (−0.30 to −0.06)	−0.028 (−0.038 to −0.017)	−0.017 (−0.025 to −0.009)	0.25 (−0.034 to 0.53)
Sedentary, min/d	0.13 (−0.094 to 0.358)	−0.043 (−0.21 to 0.20)	0.012 (0.0029 to 0.022)	0.014 (−0.0031 to 0.030)	−0.064 (−0.24 to 0.12)
MVPA, min/d[c]	−0.54 (−0.79 to −0.30)	−0.17 (−0.30 to −0.04)	−0.030 (−0.043 to −0.017)	−0.014 (−0.023 to −0.0046)	0.31 (0.036 to 0.59)
Sedentary, min/d[c]	−0.12 (−0.32 to 0.09)	−0.10 (−0.21 to 0.02)	−0.009 (−0.026, 0.008)	0.006 (−0.010 to 0.023)	0.096 (−0.098 to 0.29)

Abbreviations: HDL, high-density lipoprotein; MVPA, moderate- to vigorous-intensity physical activity; SBP, systolic blood pressure. See Table 3 for SI conversion factors.

[a]Coefficients represent the change in the outcome for a 100-cpm change in total physical activity and a 10-minute change in time spent in MVPA and a 60-minute change in time spent sedentary. Data are adjusted for age, sex, monitor wear minutes, and waist circumference (when it is not the outcome).

[b]SBP is additionally adjusted for height; and fasting insulin and triglycerides were log transformed.

[c]MVPA is additionally adjusted for sedentary time and sedentary time is mutually adjusted for MVPA.

with any outcome independent of time in MVPA. In the combined analyses, higher levels of MVPA were associated with better cardiometabolic risk factors across tertiles of sedentary time. The differences in outcomes between higher and lower MVPA were greater with lower sedentary time. Mean differences in waist circumference between the bottom and top tertiles of MVPA were 5.6 cm (95% CI, 4.8-6.4 cm) for high sedentary time and 3.6 cm (95% CI, 2.8-4.3 cm) for low sedentary time. Mean differences in systolic blood pressure for high and low sedentary time were 0.7 mm Hg (95% CI, −0.07 to 1.6) and 2.5 mm Hg (95% CI, 1.7-3.3), and for high-density lipoprotein cholesterol, differences were −2.6 mg/dL (95% CI, −1.4 to −3.9) and −4.5 mg/dL (95% CI, −3.3 to −5.6), respectively. Geometric mean differences for insulin and triglycerides showed similar variation. Those in the top tertile of MVPA accumulated more than 35 minutes per day in this intensity level compared with fewer than 18 minutes per day for those in the bottom tertile. In prospective analyses (N = 6413 at 2.1 years' follow-up), MVPA and sedentary time were not associated with waist circumference at follow-up, but a higher waist circumference at baseline was associated with higher amounts of sedentary time at follow-up.

Conclusion.—Higher MVPA time by children and adolescents was associated with better cardiometabolic risk factors regardless of the amount of sedentary time (Table 5).

▶ There has recently been a trend to examine not only habitual physical activity but also the amount of time a person spends sitting when assessing a healthy lifestyle. Perhaps because sitting time is more easily measured than the time spent in physical activity, the additional measurement has contributed to the description of cardiac risk factors in a number of studies. This meta-analysis examined this question with respect to a massive sample of children, and the data on physical activity patterns were based on accelerometry records rather than questionnaires. The accelerometer generally provides a more reliable indication of physical activity patterns than questionnaires, although it is unable to detect cycling, which may be a major source of exercise for some children. The added count used to detect an active child was a substantial 3000 impulses per day. The accelerometer gives a relatively unequivocal indication of when a child is sedentary. In opposition to some reports, the present analysis found no independent influence of sitting on cardiac risk factors (Table 5), although there did seem to be an interactive effect, with physical activity being linked to a more favorable profile in those who spent less time sitting. One issue in interpretation of the analysis is that account was only taken of total sedentary time; sitting may be much worse for cardiovascular health if it is spent in front of a television screen, watching advertisements for food and drink and thus being stimulated to ingest unneeded refreshments. Moreover, the studies considered were cross-sectional in design, so it is not possible to make causal inferences. Finally, the differences in cardiac risk factors between those classed as active and those rated as sedentary were quite small if viewed in a clinical perspective.

R. J. Shephard, MD (Lond), PhD, DPE

Body mass index, fitness and physical activity from childhood through adolescence

Pahkala K, Hernelahti M, Heinonen OJ, et al (Univ of Turku, Finland; et al)
Br J Sports Med 47:71-77, 2013

Background.—Obesity, sedentary lifestyle and poor cardiorespiratory fitness in childhood may increase the risk of health problems later in life.

Purpose.—The authors studied the association of early childhood weight status with cardiorespiratory fitness and leisure-time physical activity (LTPA) in adolescence. The stability and associations of LTPA and fitness from childhood through adolescence were also studied.

Methods.—Body mass index (BMI) was assessed annually since birth in a prospective, longitudinal study. The mean BMI between ages 2 and 7 years indicated weight status at preschool age. Fitness was studied with a shuttle run test at age 9 and with a maximal cycle ergometer test at age 17. The same questionnaire was used to assess LTPA at age 9, 13 and 17. Complete data on preschool BMI, LTPA at ages 13 and 17 and fitness at age 17 years was provided by 351 children, while fitness and LTPA data were available for 74 children at ages 9 and 17.

Results.—Preschool BMI was inversely associated with fitness in adolescence independently of adolescent LTPA ($p = 0.0001$). Children who had a high preschool BMI but whose weight status was reduced in adolescence had similar fitness in adolescence as the children with a persistently low BMI. Regardless of the fitness level in childhood, the children whose LTPA increased between age 9 and 17 had a similar adolescent fitness level as persistently active subjects.

Conclusions.—It is important to maintain a healthy body weight and a physically active lifestyle from very childhood through adolescence to improve fitness during adolescence.

▶ Before this study, little was known regarding whether weight in early childhood was linked to aerobic fitness and activity in adolescence. Throughout the world, lack of physical activity is the fourth-most important risk factor associated with mortality and this is probably based on activity habits early in life.[1] This study shows that a persistently high body mass index (BMI) from a very young age is linked to lower fitness during adolescence regardless of the level of physical activity. The novel finding of this study is that if children with a high preschool BMI reduce their BMI, their fitness level during adolescence is similar to those with a persistently low BMI. As expected, increasing physical activity levels from childhood to adolescence is associated with improved fitness independent of childhood fitness level. Overall, this study shows the importance of maintaining a healthy body weight and a physically active lifestyle throughout childhood and adolescence.

D. C. Nieman, DrPH

Reference

1. World Health Organization. Global Health Risks. Mortality and burden of disease attributable to selected major risks. WHO Library Cataloguing-in-Publication Data, 2009:10. http://www.who.int/healthinfo/global_burden_disease/GlobalHealthRisks_report_full.pdf. Accessed October 2, 2011.

Serum Vitamin D, Physical Activity, and Metabolic Risk Factors in Korean Children

Ha C-D, Cho J-K, Lee S-H, et al (Sungkyunkwan Univ, Suwon, Republic of Korea; Pohang Univ of Science and Technology, Republic of Korea)
Med Sci Sports Exerc 45:102-108, 2013

Purpose.—The purpose of this study was to investigate the relationship of serum vitamin D levels with lifestyle factors, including body fatness and physical activity (PA) parameters, and the clustering of metabolic risk factors in the Korean pediatric population.

Methods.—Serum 25-hydroxyvitamin D levels, accelerometer-based PA, and body fatness and metabolic syndrome parameters were assessed in a sample of children of Korean descent ($N = 310$). Correlation and multivariate linear regression were used to explore the relationships among serum vitamin D levels, lifestyle factors, and the clustering of metabolic risk factors in the study sample.

Results.—Serum vitamin D levels were negatively associated with body fatness parameters, including body mass index, percent body fat, and waist circumference, but positively associated with accelerometer-based PA including low, moderate, and vigorous levels. In addition, serum vitamin D levels were inversely related to total cholesterol, triglycerides, fasting glucose, and insulin. A stepwise linear regression model showed that both low serum vitamin D levels and decreased vigorous PA were independent predictors for individual variation in the clustering of metabolic risk factors in this study sample.

Conclusion.—The results of this study suggest that an increase in vigorous PA and vitamin D intake should be two major targets of public health inventions against the clustering of metabolic risk factors in the Korean pediatric population.

▶ Serum 25-hydroxyvitamin D (25[OH]D) is the best indicator and major form of vitamin D in the blood, with a circulating half-life of 2 to 3 weeks. Vitamin D deficiency is defined as a 25(OH)D level of less than 20 ng/mL, with vitamin D insufficiency defined as 21 to 29 ng/mL. Estimates are that 20% to 100% of children, young and middle-aged adults, and community-dwelling elderly men and women are vitamin D deficient.[1] The vitamin D receptor is found in most tissues of the body, and vitamin D has been linked to wide-ranging biological effects, including improved calcium absorption and bone health, blood vessel growth, muscle function, immune function, and insulin production. Low serum vitamin

D levels are associated with numerous health conditions, such as the metabolic syndrome, obesity, colon cancer (and perhaps breast cancer), infection, autoimmunity, falls, fractures, and age-related decline in cognitive function.[2] This study shows that vitamin D is linked to health, body fatness, and risk factors, even in 10- to 12-year-olds. The authors recommend that an increase in vitamin D intake and vigorous physical activity should be major targets of lifestyle interventions against the clustering of metabolic risk factors.

D. C. Nieman, DrPH

References

1. Holick MF, Binkley NC, Bischoff-Ferrari HA, et al; Endocrine Society. Evaluation, treatment, and prevention of vitamin D deficiency: an Endocrine Society clinical practice guideline. *J Clin Endocrinol Metab*. 2011;96:1911-1930.
2. Moreno LA, Valtueña J, Pérez-López F, González-Gross M. Health effects related to low vitamin D concentrations: beyond bone metabolism. *Ann Nutr Metab*. 2011;59:22-27.

Estimated Energy Expenditures for School-Based Policies and Active Living
Bassett DR, Fitzhugh EC, Heath GW, et al (Univ of Tennessee, Knoxville; Univ of Tennessee, Chattanooga)
Am J Prev Med 44:108-113, 2013

Background.—Despite overwhelming evidence of the health benefits of physical activity, most American youth are not meeting the 60 minutes per day recommendation for moderate- to vigorous-intensity physical activity (MVPA). Policy changes have the potential to bring about substantial increases in physical activity in youth, within school and community settings.

Purpose.—The purpose of this study was to quantify the increase in energy expenditure for school-based policies and built environment changes.

Methods.—Scientific literature reviews were consulted, and more than 300 published studies (1995–2011) in English were identified based on titles and abstracts. After an initial screening, 85 articles were included. Study quality was assessed, and the impact of various strategies for increasing physical activity in youth was estimated from objective measurements/ direct observation.

Results.—Within school settings, the average minutes of MVPA gained per school day for studies in each intervention category were as follows: mandatory physical education (23 minutes); classroom activity breaks (19 minutes); afterschool activity programs (10 minutes); standardized physical education curricula (6 minutes more than traditional physical education); modified playgrounds (6 minutes); and modified recess (5 minutes more than traditional recess). Within community settings, significant MVPA was associated with active commuting (16 minutes) and park renovations (12 minutes), but proximity to parks had a small effect (1 minute). No

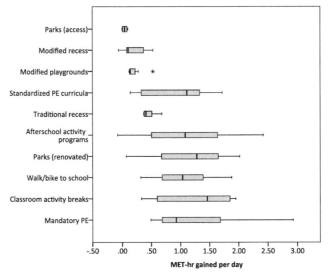

FIGURE 1.—MET-hour gained per day in response to various physical activity interventions. *Note*: The vertical lines within each box depict the medians; the boxes represent the interquartile ranges (25th—75th percentile); and the ends of the horizontal lines represent the minimums and maximums. *Study outcome was an outlier. PE, physical education. (Reprinted from American Journal of Preventive Medicine. Bassett DR, Fitzhugh EC, Heath GW, et al. Estimated energy expenditures for school-based policies and active living. *Am J Prev Med.* 2013;44:108-113, Copyright 2013, with permission from Elsevier.)

conclusions could be drawn regarding joint-use agreements, because of a lack of studies quantifying their impact on energy expenditure.

Conclusions.—Of the various policies and built environment changes examined, the largest effects were seen with mandatory physical education, classroom activity breaks, and active commuting to school. Policymakers can use this information along with estimates of the cost, feasibility, and population reach, to identify the best options for increasing physical activity in youth (Fig 1).

▶ Accelerometer data from the National Health and Nutrition Examination Survey indicate that only 42% of US children age 6 to 11 years meet the national physical activity guideline of at least 60 minutes of moderate- to vigorous-intensity physical activity per day, and fewer than 8% of US adolescents achieve this goal.[1] Physical activity levels can be influenced by policy changes affecting schoolchildren (K—12) and altering the built environment, but the relative importance of all the various options has not been ascertained. As summarized in Fig 1, this study indicates that mandating daily physical education has the greatest impact on physical activity of US youth. Although physical education classes vary, most increase physical activity and help children develop motor skills. Only a small minority of elementary, middle, and high schools offer daily physical activity, and much needs to be done to turn this around.

D. C. Nieman, DrPH

Reference

1. Troiano RP, Berrigan D, Dodd KW, Mâsse LC, Tilert T, McDowell M. Physical activity in the United States measured by accelerometer. *Med Sci Sports Exerc.* 2008;40:181-188.

Step Count Targets Corresponding to New Physical Activity Guidelines for the Early Years

Gabel L, Proudfoot NA, Obeid J, et al (McMaster Univ, Hamilton, Ontario, Canada)
Med Sci Sports Exerc 45:314-318, 2013

Purpose.—New physical activity guidelines recommend that children age 3—4 yr should accumulate at least 180 min of physical activity at any intensity spread throughout the day, including progression toward at least 60 min of energetic play by 5 yr of age. Step count targets corresponding to these recommendations will help practitioners and researchers monitor physical activity.

Methods.—One hundred thirty-three preschoolers were instructed to wear accelerometers for seven consecutive days. Activity and step count data were recorded in 3-s epochs. Step count targets equivalent to physical activity recommendations were derived using prediction equations from regression analyses. Receiver operating curve analyses were conducted to compare the sensitivity and specificity of the derived thresholds as well as a range of other targets.

Results.—The daily step count target derived for 180 min of physical activity of any intensity was 6013 ± 88, whereas the target for 180 min of physical activity of any intensity including at least 60 min of moderate-to-vigorous physical activity was 6191 ± 103. The smallest discrepancy

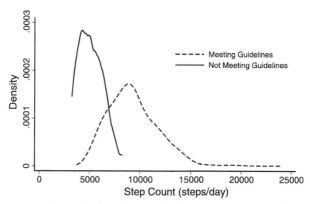

FIGURE 1.—Kernel density plot illustrating the distribution of step counts for days meeting and not meeting 180 min of physical activity of any intensity. (Reprinted from Gabel L, Proudfoot NA, Obeid J, et al. Step count targets corresponding to new physical activity guidelines for the early years. *Med Sci Sports Exerc.* 2013;45:314-318, with permission from the American College of Sports Medicine.)

between days meeting physical activity guidelines and step count targets was found with a 6000-step-per-day target. Receiver operating curves confirmed a balanced sensitivity and specificity of this target.

Conclusions.—On the basis of our data, we suggest that a new step count target of 6000 steps per day should be used to determine whether 3- to 5-yr-old children are meeting physical activity recommendations (Fig 1).

▶ Canadian physical activity guidelines recommend that children ages 3—4 years should accumulate at least 180 minutes of physical activity at any intensity spread throughout the day, including progression toward at least 60 minutes of energetic play by 5 years of age.[1] Pedometry is an inexpensive tool for counting steps, but little is known regarding how many steps by young children equate to 180 minutes of activity per day. About 12 000 steps per day are recommended for 6- to 19-year-olds and correspond to 60 minutes of physical activity.[2] As shown in Fig 1, about 6000 steps per day are recommended for preschoolers.

D. C. Nieman, DrPH

References

1. Tremblay MS, Leblanc AG, Carson V, et al. Canadian physical activity guidelines for the early years (aged 0-4 years). *Appl Physiol Nutr Metab*. 2012;37:345-356.
2. Colley RC, Janssen I, Tremblay MS. Daily step target to measure adherence to physical activity guidelines in children. *Med Sci Sports Exerc*. 2012;44:977-982.

Role of Childhood Aerobic Fitness in Successful Street Crossing

Chaddock L, Neider MB, Lutz A, et al (Univ of Illinois at Urbana—Champaign; Univ of Central Florida, Orlando)
Med Sci Sports Exerc 44:749-753, 2012

Increased aerobic fitness is associated with improved cognition, brain health, and academic achievement during preadolescence.

Purpose.—In this study, we extended these findings by examining the relationship between aerobic fitness and an everyday real-world task: street crossing. Because street crossing can be a dangerous multitask challenge and is a leading cause of injury in children, it is important to find ways to improve pedestrian safety.

Methods.—A street intersection was modeled in a virtual environment, and higher-fit ($n = 13$, 7 boys) and lower-fit ($n = 13$, 5 boys) 8- to 10-yr-old children, as determined by $\dot{V}O_{2max}$ testing, navigated trafficked roads by walking on a treadmill that was integrated with an immersive virtual world. Child pedestrians crossed the street while undistracted, listening to music, or conversing on a hands-free cellular phone.

Results.—Cell phones impaired street crossing success rates compared with the undistracted or music conditions for all participants ($P = 0.004$), a result that supports previous research. However, individual differences in aerobic fitness influenced these patterns (fitness × condition interaction, $P = 0.003$). Higher-fit children maintained street crossing success rates across all three conditions (paired *t*-tests, all $P > 0.4$), whereas lower-fit children showed decreased success rates when on the phone, relative to the undistracted ($P = 0.018$) and music ($P = 0.019$) conditions.

Conclusions.—The results suggest that higher levels of childhood aerobic fitness may attenuate the impairment typically associated with multitasking during street crossing. It is possible that superior cognitive abilities of higher-fit children play a role in the performance differences during complex real-world tasks.

▶ A few years ago, a colleague of mine and I were teaching the pediatric public health section of the medical school curriculum at our university. My colleague, who is an injury epidemiologist, started the lecture by talking about the burden that injury places on children and youth. Among his evidence he presented a study that examined pediatric pedestrian injuries and described the role that active transportation played in such injuries. I followed this with a presentation on the declining activity levels of children and youth and the negative impact this was having on their health. Among the evidence I presented was a study that showed that a lack of active transportation to school contributes to reduced physical activity levels. You can imagine the medical students' reaction to this mixed message on the health impacts of active transportation. I thought this study by Chaddock and colleagues was a bridge between the potential positive and negative aspects of active transportation.

The key finding of this study is that children with higher aerobic fitness levels have superior cognitive abilities, and that this can help attenuate the increased pedestrian injury risk faced while multitasking during street crossing. In other words, using a cell phone or listening to music in a simulated street-crossing exercise distracted the children and impaired their street crossing (eg, longer street crossing times, more time to make judgements, fewer head turns). However, aerobic fitness influenced this impairment such that street-crossing exercises were impaired to a lesser extent with fit children. The authors concluded that "childhood aerobic fitness not only relates to performance in the classroom and laboratory but also extends to childhood pedestrian-automobile accidents, and perhaps more general, multitasking." These are relevant conclusions and findings given that the current generation of young people are surrounded by technology, and multitasking with this technology is a big part of their lives.

I. Janssen, PhD

Preschoolers' Physical Activity, Screen Time, and Compliance with Recommendations

Hinkley T, Salmon J, Okely AD, et al (Univ of Wollongong, Australia; Deakin Univ, Victoria, Australia)
Med Sci Sports Exerc 44:458-465, 2012

Purpose.—Little evidence exists about the prevalence of adequate levels of physical activity and of appropriate screen-based entertainment in preschool children. Previous studies have generally relied on small samples.

This study investigates how much time preschool children spend being physically active and engaged in screen-based entertainment. The study also reports compliance with the recently released Australian recommendations for physical activity (≥ 3 h·d^{-1}) and screen entertainment (≤ 1 h·d^{-1}) and the National Association for Sport and Physical Education physical activity guidelines (≥ 2 h·d^{-1}) and American Academy of Pediatrics screen-based entertainment recommendations (≤ 2 h·d^{-1}) in a large sample of preschool children.

Methods.—Participants were 1004 Melbourne preschool children (mean age = 4.5 yr, range = 3–5 yr) and their families in the Healthy Active Preschool Years study. Physical activity data were collected by accelerometry during an 8-d period. Parents reported their child's television/video/DVD viewing, computer/Internet, and electronic game use during a typical week. A total of 703 (70%) had sufficient accelerometry data, and 935 children (93%) had useable data on time spent in screen-based entertainment.

Results.—Children spent 16% (approximately 127 min·d^{-1}) of their time being physically active. Boys and younger children were more active than were girls and older children, respectively. Children spent an average of 113 min·d in screen-based entertainment. Virtually no children (<1%) met both the Australian recommendations and 32% met both the National Association for Sport and Physical Education and American Academy of Pediatrics recommendations.

Conclusions.—The majority of young children are not participating in adequate amounts of physical activity and in excessive amounts of screen-based entertainment. It is likely that physical activity may decline and that screen-based entertainment may increase with age. Compliance with recommendations may be further reduced. Strategies to promote physical activity and reduce screen-based entertainment in young children are required.

▶ The early years are an important time to develop fundamental movement skills and appropriate physical activity behaviors. Society has traditionally thought of the early years as a time in life when children are inherently active enough. However, in recent years, researchers have started to disprove this misconception. In recognition of the low physical activity and high sedentary behavior levels of young children, Australia, Canada, and the United Kingdom have all recently released public health guidelines for physical activity and sedentary behavior for the early years. This article examined the prevalence of 3- to 5-year-old preschoolers within Australia that complied with these guidelines. The guidelines, which are quite consistent within each of the 3 countries, are that children of the early years accumulate 180 minutes or more per day of activity of any intensity and that they limit their screen time to 60 minutes of less. A combination of objective (accelerometers) and subjective (questionnaires) measures was used to measure the physical activity and sedentary behavior of approximately 1000 children aged 3-5 years.

Within this sample of preschoolers, only 127 minutes per day, or 16% of waking hours, were spent in physical activity of any intensity, with only 5 minutes per day of moderate or vigorous physical activity. Screen time levels, which included television/video viewing, electronic games, and computer use, averaged 112 minutes per day. None of the participants met the 180 min/day physical activity target on all 8 days that the accelerometers were worn, and only 5% met this target on the average day. Only 22% of children met the 60-minute-per-day or less screen time target. These are startling and troublesome figures. It is important for physicians to realize that their young patients may not be as active as they or the children's parents think. According to this research, most preschool-aged children are insufficiently active. Future research needs to more clearly identify the factors that contribute to the physical activity and sedentary behavior levels of children of the early years and the health implications of these behaviors in this age group.

I. Janssen, PhD

Step Count Targets Corresponding to New Physical Activity Guidelines for the Early Years

Gabel L, Proudfoot NA, Obeid J, et al (McMaster Univ, Hamilton, Ontario, Canada)
Med Sci Sports Exerc 45:314-318, 2013

Purpose.—New physical activity guidelines recommend that children age 3–4 yr should accumulate at least 180 min of physical activity at any intensity spread throughout the day, including progression toward at least 60 min of energetic play by 5 yr of age. Step count targets corresponding to these recommendations will help practitioners and researchers monitor physical activity.

Methods.—One hundred thirty-three preschoolers were instructed to wear accelerometers for seven consecutive days. Activity and step count data were recorded in 3-s epochs. Step count targets equivalent to physical activity recommendations were derived using prediction equations from regression analyses. Receiver operating curve analyses were conducted to compare the sensitivity and specificity of the derived thresholds as well as a range of other targets.

Results.—The daily step count target derived for 180 min of physical activity of any intensity was 6013 ± 88, whereas the target for 180 min of physical activity of any intensity including at least 60 min of moderate-to-vigorous physical activity was 6191 ± 103. The smallest discrepancy between days meeting physical activity guidelines and step count targets was found with a 6000-step-per-day target. Receiver operating curves confirmed a balanced sensitivity and specificity of this target.

Conclusions.—On the basis of our data, we suggest that a new step count target of 6000 steps per day should be used to determine whether 3- to 5-yr-old children are meeting physical activity recommendations.

▶ The Canadian physical activity guidelines for children aged 3-5 years is to accumulate at least 150 minutes of physical activity of any intensity spread throughout the day and to progress toward at least 60 min/day of energetic play by age 5 years. This study was completed to determine criteria for step counts associated with the Canadian physical activity guidelines for young children. These investigators proposed that 6000 steps per day be used as a target for children aged 3-5 years; this was the first step count target derived from evidence-based recommendations for this age group. To arrive at this conclusion, children (70 boys and 63 girls; 20% were overweight) wore pedometers and accelerometers for an average of 5.5 days throughout the waking hours except for aquatic activities. Parents recorded in journals the wear time and activities engaged in by their children. Step counts and accelerometer minutes of all physical activity and moderate- to vigorous-intensity physical activity were strong. Prediction equations, sensitivity, and specificity analyses led to the threshold of 6000 steps/day. Seventy-three percent of the children achieved the recommended 180 min/day of physical activity, 57% achieved at least 60 min/day of moderate-intensity activity, and 65% met the 6000-steps/day target. Thus, the children demonstrated a range of activity. In the United States, the current physical activity recommendations for children aged 6 and older are to accumulate at least 60 minutes of moderate to vigorous physical activity daily and to include vigorous activity on at least 3 days per week.[1] The National Association for Sport and Physical Education makes the same recommendation for toddlers and preschool children.[2] Perhaps in the near future, pediatricians will present children with their first pedometer at age 3 and step counts will be monitored as standard of care during annual pediatric health care examinations.

C. M. Jankowski, PhD

References

1. Division of Nutrition, Physical Activity, and Obesity, National Center for Chronic Disease Prevention and Health Promotion. www.CDC.gov/physicalactivity/everyone/guidelines/children. Last updated and reviewed, Accessed November 9, 2011.
2. AAHPERD. www.aahperd.org/naspe/standards/nationalguidelines/activestart.cfm. 2013. Accessed November 9, 2011.

A 4-Year Exercise Program in Children Increases Bone Mass Without Increasing Fracture Risk
Löfgren B, Dencker M, Nilsson J-Å, et al (Lund Univ, Sweden)
Pediatrics 129:e1468-e1476, 2012

Background.—Most prospective pediatric exercise intervention studies cover <1 year and use bone traits as surrogate end points for fractures. This prospective controlled exercise intervention study therefore followed not only skeletal development but also fracture incidence for 4 years.

Methods.—Fractures were prospectively registered in a cohort of children aged 7 to 9 years, 446 boys and 362 girls in the intervention group (2675 person-years) and 807 boys and 780 girls in the control group (5661 person-years). The intervention included 40 minutes per day of school

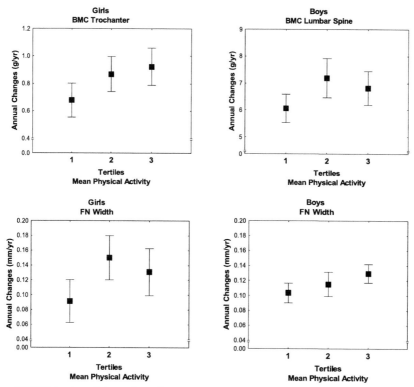

FIGURE 2.—Annual changes in trochanter BMC ($P<.05$) and FN width ($P<.05$) in girls and LS BMC ($P<.05$) and FN width ($P<.05$) in boys divided into tertiles according to weekly duration of physical activity. Data are presented as means with 95% CI. (Reprinted from Löfgren B, Dencker M, Nilsson J-Å, et al. A 4-year exercise program in children increases bone mass without increasing fracture risk. *Pediatrics.* 2012;129:e1468-e1476, Copyright 2012, with permission from the American Academy of Pediatrics.)

physical education for 4 years whereas the controls had 60 minutes per week. In a subsample, 73 boys and 48 girls in the intervention and 52 boys and 48 girls in the control group, bone mineral content (g) and bone width (cm) were followed by means of dual-energy radiograph absorptiometry.

Results.—The rate ratio for fractures was 1.11. In the dual-energy radiograph absorptiometry—measured children, there were no group differences at baseline in age, anthropometrics, or bone traits. The mean annual gain in lumbar spine bone mineral content was 7.0% higher in girls and 3.3% higher in boys and in femoral neck width 1.7% higher in girls and 0.6% higher in boys in the intervention than in the control group.

Conclusions.—A population-based moderately intense 4-year exercise program in 7- to 9-year-old children increased bone mass and size without affecting the fracture risk (Fig 2).

▶ Löfgren and colleagues reported findings from the Malmö Pediatric Osteoporosis Prevention Study, a population-based nonrandomized exercise intervention study of skeletal development and fracture risk in children. Their aim was to determine if higher levels of physical activity would produce long-term skeletal benefits without increasing fracture risk in children. In adults, fracture incidence increases with very high levels of physical activity as well as low bone mineral density. Children entered that study at age 7 to 9 years and they transitioned toward puberty during the 4-year follow-up. The importance of this age group is that pre- and peripubertal bone surfaces undergo rapid apposition when exposed to loading forces. In 1 school, the children participated in daily physical activity that accumulated to 200 min/wk. In 3 other schools, the children participated in the usual 60 min/wk of physical education. The physical activity was of a general nature (ball games, running) rather than specialized for bone loading forces. Fracture incidence was determined from approximately 2400 children. A subcohort of children (96 girls, 125 boys) completed dual-energy X-ray absorptiometry (DXA) measures at baseline and annually for 4 years. Three interesting findings emerged. First, children in the 200-minute cohort had greater increases in bone mineral content (BMC) and bone width compared with the 60-minute cohort, with more consistent effects seen in girls compared with boys. Second, fracture rate did not increase with more physical activity; neither was greater physical activity protective of fracture. Third, there was a dose-response relationship between the duration of total physical activity (school and other) and BMC of the trochanter in girls and lumbar spine in boys and FN width in boys and girls (Fig 2). A thresholdlike effect for lumbar spine BMC in boys and FN width in girls suggests the greatest skeletal benefits occurred between the lowest and middle tertiles of physical activity duration. Detecting a dose-response relationship between bone changes and exercise is rare and intriguing. Limitations to consider were that duration of physical activity was obtained from questionnaires and only about 10% of students had DXA measurements.

C. M. Jankowski, PhD

Motor Activity in Children With Autism: A Review of Current Literature
Downey R, Rapport MJK (Univ of Colorado, Denver)
Pediatr Phys Ther 24:2-20, 2012

Physical therapists have expanded their role and visibility in the treatment of children with autism spectrum disorders (ASD). Limitations in motor activity have not been considered in the assessments of core deficits of this population; however, physical therapists should be prepared to discuss and address these limitations in children with ASD.

Purpose.—The primary purposes of this review were to summarize current evidence for motor activity limitations in children with ASD and suggest further areas of research in physical therapy and autism while considering how physical therapy may benefit children with autism.

Method.—A literature search was carried out in 2009 and 2010 by using multiple search engines.

Results.—Forty-nine articles met inclusion criteria and were included in the review.

Conclusion.—Findings indicate that limitations in motor activity may be present in individuals with ASD, and further research is needed to identify specific functional limitations.

▶ Impaired motor activity is not considered one of the core deficits in autism spectrum disorder (ASD), yet motor deficits and delays clearly exist. In this extensive review, Downey and Rapport provide an overview of the existing evidence for developmental delay in prospective studies of infants at high risk for development of autism and those at low risk. In addition, this publication provides existing knowledge on differences between typically developing children and children with ASD in gestures and motor imitation, postural control, and dyspraxia (deficits in motor planning) at all ages. The information on infants and toddlers is of particular importance, and the need for early intervention is clearly being addressed. This publication would be of particular interest to physiotherapists, occupational therapists, kinesiologists, and recreational therapists who implement sensorimotor interventions and recreational activities for children both typically developing and from special populations. Although considerable improvements have been achieved in early diagnosis, children who present on the "milder" end of the spectrum may not be diagnosed as easily and therefore being aware of motor deficit may clue those practitioners who work with children in recreational settings. Of considerable scientific interest is the possible link between motor imitation and motor activity in children with ASD. The authors raise interesting questions as to whether limitations in motor activity impact on social activity and have adverse effects on motor imitation. Additionally, the evidence supporting the difficulty that children with ASD have with motor planning is and should be of considerable concern.

V. Galea, PhD

Defining the active ingredients of interactive computer play interventions for children with neuromotor impairments: A scoping review

Levac D, Rivard L, Missiuna C (McMaster Univ, Canada)
Res Dev Disabil 33:214-223, 2012

Rehabilitation researchers who investigate complex interventions are challenged to describe the "active ingredients" of their interventions: the reason(s) why a treatment is expected to be effective. Interactive Computer Play (ICP) is an emerging complex intervention in rehabilitation practice and research. The purpose of this scoping review is to identify the active ingredients of ICP interventions that are designed to improve motor outcomes in children with neuromotor impairments. Eleven potential active ingredients were identified with the following foci: ICP system or game properties; intervention effects on the user; and therapist roles. However, few studies explicitly evaluate the impact of particular ingredients on outcomes. Identification of active ingredients in ICP interventions can inform trial design and clinical decision-making. Research and clinical practice will benefit from studies that utilize a framework such as motor learning theory to guide hypotheses and measurement of the active ingredients of complex interventions.

▶ Interactive computer play (ICP) is quickly gaining acceptance among pediatric rehabilitation specialists. It is described as "any kind of computer game or virtual reality technique where the child can interact and play with virtual objects in a computer-generated environment."[1] ICP is a complex intervention and is unfortunately implemented in the absence of thorough, rigorous research into the effectiveness of the therapy. Moreover, complex interventions are often implemented without a good sense of the theoretical mechanisms through which a change in the sensory-motor function of the child might occur. These are termed "active ingredients" and may include such items as intensity or dosage. Levac and colleagues used a "scoping" review,[2] a review of the breadth and depth of a field of research in order to analyze and interpret the results and observations of the studies identified and reviewed, to define the potential active ingredients of ICP when used in children with neuromotor impairments such as cerebral palsy. In this way of defining the active ingredients, this study informs and provides support for the use of ICP by pediatric rehabilitation specialists as well as recreation specialists providing activities for children with disabilities. The information contained in this publication is quite extensive. The authors identified 9 active ingredients from various studies in which the authors linked the item to an actual outcome. These were grouped as Level 1 active ingredients and were grouped under ICP system or game properties (5 items), effect on the user (3, eg, motivation with 6 sub-items), and therapist roles.[1] Level 2a and Level 2b items from lower-quality studies were items that were either not explicitly identified by the study authors (as in Level 1) or linked to an outcome. Levac and colleagues state quite correctly that research in the use of ICP as an intervention is presently not well-grounded within a theoretical framework. They suggest the use of motor learning theory as a relevant framework for identifying active ingredients within ICP interventions because many of the active ingredients defined in this publication are inherent in motor learning theory, particularly in its application to rehabilitation. In this way, theories about the usefulness and applicability of ICP may be proven or refuted in well-designed theoretically based studies.

V. Galea, PhD

References

1. Sandlund M, McDonough S, Häger-Ross C. Interactive computer play in rehabilitation of children with sensorimotor disorders: a systematic review. *Dev Med Child Neurol.* 2009;51:173-179.
2. Levac D, Colquhoun H, O'Brien K. Scoping studies: advancing the methodology. *Implement Sci.* 2010;5:69.

Developmental Coordination Disorder: A Pilot Diffusion Tensor Imaging Study

Zwicker JG, Missiuna C, Harris SR, et al (Univ of British Columbia, Vancouver, Canada; McMaster Univ, Hamilton, Ontario, Canada)
Pediatr Neurol 46:162-167, 2012

Motor deficits associated with developmental coordination disorder are not attributable to macrostructural brain abnormalities, but differences in brain microstructure may exist. Using diffusion tensor imaging, we explored the integrity of motor, sensory, and cerebellar pathways in children with and without developmental coordination disorder. In seven children with the disorder and nine typically developing children (aged 8-12 years), we measured diffusivity and fractional anisotropy of the corticospinal tract, posterior thalamic radiation, and superior and middle cerebellar peduncles. Fractional anisotropy of motor and sensory tracts and diffusion parameters in cerebellar peduncles did not differ between groups. Mean diffusivity of the corticospinal tract and posterior thalamic radiation was lower in children with developmental coordination disorder compared with control children ($P < 0.04$ and $P < 0.06$, respectively). Results were driven by lower axial diffusivity, which was significantly correlated with motor impairment scores on the Movement Assessment Battery for Children-2 for both the corticospinal tract ($r = 0.56$, $P = 0.03$) and posterior thalamic radiation ($r = 0.70$, $P = 0.003$). Reduced axial diffusivity in motor and sensory tracts may be implicated in developmental coordination disorder, but replication in a larger study is needed to confirm these findings.

▶ Developmental coordination disorder (DCD) is an outwardly motor disorder of yet-to-be defined etiology. It manifests as difficulties in the performance of complex tasks such as doing up buttons or writing; however, children with this condition also may have difficulty performing gross motor tasks such as riding a bicycle. Although current thinking points to central nervous system pathology and recent functional magnetic resonance imaging (MRI) studies have pointed out differences in children with DCD compared with typically developing children,[1] these studies are few and quite recent. Zwicker and colleagues took advantage of a type of structural MRI methodology, termed diffusion tensor imaging (DTI), where explorations at the microstructural level are possible. This technique takes advantage of the diffusion of water molecules in brain white matter and their interaction with those fibers along the way. Additionally, diffusion is a 3-dimensional phenomenon with molecular mobility in various tissues not being the same in all directions and therefore termed "anisotropic."[2] Using DTI, Zwicker and colleagues investigated the integrity of motor, sensory, and cerebellar pathways in children with DCD and in typically developing age-matched controls using 2 diffusion statistics, mean diffusivity and fractional anisotropy. Mean diffusivity is reflective of the overall mean-squared displacement of molecules and the presence of obstacles to diffusion. A complete explanation of fractional anisotropy is beyond the limitations of this critique,[2] but simply speaking is reflective of the variance of the three Eigen values characterizing anisotropy and represents the direction of water diffusion. Interestingly and paradoxically, no differences were found in the cerebellar pathways (as observed from cerebellar peduncles) between children with DCD and controls. Differences were found in the mean diffusivity of the corticospinal tract and that did correlate with measures of motor impairment. Lower diffusivity, in this case in the axial direction, may reflect that in DCD there may be alterations in axonal microstructure or differences in water content. This is one of the first studies of this kind to investigate connectivity in children with DCD and therefore important to practitioners working with children for that reason. However, the sample was quite small (DCD, n = 7; controls, n = 9) and therefore this was quite rightly termed a pilot study. Nevertheless, DTI remains a very powerful technique for determining effectiveness of intervention programs designed to improve sensorimotor function, hopefully through improved connectivity, through pre- and post-intervention measures of white matter tract characteristics.

V. Galea, PhD

References

1. Kashiwagi M, Iwaki S, Narumi Y, Tamai H, Suzuki S. Parietal dysfunction in developmental coordination disorder: a functional MRI study. *Neuroreport.* 2009;20:1319-1324.
2. Le Bihan D, Mangin JF, Poupon C, et al. Diffusion tensor imaging: concepts and applications. *J Magn Reson Imaging.* 2001;13:534-546.

Mental Health Difficulties in Children With Developmental Coordination Disorder

Lingam R, Jongmans MJ, Ellis M, et al (Univ of Bristol, UK; Univ Med Centre Utrecht, Netherlands)
Pediatrics 129:e882-e891, 2012

Objective.—To explore the associations between probable developmental coordination disorder (DCD) defined at age 7 years and mental health difficulties at age 9 to 10 years.

Methods.—We analyzed of prospectively collected data (N = 6902) from the Avon Longitudinal Study of Parents and Children. "Probable" DCD was defined by using *Diagnostic and Statistical Manual of Mental Disorders, Fourth Edition, Text Revision* criteria as those children below the 15th centile of the Avon Longitudinal Study of Parents and Children Coordination Test, with functional limitations in activities of daily living or handwriting, excluding children with neurologic difficulties or an IQ <70. Mental health was measured by using the child-reported Short Moods and Feelings Questionnaire and the parent-reported Strengths and Difficulties Questionnaire. Multiple logistic regression models, with the use of multiple imputation to account for missing data, assessed the associations between probable DCD and mental health difficulties. Adjustments were made for environmental confounding factors, and potential mediating factors such as verbal IQ, associated developmental traits, bullying, self-esteem, and friendships.

Results.—Children with probable DCD ($N = 346$) had an increased odds of self-reported depression, odds ratio: 2.08 (95% confidence interval: 1.36—3.19) and parent-reported mental health difficulties odds ratio: 4.23 (95% confidence interval: 3.10—5.77). The odds of mental health difficulties significantly decreased after accounting for verbal IQ, social communication, bullying, and self-esteem.

Conclusions.—Children with probable DCD had an increased risk of mental health difficulties that, in part, were mediated through associated developmental difficulties, low verbal IQ, poor self-esteem, and bullying. Prevention and treatment of mental health difficulties should be a key element of intervention for children with DCD.

▶ Children with developmental coordination disorder (DCD) are at high risk for developing mental health difficulties such as anxiety and depression with the risk increasing when there is also evidence of attention deficit hyperactivity disorder.[1] Lingham and colleagues sought to explore this association using data prospectively collected in a large cohort (n = 14062 live births) from the Avon Longitudinal Study of Parents and Children (ALSPAC). Children between 7 and 8 years of age were tested for their motor skills (n = 6902) and were identified as probable DCD if they scored below the 15th percentile of the ALSPAC coordination test derived from 3 subtests from the Movement Assessment Battery for Children. In those in whom functional limitations were identified, failure on standardized writing assessments as well as scores below the 15th percentile of an activities of daily living scale were then included. The outcome variable of interest was the Short Mood and Feelings Questionnaire, a 13-item instrument used to report depressive symptoms when children turn 10 years old, as well as the Strengths and Difficulties Questionnaire completed by the child's parents at 9.5 years old. The result of this careful screening yielded a final sample of 346 children. Other studies showing this relationship tend to be cross-sectional[2] in nature with longitudinal studies being relatively rare. Because of the longitudinal research used in this publication, Lingham and colleagues were able to control for several confounding factors as well as identifying and assessing potential mediators such as verbal IQ. Examples of actors that increased the risk of developing mental health difficulties were decreased verbal IQ, lower global self-esteem, lower scholastic competence, and being bullied. On the other hand, examples of protective factors were high verbal IQ and high self-esteem. This publication is of interest to the readers of the YEAR BOOK OF SPORTS MEDICINE because of the importance of pediatric health care practitioners recognizing children with moderate to severe motor coordination deficits and encouraging the need for mental health screening particularly if the child experienced bullying and has low self-esteem. The inclusion of these children, early in life, in targeted recreational activities and interventions designed to increase self-esteem and social interaction, as well as giving the child strategies to deal with bullying, may obviate the risk of depression later on in life.

V. Galea, PhD

References

1. Sigurdsson E, Van Os J, Fombonne E. Are impaired childhood motor skills a risk factor for adolescent anxiety? Results from the 1958 U.K. birth cohort and the National Child Development Study. *Am J Psychiatry.* 2002;159:1044-1046.
2. Chen YW, Tseng MH, Hu FC, Cermak SA. Psychosocial adjustment and attention in children with developmental coordination disorder using different motor tests. *Res Dev Disabil.* 2009;30:1367-1377.

Women

Female Athlete Triad Screening in National Collegiate Athletic Association Division I athletes: Is the Preparticipation Evaluation Form Effective?

Mencias T, Noon M, Hoch AZ (Med College of Wisconsin, Milwaukee)
Clin J Sport Med 22:122-125, 2012

Objective.—To evaluate the screening practices and preparticipation evaluation (PPE) forms used to identify college athletes at risk for the female athlete triad (triad).

Design.—Phone and/or e-mail survey.

Setting.—National Collegiate Athletic Association (NCAA) Division I universities.

Participants.—All 347 NCAA Division I universities were invited to participate in a survey, with 257 participating in the survey (74%) and 287 forms collected (83%).

Main Outcome Measures.—Information about the nature of the PPE was requested from team physicians and certified athletic trainers during a phone or e-mail survey. In addition, a copy of their PPE form was requested

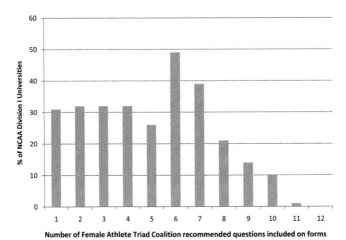

FIGURE.—Combined assessment of PPE forms used at 287 Division I universities. (Reprinted from Mencias T, Noon M, Hoch AZ. Female athlete triad screening in National Collegiate Athletic Association Division I athletes: is the preparticipation evaluation form effective? *Clin J Sport Med.* 2012;22:122-125, with permission from Lippincott Williams & Wilkins.)

TABLE 1.—Items Recommended by the Female Athlete Triad Coalition to Screen for the Triad on PPE Forms

Items Recommended by the Female Athlete Triad Coalition to Screen for the Triad on PPE Forms	Included in Screening Forms, No. (%) (N = 287)
Disordered eating	
Do you worry about your weight?	164 (57)
Do you limit the foods you eat?	131 (46)
Do you lose weight to meet image requirements for your sport?	121 (42)
Does your weight affect the way you feel about yourself?	4 (1)
Do you feel you have lost control over what you eat?	17 (6)
Do you make yourself vomit; use diuretics or laxatives after you eat?	36 (13)
Have you ever suffered from an eating disorder?	176 (61)
Do you ever eat in secret?	7 (2)
Menstrual dysfunction	
What age was your first menstrual period?	167 (58)
Do you have monthly menstrual cycles?	210 (73)
How many menstrual cycles have you had in the last year?	151 (53)
Bone health	
Have you ever had a stress fracture?*	237 (83)

*A point was awarded for asking about any fracture, but many schools specifically asked about lower extremity stress fractures (N = 287).

to evaluate for inclusion of the 12 items recommended by the Female Athlete Triad Coalition for primary screening for the triad.

Results.—All 257 universities (100%) required a PPE for incoming athletes; however, only 83 universities (32%) required an annual PPE for returning athletes. Screening was performed on campus at 218 universities (85%). Eleven universities (4%) were using the recently updated fourth edition PPE. Only 25 universities (9%) had 9 or more of the 12 recommended items included in their forms, whereas 127 universities (44%) included 4 or less items. Relevant items that were omitted from more than 40% of forms included losing weight to meet the image requirements of a sport; using vomiting, diuretics, and/or laxatives to lose weight; and the number of menses experienced in the past 12 months.

Conclusions.—The current PPE forms used by NCAA Division I universities may not effectively screen for the triad (Fig, Table 1).

▶ This study is similar to previous surveys conducted in United States[1] and Canadian[2] universities, but explores the topic in further detail in a much larger cohort in 347 National Collegiate Athletic Association (NCAA) Division I universities. Specifically, the most current versions of their athlete history questionnaires used for their preparticipation evaluation (PPE) form were analyzed for inclusion of the 12 items that the Female Athlete Triad Coalition recommends for preparticipation triad screening of female athletes. The Female Athlete Triad Coalition is a group of representatives from member universities and organizations, including the American College of Sports Medicine (ACSM), International Olympic Committee (IOC), American Medical Society for Sports Medicine, American Academy of Orthopedic Surgeons, American Academy of Pediatrics, NCAA, American Dietetic Association, and National Athletic Trainers Association, among others. The Female

Athlete Triad Coalition used the third edition PPE, the IOC Female Athlete Triad PPE, and the ACSM Female Athlete Triad Position Stand to generate its original questionnaire, which consists of 8 questions on disordered eating, 3 questions on menstrual dysfunction, and 1 question on bone health (Table 1). The PPE forms received through this survey were also evaluated for inclusion of a nutritional assessment in the form of a record of food and energy expenditure to calculate energy availability. With a 74% response rate (257/347 NCAA Division I universities) and 83% of the surveyed universities (287/347) returning a copy of their PPE form, a reasonably thorough snapshot of current practices was generated.

Although all 257 universities required a PPE and physical evaluation for incoming freshman and transfer athletes, only 83 (23%) required an annual PPE for returning athletes. Interestingly, at the 218 universities (85%) where screening was performed on campus, the history portion of the questionnaire was typically reviewed by an athletic trainer and signed off on by a physician; of these, 45% had completed a sports medicine fellowship. Analysis of the various PPE forms revealed that relevant questions to screen for disordered eating were omitted from more than 50%, and questions to screen for menstrual dysfunction from more than 40% of the forms (Fig); only 20 universities (7%) included a nutritional assessment.

Although some advancement in awareness of and screening for components of the female athlete triad in Division 1 NCAA schools was found, in comparison to the earlier studies, there is still an obvious need to develop effective preparticipation screening tools and to explore the most sensitive and specific items to include. Further research is warranted on this important topic, as is education and wider implementation of recommendations.

C. Lebrun, MDCM, MPE, CCFP, Dip Sport Med, FACSM

References

1. Beals K. Eating disorder and menstrual dysfunction screening, education and treatment programs. *Phys Sportsmed.* 2003;31:33-38.
2. Rumball JS, Lebrun CM. Use of the preparticipation physical examination form to screen for the female athlete triad in Canadian interuniversity sport universities. *Clin J Sport Med.* 2005;15:320-325.

Eating Disorder Risk and the Role of Clothing in Collegiate Cheerleaders' Body Images
Torres-McGehee TM, Monsma EV, Dompier TP, et al (Univ of South Carolina, Columbia; Datalys Ctr, Indianapolis, IN)
J Athl Train 47:541-548, 2012

Context.—With increased media coverage and competitive opportunities, cheerleaders may be facing an increase in eating disorder (ED) prevalence linked to clothing-related body image (BI).

Objective.—To examine ED risk prevalence, pathogenic weight control behaviors, and variation in clothing-specific BI across position and academic status among collegiate cheerleaders.

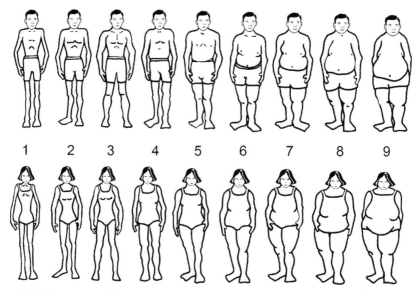

FIGURE.—Standard figural stimuli reprinted with permission from Stunkard et al.[16] Body mass anchors: silhouette $1 = 18.3$, $2 = 19.3$, $3 = 20.9$, $4 = 23.1$, $5 = 26.2$, $6 = 29.9$, $7 = 34.3$, $8 = 38.6$, $9 = 45.4$.[17] *Editor's Note*: Please refer to original journal article for full references. (Reprinted from Torres-McGehee TM, Monsma EV, Dompier TP, et al. Eating disorder risk and the role of clothing in collegiate cheerleaders' body images. *J Athl Train.* 2012;47:541-548, © 2012, Allen Press, Inc.)

Design.—Cross-sectional study.

Setting.—National Collegiate Athletic Association Division I and II institutions.

Patients or Other Participants.—Female collegiate cheerleaders (n = 136, age = 20.4 ± 1.3 years, height = 160.2 ± 8.1 cm, weight = 57.2 ± 8.3 kg).

Main Outcome Measure(s).—Participants self-reported height, weight, and desired weight and completed the Eating Attitudes Test. Body image perceptions in 3 clothing types (daily clothing, midriff uniform, full uniform) were assessed using sexbased silhouettes (body mass index = 18.3 kg/m^2 for silhouette 1, 23.1 kg/m^2 for silhouette 4).

Results.—The ED risk for cheerleaders was estimated at 33.1%. However, when body mass index was controlled using backward stepwise logistic regression, flyers had greater odds (odds ratio = 4.4, 95% confidence interval = 1.5, 13.2, $P = .008$) of being at risk compared with bases, but no difference was noted between the base and back-spot positions (odds ratio = 1.9, 95% confidence interval = 0.5, 6.6, $P = .333$). A main effect of BI perceptions was seen ($P < .001$), with a significant interaction by clothing type ($F_{2,133} = 22.5$, $P < .001$, $\eta^2 = 0.14$). Cheerleaders desired to be smaller than their perceived BIs for each clothing type, with the largest difference for midriff uniform (2.6 ± 0.8 versus 3.7 ± 0.9), followed by full uniform (2.7 ± 0.8 versus 3.5 ± 0.9) and daily clothing (2.8 ± 0.8 versus 3.5 ± 0.9).

TABLE 3.—Comparison of Prevalence Rates (Proportions, %) of Pathogenic Behaviors Among Cheerleaders and Other Female Athletes

	Current Study	Torres-McGehee et al, 2011[20]	Torres-McGehee et al, 2009[7]	Greenleaf et al, 2009[2]	Carter and Rudd, 2005[12]	Johnson et al, 1999[3]	Black and Burckes-Miller, 1988[23]
Sample size	136	138	101	204	2001: 353 2002: 355	562	382
Athletes	Cheerleaders	Equestrian	Auxiliary Units	Mixed	Mixed	Mixed	Mixed
Pathogenic behavior							
Binge eating	11.8	24.6	14.9	15.2	7.1–6.2	16.2	NA
Vomiting	9.6	11.6	9.9	2.9	1.7–2.8	6.4	7.3
Laxatives	19.9[a]	15.2[a]	18.9[a]	0.98	4.6–2.3	1.78	4.5
Diet pills, dieting	NA	NA	NA	15.7	NA	1.42	15.3
Diuretics	NA	NA	NA	1.5	NA	0.53	4.2
Exercise	1.5	NA	NA	25.5	NA	NA	53.1
Thoughts of suicide[b]	NA	NA	0.0	NA	NA	NA	NA
Lost 20 lb or more	2.2	NA	NA	NA	NA	NA	NA

Abbreviation: NA indicates no reported measures for these variables.
Editor's Note: Please refer to original journal article for full references.
[a]Included laxatives, diet pills, and diuretics in 1 question.
[b]The previous version of the Eating Attitudes Test-26 included the question "Have you ever thought of or attempted suicide"? The question is not included in the current version, which we used in our study.

Conclusions.—Cheerleaders, especially flyers, appear to be at risk for EDs, with greatest BI dissatisfaction when wearing their most revealing uniforms (ie, midriffs). Universities, colleges, and the national governing bodies of these squads need to focus on preventing eating disorders and BI dissatisfaction and promoting self-esteem (Fig, Table 3).

▶ Although the incidence of components of the female athlete triad has been researched extensively in other collegiate sports, cheerleading is not considered a National Collegiate Athletic Association (NCAA) varsity sport, and as such, is not regulated under the NCAA rules, especially as they pertain to the use of dietary supplements or weight loss agents. Neither are the athletes required to have annual preparticipation physical evaluations (PPEs) as a prerequisite for participation.

This cross-sectional study represents the largest group of cheerleaders investigated for eating disorder (ED) risk. Using the Eating Attitudes Test (EAT), including the subscales, and the subjects' self-reported height, weight, and desired weight, the ED risk was estimated at 33% overall, with "flyers" being at slightly higher risk than "bases" or "back" spots. The gender-specific body mass index Figural Stimuli Silhouette (Fig) was used to assess body disturbance based on perceived and desired body images in 3 situations: normal daily clothing, midriff uniform, and full-length uniform. Not surprisingly, cheerleaders desired to be smaller than their perceived body image for each of these types, with the largest difference for midriff uniform. This is an added pressure brought to the sport by the increasing competitiveness of the sport itself as well as by the presence of media (nationwide in many cases), which tends to "add 10 pounds." A comparison of prevalence rates of pathogenic behaviors among cheerleaders and other female athletes (Table 3) shows the rates to be similar or greater than other activities such as equestrian, auxiliary units, and mixed groups of athletes. The findings of this research suggest that more attention should be paid to risk factors and unhealthy behaviors in these female athletes, with more medical supervision and help, as needed. Coaches, universities, and colleges as well as national governing bodies of these squads need to focus on programs for preventing body image dissatisfaction and disordered eating and promoting self-esteem. In addition, very little research has been done in the population of male cheerleaders, who may have similar issues.

C. Lebrun, MDCM, MPE, CCFP, Dip Sport Med, FACSM

Are Under- and Overweight Female Elite Athletes Thin and Fat? A Controlled Study
Torstveit MK, Sundgot-Borgen J (Univ of Agder, Kristiansand, Norway; Norwegian School of Sport Sciences, Oslo, Norway)
Med Sci Sports Exerc 44:949-957, 2012

Purpose.—The study's purpose was to relate body mass index (BMI) to body fat percentage as measured by dual-energy X-ray absorptiometry in female elite athletes from different sports and nonathletic controls and to investigate what characterizes the athletes with unhealthy low and high body fat values.

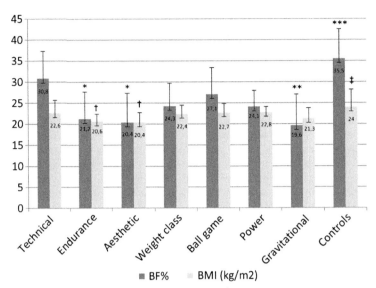

FIGURE 1.—Body fat percentage (%BF) and BMI (kg·m^{-2}) among athletes representing the different sport groups—technical sports ($n = 15$), endurance sports ($n = 41$), aesthetic sports ($n = 38$), weight class sports ($n = 6$), ball game sports ($n = 70$), power sports ($n = 11$), and gravitational sports ($n = 5$)—and controls ($n = 145$). Values are given as mean T SD. *$P < 0.001$ compared with ball game sports and technical sports; **$P < 0.05$ compared with technical sports; ***$P < 0.001$ compared with endurance, aesthetic, ball game, power, and gravitational sports, and $P < 0.05$ compared with weight class sports. †$P < 0.05$ compared with ball game sports; ‡$P < 0.001$ compared with endurance and aesthetic sports. (Reprinted from Torstveit MK, Sundgot-Borgen J. Are under-and overweight female elite athletes thin and fat? A controlled study. *Med Sci Sports Exerc.* 2012;44:949-957, the American College of Sports Medicine.)

Methods.—This study was conducted in three phases: 1) screening with a detailed questionnaire, 2) body composition measurement (dual-energy x-ray absorptiometry), and 3) clinical interview. All female elite athletes representing national teams at the junior or senior level age 13–39 yr ($n = 938$) and an age group—matched randomly selected population-based control group ($n = 900$) were invited to participate. A stratified random sample was invited to participate in parts 2 and 3. A total of 186 athletes (62%) and 145 controls (48%) participated in all three phases.

Results.—Of those athletes with normal BMI values (18.5–24.9 kg·m^{-2}) ($n = 150$), 2.0% were classified with low body fat levels (<12%), and 6.7% were classified with obese body fat levels ($\geq 33\%$). The median value for the entire group was 24.3% body fat. For the controls with normal BMI values ($n = 96$), none was classified with low body fat levels, and 50% were classified with obese body fat levels (median = 33.1%). The correlation between BMI and body fat percentage was 0.671 ($P < 0.01$) (SEE = 5.3%) for the athletes and 0.813 ($P < 0.01$) (SEE = 4.1%) for the controls. Both under- and overfat athletes self-reported menstrual dysfunction, stress fractures, history of weight fluctuation, and use of pathogenic weight control methods and were diagnosed with clinical eating disorders and/or low bone density.

Conclusions.—Our data show that BMI is not a valid measure for assessing or monitoring body composition in female elite athletes, and it should be used carefully in female nonathletes (Fig 1).

▶ This study addresses the pitfalls of using body mass index (BMI) as a surrogate measure of body composition to classify elite female athletes for sports with weight class restrictions, prediction of performance, and for identifying athletes with eating disorders. The authors measured BMI and percentage of body fat by dual-energy x-ray absorptiometry in 186 athletes and 145 controls aged 13 to 39 years. The World Health Organization criteria for BMI were used to classify women as underweight, normal weight, or overweight. Body fat of 12% and 33% classified the women as underfat and overfat, respectively. The athletes were elite, defined as membership on junior or senior national sport teams (eg, Olympics or World Cup) or recruitment squads competing in leanness (endurance, aesthetic, weight class, and gravitational) and nonleanness (technical, ball game, and power) sports (Fig 1). Training or physical activity habits, menstrual, dietary, and weight history, and disordered eating behavior questionnaires were administered to athletes and controls. The correlation between BMI and body fat was 0.67 for athletes compared with 0.81 for controls. Of athletes classified as overweight, 60% had a body fat that was over 33%, whereas 97% of overweight controls were classified as high fat. Seven athletes were underfat, but only 3 of them were classified as underweight. Traits associated with the female athlete triad were prevalent in athletes classified as overfat and underfat. In a cohort of athletes with triad traits, 48% of overfat and 57% of underfat athletes were diagnosed with a clinical eating disorder.

These data support the recommendation that BMI should not be used for assessing the body composition, competitive eligibility, or health status of elite female athletes. Further, coaches and trainers should not permit BMI or the appearance of thinness to cloud their judgment about eating disorders in their athletes. At the elite level, sport performance, training, and equipment have become extremely technical. It is unfortunate that BMI remains an acceptable measure of body composition.

C. M. Jankowski, PhD

Exercise Performance over the Menstrual Cycle in Temperate and Hot, Humid Conditions
Janse De Jonge XAK, Thompson MW, Chuter VH, et al (Univ of Newcastle, Australia; The Univ of Sydney, Australia; et al)
Med Sci Sports Exerc 44:2190-2198, 2012

Purpose.—This study investigated the effects of the menstrual cycle on prolonged exercise performance both in temperate (20°C, 45% relative humidity) and hot, humid (32°C, 60% relative humidity) conditions.
Methods.—For each environmental condition, 12 recreationally active females were tested during the early follicular (day 3—6) and midluteal

TABLE 2.—Individual Times to Exhaustion (Minutes) and Percentage Change for Participants During the Follicular and Luteal Phase of the Menstrual Cycle in Both Temperate and Hot, Humid Conditions

Participant	Temperate Conditions			Hot, Humid Conditions		
	Follicular (Min)	Luteal (Min)	% Change	Follicular (Min)	Luteal (Min)	% Change
1	70.2	64.3	−9.2%	49.8	45.0	−10.7%
2	71.8	71.7	−0.1%	70.8	68.8	−2.9%
3	67.4	67.3	−0.1%	60.0	49.0	−22.4%
4	73.0	72.3	−1.0%	70.7	69.1	−2.3%
5	75.7	74.8	−1.2%	68.3	67.7	−0.9%
6	76.2	76.8	0.8%	74.6	71.5	−4.3%
7	75.0	74.9	−0.1%	71.9	70.1	−2.6%
8	72.8	72.9	0.1%		Excluded	
9		Excluded		67.4	67.8	0.6%
Mean	72.8	71.9	−1.4%	66.7*	63.6*	−5.7%*
SD	3.0	4.2	3.2%	8.1	10.4	7.5%

*Significant difference between the menstrual cycle phases ($P < 0.05$).

(day 19–25) phases, verified by measurement of estradiol and progesterone. For all four tests, thermoregulatory, cardiorespiratory, and perceptual responses were measured during 60 min of exercise at 60% of maximal oxygen consumption followed by an incremental test to exhaustion.

Results.—No differences in exercise performance between menstrual cycle phases were found during temperate conditions ($n = 8$) despite a higher resting and submaximal exercise core temperature (T_c) in the luteal phase. In hot, humid conditions ($n = 8$), however, prolonged exercise performance, as exercise time to fatigue, was significantly reduced during the luteal phase. This finding was not only accompanied by higher resting and submaximal exercise T_c but also a higher rate of increase in T_c during the luteal phase. Furthermore, submaximal exercise HR, minute ventilation, and RPE measures were higher during the luteal phase in hot, humid conditions. No significant differences were found over the menstrual cycle in heat loss responses (partitional calorimetry, sweat rate, upper arm sweat composition) and T_c at exhaustion.

Conclusion.—In temperate conditions, no changes in prolonged exercise performance were found over the menstrual cycle, whereas in hot, humid conditions, performance was decreased during the luteal phase. The combination of both exercise and heat stress with the elevated luteal phase T_c at the onset of exercise resulted in physiological and perceptual changes and a greater thermosensitivity, which may explain the decrease in performance (Table 2).

▶ Given that the resting body temperature is 0.3 to 0.5°C higher during the luteal phase of a woman's menstrual cycle, one might anticipate an associated deterioration of endurance performance, particularly under hot environmental conditions. Some previous reports have found no differences in the time to exhaustion over the menstrual cycle,[1-3] but these studies were conducted under temperate conditions, where a rising core temperature was less likely to be the main factor limiting performance. The present study compared responses to an hour of endurance exercise under temperate and hot, humid conditions, demonstrating that although the menstrual cycle had no influence on time to exhaustion in the temperate environment, there was a substantial impact in the heat (Table 2). Not only did subjects begin their exercise bout at a higher core temperature during the luteal phase, but their core temperatures also rose faster as the exercise progressed. The critical temperature for both exhaustion and dangerous heat stress would thus be reached more quickly in the luteal phase. There were considerable intersubject differences in response, and it would be interesting to explore the reasons for this. In 1 previous investigation that found no effect of the menstrual cycle on shuttle running under hot conditions,[4] the average luteal phase progesterone concentration was low and there was no significant change of resting core endurance during the luteal phase. In the present study, subjects were excluded from analysis if their progesterone levels did not rise to 16 nmol/L, but nevertheless the person with the greatest luteal phase impairment (−22.4%) also had the highest luteal progesterone level (57.1 nmol/L). The practical implication is that endurance competitors will find it advantageous to align their menstrual cycles so that they can compete during the follicular phase of their menstrual cycle.

R. J. Shephard, MD (Lond), PhD, DPE

References

1. Lebrun CM, McKenzie DC, Prior JC, Taunton JE. Effects of menstrual cycle phase on athletic performance. *Med Sci Sports Exerc.* 1995;27:437-444.
2. Beidleman BA, Rock PB, Muza SR, Fulco CS, Forte VA, Cymerman A. Exercise VE and physical performance at altitude are not affected by menstrual cycle phase. *J Appl Physiol.* 1999;86:1519-1526.
3. Bailey SP, Zacher CM, Mittleman KD. Effect of menstrual cycle phase on carbohydrate supplementation during prolonged exercise to fatigue. *J Appl Physiol.* 2000;88:690-697.
4. Sunderland C, Nevill M. Effect of the menstrual cycle on performance of intermittent, high-intensity shuttle running in a hot environment. *Eur J Appl Physiol.* 2003;88:345-352.

Former Premenarcheal Gymnasts Exhibit Site-Specific Skeletal Benefits in Adulthood After Long-Term Retirement

Erlandson MC, Kontulainen SA, Chilibeck PD, et al (Univ of Saskatchewan, Saskatoon, Canada)

J Bone Miner Res 27:2298-2305, 2012

Young female gymnasts have greater bone strength compared to controls; although possibly due to selection into gymnastics, it is thought that their loading activity during growth increases their bone mass, influencing both bone geometry and architecture. If such bone mass and geometric adaptations are maintained, this may potentially decrease the risk of osteoporosis and risk of fracture later in life. However, there is limited evidence of the persisting benefit of gymnastic exercise during growth on adult bone geometric parameters. Therefore, the purpose of this study was to determine whether adult bone geometry, volumetric density, and estimated strength were greater in retired gymnasts compared to controls, 10 years after retirement from the sport. Bone geometric and densitometric parameters, measured by peripheral quantitative computed tomography (pQCT) at the radius and tibia, were compared between 25 retired female gymnasts and 22 controls, age range 22 to 30 years, by multivariate analysis of covariance (covariates: age, height, and muscle cross-sectional area). Retired gymnasts had significantly greater adjusted total and trabecular area (16%), total and trabecular bone mineral content (BMC) (18% and 22%, respectively), and estimated strength (21%) at the distal radius ($p < 0.05$) than controls. Adjusted total and cortical area and BMC, medullary area, and estimated strength were also significantly greater (13% to 46%) in retired gymnasts at the 30% and 65% radial shaft sites ($p < 0.05$). At the distal tibia, retired gymnasts had 12% to 13% greater total and trabecular BMC and volumetric bone mineral density as well as 21% greater estimated strength; total and cortical BMC and estimated strength were also greater at the tibial shaft (8%, 11%, and 10%, respectively) ($p < 0.05$). Former female gymnasts have significantly better geometric and densitometric properties, as well as estimated strength, at the radius and tibia 10 years after retirement from gymnastics compared to females who did not participate in gymnastics in childhood and adolescence.

▶ Weight-bearing physical activity during childhood and adolescence is associated with site-specific increases in bone mass, which may theoretically decrease the risk of osteoporosis and fractures in later life. In gymnastics, in particular, athletes experience forces 3 to 10 times their body weight on their hands and feet. Most previous studies in competitive adolescent female gymnasts have used dual-energy X-ray absorptiometry—derived bone mineral density (BMD) and bone mineral content and have shown an 8% to 23% increase in these measures compared with controls. What is unique about the current study is that the researchers have used peripheral quantitative computed tomography at the radius and tibia to assess bone geometric and densitometric parameters 10 years after retirement from the sport. Furthermore, these women were recruited as premenarchal gymnasts in 1995, and each of them were matched at that time by size, maturity, and chronological age to a nongymnastic premenarchal control. Of the initial 30 matched pairs, the researchers were able to recontact and assess 25 retired female gymnasts and 22 controls. They measured anthropometric characteristics, and by questionnaires determined habitual physical activity and calcium and vitamin D intake as well as menstrual history, including age at menarche and use of contraceptives. In the gymnasts, further questions focused on age of onset of gymnastics activity, intensity and duration of training (number of sessions/hours of training per week, and level of competition), and reasons for retirement from gymnastics activity. Using multivariate analysis of covariance, it was shown that the former female gymnasts had significantly better site-specific geometric and densitometric properties, as well as estimated strength, 10 years after retirement from gymnastics compared with control subjects who did not participate in gymnastics in childhood and adolescence. Skeletal adaptations were geometric in nature at the radius, resulting in 22% to 32% greater estimated bone strength in retired gymnasts. At the tibia, greater volumetric BMD, without an increase in bone size, resulted in 24% greater estimated bone strength. It remains to be seen (and will likely be further investigated as part of this longitudinal study) if these benefits will persist through to menopause and have any impact on fracture risk.

C. Lebrun, MDCM, MPE, CCFP, Dip Sport Med, FACSM

Pharmacokinetics and adhesion of the Agile transdermal contraceptive patch (AG200-15) during daily exposure to external conditions of heat, humidity and exercise

Archer DF, Stanczyk FZ, Rubin A, et al (Eastern Virginia Med School, Norfolk; Univ of Southern California, Los Angeles; Agile Therapeutics Inc, Princeton, NJ)
Contraception 87:212-219, 2013

Background.—This study compares the pharmacokinetic profile, adhesion and safety of the AG200-15 Agile Patch (AP), a novel contraceptive patch releasing low-dose ethinyl estradiol (EE) and levonorgestrel (LNG), during wear under external conditions of heat, humidity and exercise versus normal activities.

Study Design.—This open-label, three-period, five-Treatment, crossover study randomized 24 healthy women to one of six external condition sequences. Each sequence included one normal wear and two external conditions periods. Participants wore the AP for 7 days under normal conditions or conditions of daily sauna, treadmill, whirlpool or cool water immersion, with a 7-day washout between treatments. Blood samples were collected for pharmacokinetic evaluations.

Results.—Twenty-four subjects completed the study. For EE, the mean maximum concentration level (C_{max}), area under the plasma concentration—Time curve from time 0 to 168 h (AUC_{0-168}) and area under the plasma concentration—Time curve from time 0 to infinity (AUC_{0-inf}) were higher during normal conditions compared with all external conditions (geometric means ratio range: 80%—93%), except cool water. Mean steady-state concentrations (C_{ss}) of EE were highest under normal conditions, followed by cool water, sauna, whirlpool and treadmill. The LNG mean C_{max}, AUC_{0-168}, AUC_{0-inf} and C_{ss} were higher under normal wear versus all other conditions (geometric means ratios: 75%—82%), with the exception of AUC_{0-168}, AUC0-inf and C_{ss} for cold water. Median times to maximum concentration (T_{max}) for EE and LNG were comparable across conditions. Patch adhesion was excellent under all conditions. Adverse events were mild, with none serious or leading to discontinuation.

Conclusions.—Although slightly lower mean drug concentration levels were observed for whirlpool, treadmill and sauna, drug concentrations under all conditions were well within therapeutic ranges established for the AP during normal wear and within ranges reported for low-dose

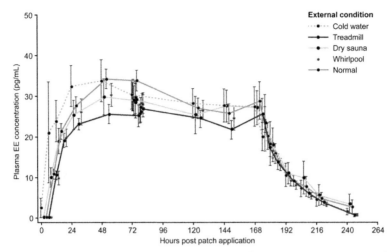

FIGURE 1.—Plasma concentrations (mean ± standard error) of EE during 7 days of treatment with the Agile Patch under normal conditions or conditions of daily exposure to cool water immersion, treadmill, dry sauna or whirlpool. (Reprinted from Contraception. Archer DF, Stanczyk FZ, Rubin A, et al. Pharmacokinetics and adhesion of the Agile transdermal contraceptive patch (AG200-15) during daily exposure to external conditions of heat, humidity and exercise. *Contraception.* 2013;87:212-219, Copyright 2013, with permission from Elsevier.)

combination oral contraceptives. Patch adhesion was excellent; the AP was safe and well tolerated under all conditions (Fig 1).

▶ An increasing number of pharmaceutical products are now being delivered by means of skin patches, raising the question of their efficacy when used by a person with an active lifestyle. Does sweating or swimming compromise the safety or the efficacy of a patch? If the blood flow to the skin is increased, absorption of a drug may be increased, as has sometimes been observed with nicotine and trinitrin patches.[1,2] There have also been concerns that increased absorption from contraceptive patches could provoke venous thrombo-embolism.[3,4] This study evaluated the drug delivery of one of the latest types of patch intended for active subjects under various challenging conditions such as 30 minutes of daily treadmill walking, 10 minutes per day in a hot whirlpool, or use of a sauna. Few of the patches showed any tendency to become detached, and the drug dosage remained closely within the intended therapeutic profile (Fig 1). It would be interesting to repeat these observations using other commonly available types of patches.

R. J. Shephard, MD (Lond), PhD, DPE

References

1. Vanakoski J, Seppälä T, Sievi E, Lunell E. Exposure to high ambient temperature increases absorption and plasma concentrations of transdermal nicotine. *Clin Pharmacol Ther.* 1996;60:308-315.
2. Barkve TF, Langseth-Manrique K, Bredesen JE, Gjesdal K. Increased uptake of transdermal glyceryl trinitrate during physical exercise and during high ambient temperature. *Am Heart J.* 1986;112:537-541.

3. Burkman RT. Transdermal hormonal contraception: benefits and risks. *Am J Obstet Gynecol.* 2007;197:134.e1-134.e6.
4. Cole JA, Norman H, Doherty M, Walker AM. Venous thromboembolism, myocardial infarction, and stroke among transdermal contraceptive system users. *Obstet Gynecol.* 2007;109:339-346.

Lipid Peroxidation in Judoists Using Oral Contraceptives

Massart A, Portier H, Rosado F, et al (CIDAF, STAPS, Orleans, France; Université d'Orleans, France; Centro de Investigação, Coimbra, Portugal; et al)
Int J Sports Med 33:781-788, 2012

12 female judoists using oral contraceptives (OCU) containing 0.03 mg ethinylestradiol and 3 mg drospirenone for 20 ± 12 months (mean ± SD) were compared with a control group of 14 judoist noncontraceptive users (NCU) in order to evaluate resting (T_1) and postexercise (T_2) lipid peroxidation (LPO) and antioxidant parameters. Data were collected 20 min before and 10 min after a morning session of judo training and included determination of lag phase (Lp) before free radical-induced oxidation, glutathione peroxidase (GPx), α-tocopherol, retinol, and oxidative stress markers related to LPO. Significantly higher resting oxidative stress (+125.8 and +165.2% for malondialdehyde and lipid peroxides, respectively) and lower values of Lp and GPx (−23.4 and −12.1%, respectively) were observed in the OCU compared with NCU. The judo training session induced an increase in plasma LPO whatever the treatment. We noted significant increases in Lp (+14.7%; $p < 0.05$ vs. preexercise) and GPx (22.1%; $p < 0.05$ vs. preexercise) only in the NCU group. We suggest

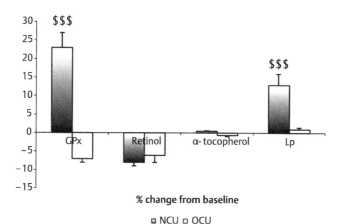

% change from baseline

□ NCU □ OCU

FIGURE 2.—Effects of exercise on antioxidant parameters expressed in percent change from baseline. NCU: non-contraception users; OCU: oral contraception users. GPx: Glutathione peroxidase; Lp: lag phase. $$$: $p < 0.001$: OCU vs. NCU. (Reprinted from Massart A, Portier H, Rosado F, et al. Lipid peroxidation in judoists using oral contraceptives. *Int J Sports Med.* 2012;33:781-788, Copyright 2012, with permission from Georg Thieme Verlag KG Stuttgart.)

that a judo training session favourably altered some antioxidants in NCU but not in OCU. As excessive oxidative stress is linked to the development of several chronic diseases, the use of agents to reduce antioxidants may be reasonable in OCU (Fig 2).

▶ There has been some previous discussion concerning the impact of oral contraceptives on oxidant stress.[1,2] Estrogens are known to have both antioxidant and pro-oxidant effects,[3-5] although the pro-oxidant effects appear to be dominant. The present cross-sectional study on a small group of judoists demonstrates that relative to nonusers, there was a substantially greater resting oxidative stress in those taking oral contraceptive medications (a combination of ethinyl estradiol and drospirenone). The users also showed a smaller stimulation of peroxidase activity during and following exercise (Fig 2). These observations suggest that female athletes who are taking oral contraceptives might profit from an increased intake of antioxidants. There is also scope for long-term evaluation of differences in health between users and nonusers in terms of such items as atherogenesis and cardiovascular disease.[6]

R. J. Shephard, MD (Lond), PhD, DPE

References

1. Pincemail J, Vanbelle S, Gaspard U, et al. Effect of different contraceptive methods on the oxidative stress status in women aged 40−48 years from the ELAN study in the province of Liege, Belgium. *Hum Reprod.* 2007;22:2335-2343.
2. De Groote D, d'Hauterive SP, Pintiaux A, et al. Effects of oral contraception with ethynilestradiol and drospirone on oxidative stress in women 18−35 years old. *Contraception.* 2009;80:187-193.
3. Chambliss KL, Shaul PW. Estrogen modulation of endothelial nitric oxide synthase. *Endocr Rev.* 2002;23:665-686.
4. Wagner AH, Schroeter MR, Hecker M. 17 beta-estradiol inhibition of NADPH oxidase expression in human endothelial cells. *FASEB J.* 2001;15:2121-2130.
5. Gordon KB, Macrae IM, Carswell HV. Effects of 17 beta-oestradiol on cerebral ischaemic damage and lipid peroxidation. *Brain Res.* 2005;1036:155-162.
6. Singh U, Jialal I. Oxidative stress and atherosclerosis. *Pathophysiology.* 2006;13:129-142.

Hormonal contraception and bone metabolism: a systematic review
Nappi C, Bifulco G, Tommaselli GA, et al (Univ of Naples "Federico II," Italy)
Contraception 86:606-621, 2012

Background.—Although a large amount of studies in the literature evaluated the effects of hormonal contraception on bone, many questions remained still unclear, such as the effect of these therapies on fracture risk.

Study Design.—We performed a systematic search of the published studies from January 1975 through January 2012 on the effects of hormonal contraceptives on bone metabolism. We analyzed the overall effect on bone mineral density (BMD) and on fracture risk of combined oral contraceptives (COCs), progestogen-only contraceptives, transdermal contraceptives and vaginal ring.

Results.—COC therapy does not seem to exert any significant effect on BMD in the general population. In adolescents, the effects of COCs on BMD seem to be mainly determined by estrogen dose. The use of COCs in perimenopausal women seems to reduce bone demineralization and may significantly increase BMD even at a 20-mcg dose. Use of depot medroxy-progesterone acetate is associated with a decrease in BMD, although this decrease seems to be partially reversible after discontinuation. Data on other progestogen-only contraceptives, transdermal patch and vaginal ring are still limited, although it seems that these contraceptive methods do not exert any influence on BMD.

Conclusions.—Hormonal contraceptives do not seem to exert any significant effect on bone in the general population. However, other randomized controlled trials are needed to evaluate the effects on fracture risk since the data available are derived from studies having the effects on BMD as the primary end point, and BMD may not accurately reflect the real fracture risk.

▶ This manuscript is a comprehensive systematic review of the effects of different forms of hormonal contraception on bone. The actions of sex steroids on the basic process of bone formation and readsorption are discussed, and several animal studies are summarized. However, the main strength of this publication lies in its rigor in database searching (which identified 1881 potentially relevant records), retrieval of records, and application of exclusion criteria and qualitative synthesis of a final 129 published human studies. Most of these, particularly the randomized controlled trials, focused on bone mineral density (BMD), which is really a surrogate marker for fracture risk. Some measured urinary and serum markers of bone turnover. In general, it appears that the use of combined oral contraceptives (COCs) does not exert any clinically significant effect on BMD in the general population. In adolescents, the dose of ethinyl estradiol (EE) is critical, with 30 mcg of EE being adequate to ensure sufficient bone accrual during these formative years, whereas COCs with only 20 mcg of EE may not be sufficient to support peak bone mass acquisition. In perimenopausal women, the use of COCs reduces bone demineralization and may significantly increase BMD even at a 20-mcg dose and is also associated with a reduction in fracture risk (based on retrospective studies only). The use of injectable depot medroxy-progesterone acetate has been shown to be detrimental to BMD, particularly in adolescents, with one particular study demonstrating a 1.5% and 3.1% decrease in lumbar spine BMD in adolescents after 1 and 2 years of use, compared with a 2.9% and 9.5% BMD increase in controls over the same period. There are insufficient data to draw any significant conclusions about the use of progestogen-only contraceptives, transdermal patch, and vaginal ring. Further studies are warranted.

C. Lebrun, MDCM, MPE, CCFP, Dip Sport Med, FACSM

Fetal wellbeing may be compromised during strenuous exercise among pregnant elite athletes

Salvesen KÅ, Hem E, Sundgot-Borgen J (Trondheim Univ Hosp (St Olav's Hosp), Norway; The Norwegian School of Sport Sciences, Oslo, Norway)
Br J Sports Med 46:279-283, 2012

Objectives.—To study fetal wellbeing and uteroplacental blood flow during strenuous treadmill running in the second trimester.

Methods.—Six pregnant Olympic-level athletes in endurance events aged 28–37 years and training 15–22 h per week before the pregnancy were tested once at 23–29 weeks of pregnancy. The women ran three to five submaximal workloads on a treadmill with approximately 60–90% of maximal oxygen consumption. The maternal—fetal circulation was assessed with Doppler ultrasound of the uterine and umbilical arteries before, during and after exercise.

Results.—Mean uterine artery volume blood flow was reduced to 60–80% after warming up and stayed at 40–75% of the initial value during exercise. Fetal heart rate (FHR) was within the normal range (110–160 bpm) as long as the woman exercised below 90% of maximal maternal heart rate (MHR). Fetal bradycardia and high umbilical artery pulsatility index (PI) occurred when the woman exercised more than 90% of maximal MHR and the mean uterine artery volume blood flow was less than 50% of the initial value. FHR and umbilical artery PI normalised quickly after stopping the exercise.

Conclusions.—Exercise at intensity above 90% of maximal MHR in pregnant elite athletes may compromise fetal wellbeing.

▶ Most women seem likely to engage in moderate rather than intense levels of physical activity during the later stages of pregnancy, and such activity is generally regarded as both a safe and a desirable practice.[1,2] If a woman is already well trained, more vigorous exercise bouts of exercise may still be acceptable,[3-6] but there has been controversy about top-level competitors who are pregnant and wish to remain in peak form, for instance between Olympic and world championships. These authors were able to obtain some estimates of uterine blood flow and fetal heart rates in a small group of Olympic athletes who were at times reaching exercise intensities higher than 90% of maternal heart rate. Adverse effects were limited if activity was kept below 90% of maternal peak heart rate, but above 90% there was a 50% drop in uterine artery blood flow and an associated fetal bradycardia, suggesting a possible impact on fetal health.

R. J. Shephard, MD (Lond), PhD, DPE

References

1. Kramer MS, McDonald SW. Aerobic exercise for women during pregnancy. *Cochrane Database Syst Rev.* 2006;(3):CD000180.
2. Barakat R, Stirling JR, Lucia A. Does exercise training during pregnancy affect gestational age? A randomised controlled trial. *Br J Sports Med.* 2008;42:674-678.

3. Kardel KR, Kase T. Training in pregnant women: effects on fetal development and birth. *Am J Obstet Gynecol.* 1998;178:280-286.
4. Penttinen J, Erkkola R. Pregnancy in endurance athletes. *Scand J Med Sci Sports.* 1997;7:226-228.
5. Webb KA, Wolfe LA, McGrath MJ. Effects of acute and chronic maternal exercise on fetal heart rate. *J Appl Physiol.* 1994;77:2207-2213.
6. Kardel KR. Effects of intense training during and after pregnancy in top-level athletes. *Scand J Med Sci Sports.* 2005;15:79-86.

Maternal Physical Activity and Insulin Action in Pregnancy and Their Relationships With Infant Body Composition

Pomeroy J, Renström F, Gradmark AM, et al (Lund Univ, Malmö, Sweden; Natl Insts of Health, Phoenix, AZ; Umeå Univ, Sweden; et al)
Diabetes Care 36:267-269, 2013

Objective.—We sought to assess the association between maternal gestational physical activity and insulin action and body composition in early infancy.

Research Design and Methods.—At 28–32 weeks' gestation, pregnant women participating in an observational study in Sweden underwent assessments of height, weight, and body composition, an oral glucose tolerance test, and 10 days of objective physical activity assessment. Thirty mothers and infants returned at 11–19 weeks postpartum. Infants underwent assessments of weight, length, and body composition.

Results.—Early insulin response was correlated with total physical activity ($r = -0.47$; $P = 0.007$). Early insulin response ($r = -0.36$; $P = 0.045$) and total physical activity ($r = 0.52$; $P = 0.037$) were also correlated with infant fat-free mass. No maternal variable was significantly correlated with infant adiposity.

TABLE 1.—Relationships between Maternal Physical Activity and Metabolic Characteristics and Infant Body Composition 4 Months Postpartum

Maternal Variables	Infant Body Composition (n = 30)		
	Fat Mass	Percent Fat	Fat-free Mass
Fasting glucose	0.01 (−0.34 to 0.37)	0.04 (−0.31 to 0.39)	0.23 (−0.14 to 0.54)
60-min glucose	0.05 (−0.31 to 0.39)	−0.04 (−0.39 to 0.32)	0.17 (−0.20 to 0.49)
120-min glucose	0.002 (−0.35 to 0.36)	−0.02 (−0.37 to 0.34)	0.02 (−0.34 to 0.37)
Early insulin response*	−0.01 (−0.37 to 0.34)	0.10 (−0.27 to 0.44)	**−0.36 (−0.63 to −0.003)**
Insulin sensitivity index	0.04 (−0.32 to 0.39)	−0.04 (−0.38 to 0.32)	0.09 (−0.27 to 0.43)
Fat mass	−0.09 (−0.43 to 0.27)	−0.11 (−0.45 to 0.25)	0.11 (−0.25 to 0.45)
Percent fat	0.005 (−0.35 to 0.36)	0.001 (−0.34 to 0.37)	0.02 (−0.35 to 0.36)
Fat-free mass	−0.10 (−0.44 to 0.27)	−0.15 (−0.48 to 0.22)	0.28 (−0.09 to 0.57)
Physical activity	0.31 (−0.07 to 0.61)	0.19 (−0.23 to 0.52)	**0.52 (0.17 to 0.74)****

Statistics are Spearman correlation coefficients (95% CI). All infant body composition variables are age- and sex-standardized scores. All correlations were partialled for gestational week, age, infant feeding, and parity. Maternal physical activity is counts per day from a chest-worn activity monitor adjusted for wear time. Results in boldface are statistically significant at P value < 0.05.
*Estimated by 30-min insulin levels.
**Retains statistical significance after Bonferroni correction.

Conclusions.—The relationships between maternal physical activity, insulin response, and infant fat-free mass suggest that physical activity during pregnancy may affect metabolic outcomes in the mother and her offspring (Table 1).

▶ There is growing recognition that the exercise behavior of pregnant women can influence not only her health, but also that of the fetus. The present study by Pomeroy et al is based on 35 mothers and shows that the lean tissue mass as estimated by doubly-labeled water (but interestingly, not the body fat content) of the young child is linked to an accurate measurement of habitual activity (a 10-day heart rate/movement sensor record) and an early insulin response to a glucose tolerance test (Table 1). The main limitation is the small sample size, necessitated because of the sophisticated tests that were used. It would be interesting to know not only the correlations with lean tissue mass, but also the size of the advantage gained by any given level of weekly activity.

R. J. Shephard, MD (Lond), PhD, DPE

Exercise during Pregnancy and the Gestational Age Distribution: A Cohort Study

Owe KM, Nystad W, Skjaerven R, et al (Norwegian School of Sport Sciences, Oslo, Norway; Norwegian Inst of Public Health, Oslo, Norway; Univ of Bergen, Norway)
Med Sci Sports Exerc 44:1067-1074, 2012

Purpose.—The study's purpose was to examine the associations between exercise performed at different time points during pregnancy and gestational age (GA) in a population-based cohort study.

Methods.—Data included 61,098 singleton pregnancies enrolled between 2000 and 2006 in the Norwegian Mother and Child Cohort Study, conducted by the Norwegian Institute of Public Health. Self-reported exercise was collected from two questionnaires in pregnancy weeks 17 and 30. GA was determined on the basis of the expected date of delivery according to ultrasound, as registered in the Medical Birth Registry of Norway. We used logistic regression to analyze preterm (< 37 completed weeks) and post-term births ($\geq$ 42 wk). Comparison of mean GA by exercise levels was estimated by a general linear model.

Results.—Mean GA for women exercising three to five times a week in week 17 was 39.51 (95% confidence interval [CI] = 39.48−39.54) compared with 39.34 (95% CI = 39.30−39.37) completed weeks for non-exercisers ($P < 0.001$). Mean differences remained for all categories of exercise after adjusting for confounding with the greatest mean difference between exercising three to five times per week in week 17 and nonexercisers (equals 1 d). Similar mean differences in GA were observed by exercise levels in week 30. The greatest protective effect on risk of preterm birth was observed for women exercising three to five times a week in week 17 or 30 (adjusted odds ratio (aOR) = 0.82, 95% CI = 0.73−0.91

TABLE 2.—Crude and Adjusted Risk of Preterm Birth by Level of Exercise During Pregnancy

		Preterm Birth (<37 Completed Weeks)		
	n (%)	cORª (95% CI)	aORᵇ (95% CI)	aORᵇ (95% CI)
Exercise frequency for week 17 (*n* = 61,098)				
Never	789 (5.9)	Ref	Ref	Ref
One to three times per month	661 (5.2)	0.88 (0.79−0.98)	0.92 (0.82−1.02)	0.91 (0.82−1.02)
One to two times per week	923 (5.1)	0.85 (0.77−0.94)	0.87 (0.79−0.97)	0.89 (0.80−0.98)
Three to five times per week	670 (4.8)	0.80 (0.72−0.89)	0.82 (0.73−0.91)	0.84 (0.75−0.93)
Six or more times per week	138 (5.0)	0.84 (0.69−1.01)	0.83 (0.68−1.00)	0.86 (0.73−1.07)
Exercise frequency for week 30 (*n* = 56,853)				
Never	1028 (5.3)	Ref	Ref	Ref
One to three times per month	534 (4.8)	0.89 (0.80−0.99)	0.88 (0.79−0.99)	0.90 (0.81−1.01)
One to two times per week	631 (4.3)	0.79 (0.71−0.88)	0.77 (0.69−0.86)	0.81 (0.73−0.89)
Three to five times per week	412 (4.1)	0.75 (0.67−0.85)	0.74 (0.65−0.83)	0.76 (0.68−0.86)
Six or more times per week	62 (4.3)	0.80 (0.62−1.04)	0.75 (0.57−0.99)	0.81 (0.62−1.05)

ªcOR indicates crude odds ratios.
ᵇAdjusted for maternal age, prepregnancy BMI, education, smoking, and parity.
ᶜAdjusted for working hours, spontaneous abortions, assisted reproduction, vaginal bleeding before the 20th week (week 17), preexisting high blood pressure (week 17), vaginal bleeding after the 20th week (week 30), and predominantly standing/walking at work (week 30).

and aOR = 0.74, 95% CI = 0.65−0.83, respectively) compared with non-exercisers. On the other hand, women exercising one to two or three to five times per week in week 17 were slightly more likely to have a postterm birth (aOR = 1.14, 95% CI = 1.04−1.24 and aOR = 1.15, 95% CI = 1.04−1.26, respectively). Mean GA did not differ by type of exercise performed during pregnancy.

Conclusions.—Exercise performed during pregnancy shifted the GA distribution slightly upward resulting in reduced preterm births and slightly increased postterm births (Table 2).

▶ It is now widely agreed that the optimal regimen for pregnant women should include moderate aerobic exercise on most days of the week[1,2] together with muscle-strengthening and flexibility exercises.[3,4] Many athletes continue to exercise very vigorously even during their third trimester, but a nagging question has been whether high levels of physical activity late during pregnancy increase the risk of preterm delivery, with the associated risks of neonatal morbidity and mortality.[5] A recent Cochrane review of this question found no evidence of increased preterm delivery when exercise was initiated by previously sedentary women, but the studies on which this conclusion was based were small and few in number.[6]

It is thus helpful to have the results of this large-scale Norwegian trial, which also indicate an association between a reduced risk of preterm delivery and all frequencies of leisure-time physical activity, whether such activity was being undertaken early or late during pregnancy (Table 2). On average, gestational age was 1 day longer in the exercisers. Moreover, the type of exercise (walking, low-impact or high-impact exercise, or horseback riding) did not seem to influence this outcome. The main weaknesses, as in most studies of this sort, were the self-assignment of exercise programs and the reliance on self-reports of activity (although a correlational-type assessment of the questionnaire's validity was made against an accelerometer). Moreover, no account was taken of activities outside of leisure, such as occupation, transportation, and caregiving. Finally, it is possible that the most vulnerable group of women (those with a history of persistent vaginal bleeding or previous miscarriages) may have been advised against exercising by their physicians. However, the overall message seems to encourage the pregnant woman to exercise.

R. J. Shephard, MD (Lond), PhD, DPE

References

1. ACOG Committee Obstetric Practice. ACOG Committee opinion. Number 267, January 2002: exercise during pregnancy and the postpartum period. *Obstet Gynecol*. 2002;99:171-173.
2. US Department of Health and Human Services. *2008 Physical Activity Guidelines for Americans*. Washington, DC: Department of Health and Human Services; 2008. 76.
3. Davies GA, Wolfe LA, Mottola MF, MacKinnon C. Joint SOGC/CSEP clinical practice guideline: exercise in pregnancy and the postpartum period. *Can J Appl Physiol*. 2003;28:330-341.
4. Royal College of Obstetrics and Gynaecology; Guidelines and audit committee of the Royal College of Obstetricans and Gynaecologists. Dorset, UK. Statement No. 4. Exercise in Pregnancy. 2006. p. 1–7.
5. Goldenberg RL, Culhane JF, Iams JD, Romero R. Epidemiology and causes of preterm birth. *Lancet*. 2008;371:75-84.
6. Kramer MS, McDonald SW. Aerobic exercise for women during pregnancy. *Cochrane Database Syst Rev*. 2006;3:CD000180.

Maternal Exercise and Growth in Breastfed Infants: A Meta-analysis of Randomized Controlled Trials

Daley AJ, Thomas A, Cooper H, et al (Univ of Birmingham, UK)
Pediatrics 130:108-114, 2012

Background and Objectives.—Studies have revealed that women who breastfeed their infants may be reluctant to exercise due to concerns that to do so would adversely affect their breast milk and consequently the growth of their infants. In this review, we seek to systematically review and statistically synthesize evidence from randomized controlled trials (RCTs) that have assessed the effects of maternal exercise on breastfed infant growth (weight gain and gain in length).

Methods.—Searches of the following electronic bibliographic databases were performed to identify RCTs: Cochrane Library (CENTRAL), Medline/PubMed, Embase, Cumulative Index to Nursing and Allied Health Literature, and SPORT Discus. RCTs that compared any type of exercise intervention with other treatments or no treatment in women exclusively or predominately breastfeeding were eligible for inclusion, as were trials involving exercise as a cointervention. Two authors extracted data from studies independently.

Results.—Four RCTs (5 comparisons) were included in the metaanalysis of infant weight gain that incorporated 170 participants. In breastfed infants, maternal exercise did not significantly affect infant weight gain (difference in mean weight gain = 18.6 g [95% confidence interval: −113.52 to 150.80, $P = .73$]). Only 1 trial assessed infant gain in length; no difference between the exercise and control groups was reported. Trials were classified as moderate or good methodological quality (moderate risk of bias).

Conclusions.—It appears that mothers can exercise and breastfeed without detriment to the growth of their infants, but this is based on limited evidence, and more research is required before this finding is confirmed.

▶ Some women who breastfeed their infants are reluctant to exercise because of concerns regarding the composition of their breast milk, breastfeeding performance, and the growth of their infant.

Some early studies suggested that lactic acid concentrations may increase in the breast milk of exercising women, lowering infant milk acceptance scores.[1] Research on dairy cows suggested that short bouts of aerobic exercise may reduce body fluid and energy levels, resulting in reduced milk volumes.[2] This meta-analysis was based on a small number of available studies but provides initial support that exercise participation while breastfeeding does not adversely affect infant weight gain. There are many exercise-related health and fitness benefits for the breastfeeding mother, and this meta-analysis provides support for clinicians to recommend that exercise training is compatible with mother and infant health.

D. C. Nieman, DrPH

References

1. Wallace JP, Inbar G, Ernsthausen K. Infant acceptance of postexercise breast milk. *Pediatrics*. 1992;89:1245-1247.
2. Lamb R, Anderson M, Walters J. Effects of forced exercise on two-year-old Holstein heifers. *J Dairy Sci*. 1979;62:699-702.

Strenuous exercise during pregnancy: is there a limit?
Szymanski LM, Satin AJ (Johns Hopkins Univ School of Medicine, Baltimore, MD)
Am J Obstet Gynecol 207:179.e1-179.e6, 2012

Objective.—The purpose of this study was to evaluate fetal responses to strenuous exercise in physically active and inactive women.

Study Design.—Forty-five healthy women (15 who were nonexercisers, 15 who were regularly active, 15 who were highly active) underwent a peak treadmill test at 28 weeks' gestation to 32 weeks 6 days' gestation. Fetal well-being (umbilical artery Doppler indices, fetal heart tracing/rate, biophysical profile [BPP]) was evaluated before and after exercise. Uterine artery Doppler scans were also obtained.

Results.—Umbilical and uterine artery Doppler indices were similar among activity groups and did not change with exercise ($P > .05$). BPP and fetal heart tracings were reassuring in all groups. However, subgroup analyses showed transient fetal heart rate decelerations after exercise and elevated umbilical and uterine artery Doppler indices in 5 highly active women. After this, BPP and fetal heart tracings were reassuring.

Conclusion.—Overall fetal well-being is reassuring after short-duration, strenuous exercise in both active and inactive pregnant women. A subset of highly active women experienced transient fetal heart rate decelerations and Doppler changes immediately after exercise. Athletes may push beyond a threshold intensity at which fetal well-being may be compromised. However, potential impact on neonatal outcomes is unknown.

▶ The 2008 Physical Activity Guidelines for Americans concluded that little is known regarding vigorous intensity aerobic activity during pregnancy and that women without an exercise history should not begin vigorous exercise during pregnancy.[1] Animal studies and limited human data on female athletes have raised concerns about fetal health during high-intensity exercise.[2] And the data from this study indicate that a subset of highly active women experienced transient fetal heart rate bradycardia immediately after exercise. The authors urge that "further research is needed on exercise in pregnant athletes to determine whether an upper limit of exercise exists that, if exceeded, places the fetus at risk." At this time, female athletes should err on the side of caution and avoid following the examples of some pregnant women who have run marathons within days and weeks of giving birth.

D. C. Nieman, DrPH

References

1. US Department of Health and Human Services. *2008 Physical Activity Guidelines for Americans*. Washington, DC: Department of Health and Human Services; 2008.
2. Salvesen KÅ, Hem E, Sundgot-Borgen J. Fetal wellbeing may be compromised during strenuous exercise among pregnant elite athletes. *Br J Sports Med.* 2012; 46:279-283.

Daily physical activity and menopausal hot flashes: Applying a novel within-person approach to demonstrate individual differences
Elavsky S, Molenaar PCM, Gold CH, et al (The Pennsylvania State Univ)
Maturitas 71:287-293, 2012

Background.—Physical activity (PA) may be a useful tool in the management of menopausal hot flashes (HFs) but findings are generally inconsistent. There are few well-designed and sufficiently powered RCTs. Applying a longitudinal within-person approach offers an alternative way to examine the PA-HFs relationship which enables complete accommodation of inter-individual differences.

Objectives.—A prospective daily diary study which applied experience sampling methods and time series modeling techniques investigated, at the within-person level, the relationship between objectively measured daily PA of varying intensities and self-reported menopausal HFs.

Methods.—Twenty-four symptomatic middle-aged women (*M* age = 50.4; SD = 4.9) completed fitness, body composition and hormonal status screening, and reported on daily HFs using an electronic PDA device across one menstrual cycle or for 30 days (if postmenopausal). Daily PA and PA intensity was measured using accelerometry and subjects completed a battery of psychological measures.

Results.—Within person analysis identified significant relations between PA and HFs in 50% of subjects, although the specific PA indicators that predicted HFs varied, both in terms of direction and magnitude. Perceived control over HFs was the variable that most consistently differentiated between women for whom more PA was associated with fewer HFs as compared to those for whom more PA was associated with more HFs, but other individual difference characteristics such as affect, depressive symptoms, and anxiety were identified.

Conclusions.—There is great individual variation in the way daily PA impacts self-reported HFs. Affective outcomes and perceived control may help potentially explain this variability.

▶ This is the first study to link objectively measured physical activity (PA) to self-report of vasomotor symptoms in women during the menopausal transition. Several methodological strengths elevate the importance of this study. For example, menopausal status was classified using the Stages of Reproductive Aging Workshop criteria (60% of the women) as well as by serum follicle-stimulating hormone levels (40% of the women) and validated psychosocial questionnaires were used. Participants recorded hot flash occurrence and contextual data into electronic personal digital assistant devices to capture "real time," as opposed to retrospective, data, and physical activity was measured using uniaxial accelerometers worn for the entire data collection phase (30 days or 1 menstrual cycle). Using a longitudinal within-person design, the investigators determined the number of unique daily hot flashes for each of 5 PA measures for each woman separately. Two different temporal analyses were performed for cross-lagged (the previous day's PA on the next day's hot flashes) and simultaneous effects (relation between PA and hot flashes on the same day). Statistically significant associations between PA and hot flash frequency (cross-lagged or same-day) were found in 10 of the 20 evaluable cases, but the direction of the associations was highly variable. For half of the women, PA was negatively associated with hot flash frequency in both the cross-lagged and real-time analyses. Perceived control over hot flashes was the most distinguishing trait between positive and negative associations of hot flash with PA. Women for whom more PA was associated with fewer hot flashes perceived more control over their hot flashes. Depression was a distinguishing characteristic of the PA and hot flash relation but was inconsistent across PA intensity levels. For example, fewer depressive symptoms were reported in women with a negative association between vigorous PA and subsequent hot flashes as well as in women who had a positive association between moderate PA and hot flashes. The authors concluded that the high subject-specificity in the relation of PA with hot flashes suggests that some subgroups of women may have PA-sensitive hot flashes. PA could be used to manage this common and disruptive symptom of the menopausal transition, but women may need to accept some trial and error to determine if and how PA relieves hot flashes. A 1-size-fits-all recommendation cannot be made for the management of hot flashes by PA. Furthermore, some women may need additional encouragement to become physically active or maintain PA if their hot flashes are worsened by PA.

C. M. Jankowski, PhD

Effect of supervised and home exercise training on bone mineral density among breast cancer patients. A 12-month randomised controlled trial
Saarto T, Sievänen H, Kellokumpu-Lehtinen P, et al (Helsinki Univ Central Hosp, Finland; The UKK Inst for Health Promotion Res, Tampere, Finland; Tampere Univ Central Hosp, Finland; et al)
Osteoporos Int 23:1601-1612, 2012

Summary.—The ability of combined step aerobic- and circuittraining to prevent bone loss after breast cancer treatments was related to skeletal site and patients' menopausal status. Among premenopausal breast cancer survivors, a 12-month exercise intervention completely prevented bone loss at the femoral neck, whereas no exercise effect was seen at lumbar spine or at neither site in postmenopausal women.

Introduction.—The primary objective of this randomised clinical trial was to determine the preventive effect of supervised weight-bearing jumping exercises and circuit training on bone loss among breast cancer patients.

Methods.—Of 573 breast cancer survivors aged 35−68 years randomly allocated into exercise or control group after adjuvant treatments, 498 (87%) were included in the final analysis. The 12-month exercise intervention comprised weekly supervised step aerobic- and circuit-exercises and similar home training. Bone mineral density (BMD) at lumbar spine and femoral neck were measured by dualenergy X-ray absorptiometry. Physical performance was assessed by 2-km walking and figure-8 running tests, and the amount of physical activity was estimated in metabolic equivalent-hours/week.

Results.—In premenopausal women, bone loss at the femoral neck was prevented by exercise, the mean BMD changes being -0.2% among the trainees vs. -1.4% among the controls ($p = 0.01$). Lumbar bone loss could not be prevented (-1.9% vs. -2.2%). In postmenopausal women, no significant exercise-effect on BMD was found either at the lumbar spine (-1.6% vs. -2.1%) or femoral neck (-1.1% vs. -1.1%).

Conclusions.—This 12-month aerobic jumping and circuit training intervention completely prevented femoral neck bone loss in premenopausal

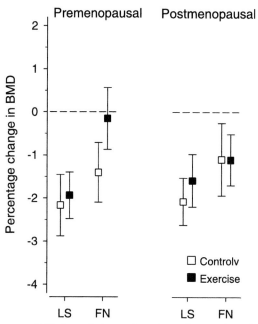

FIGURE 2.—Percentage BMD changes in the exercise and control groups during the 12-month intervention. a Premenopausal women, b postmenopausal women. (Reprinted from Saarto T, Sievänen H, Kellokumpu-Lehtinen P, et al. Effect of supervised and home exercise training on bone mineral density among breast cancer patients. A 12-month randomised controlled trial. *Osteoporos Int*. 2012;23:1601-1612, with permission from International Osteoporosis Foundation and National Osteoporosis Foundation.)

breast cancer patients, whereas no effect on BMD was seen in postmenopausal women (Fig 2).

▶ The BREX study stands out because it is the largest to date on the effects of an osteogenic exercise intervention on bone mineral density (BMD) in women with newly diagnosed invasive breast cancer. The 12-month training included circuit training and progressive jumping movements that induced impacts of 4 times body weight. Baseline BMD was measured within 4 months of the completion of chemotherapy or radiotherapy and endocrine therapy had started. Randomization to the exercise or nonexercise control group was stratified by menopausal status, age in premenopausal women, endocrine therapy in postmenopausal women, and study site. The key finding was that loss of femoral neck BMD was mitigated by the exercise training in premenopausal women but not in postmenopausal women (Fig 2). There was no protective effect of exercise on lumbar spine BMD in premenopausal or postmenopausal women. About half of the premenopausal women developed permanent amenorrhea during the training. Bone loss in the lumbar spine was significantly greater in the amenorrheic women compared with those with preserved menses (−2.6% vs −0.8%; *P* < .001). Self-reported physical activity increased in the control groups, potentially diminishing the exercise effect. The study could not address a dose response for the exercise effect on femoral neck BMD in premenopausal women. Tamoxifen use by about 75% of the premenopausal women may have contributed to the exercise-induced protection of femoral neck BMD.

C. M. Jankowski, PhD

Aging and the Elderly

A Randomized Controlled Study Investigating Static and Dynamic Balance in Older Adults After Training with Pilates

Bird M-L, Hill KD, Fell JW (Univ of Tasmania, Launceston, Australia; La Trobe Univ and Northern Health, Bundoora, Victoria, Australia)
Arch Phys Med Rehabil 93:43-49, 2012

Objective.—To evaluate effects of a Pilates intervention on balance and function in community-dwelling older (aged >60y) adults.

Design.—Randomized crossover study design lasting 16 weeks.

Setting.—University exercise clinic.

Participants.—Ambulatory older community-dwelling adults (N=32) were recruited, and 27 (mean ± SD age, $67.3 \pm 6.5y$) completed the program.

Intervention.—Participants were allocated to either 5 weeks of a group Pilates training intervention or 5 weeks of usual activity (control). After a 6-week washout period, participants performed the alternate intervention.

Main Outcome Measures.—Static and dynamic balance measures (mediolateral sway range, Four Square Step Test, Timed Up and Go Test) and leg strength were recorded at 4 times before and after each intervention (baseline [t1], interim time immediately after the first group intervention [t2], after 5-week washout [before the second intervention period] [t3], and at study conclusion after the second group intervention [t4]).

Results.—There were no significant differences between the Pilates and control groups for any measured variables ($P>.05$) despite static and dynamic balance significantly improving during the study and from pre- to post-Pilates ($P<.05$) without significant changes occurring during the control phase. Improvements that occurred during Pilates between t1 and t2 did not return to baseline after the washout period (t3). There were no changes in leg strength. Mediolateral sway range standing on a foam cushion with eyes closed improved -1.64 cm (95% confidence interval, -2.47 to -0.82) and had the largest effect size post-Pilates ($d=.72$).

Conclusions.—Although there were no significant between-group differences, participation in the Pilates component of the study led to improved static and dynamic balance. The absence of differences between conditions may be a result of small sample size or the crossover study design because Pilates may produce neuromuscular adaptations of unknown resilience (Figs 2 and 3).

▶ Pilates exercise includes muscle strengthening and flexibility components that could improve balance ability in older adults. The research on Pilates has been

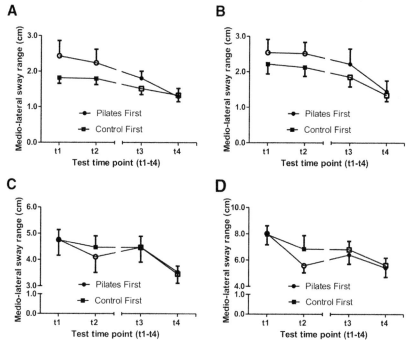

FIGURE 2.—Force platform determined mediolateral sway range (centimeters) with (A, C) eyes open and (B, D) closed and while (C, D) standing on a 65-mm foam cushion over 4 time points (t1—t4) before and after either Pilates training or usual activity (control). Data presented as mean and SE (n=27 at all times). (Reprinted from Bird M-L, Hill KD, Fell JW. A randomized controlled study investigating static and dynamic balance in older adults after training with Pilates. *Arch Phys Med Rehabil.* 2012;93:43-49, with permission from the American Congress of Rehabilitation Medicine.)

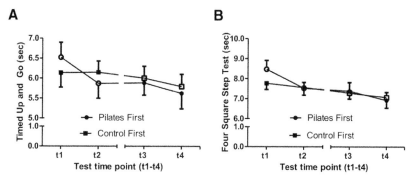

FIGURE 3.—(A) TUG Test and (B) FSST values (seconds) over 4 times (t1—t4) before and after either Pilates training or usual activity (control). Data presented as mean and SE (n=27 at all times). (Reprinted from Bird M-L, Hill KD, Fell JW. A randomized controlled study investigating static and dynamic balance in older adults after training with Pilates. *Arch Phys Med Rehabil.* 2012;93:43-49, with permission from the American Congress of Rehabilitation Medicine.)

limited by a small number of studies and lack of scientific rigor. These authors designed a higher-quality, randomized control trial of the effects of Pilates training on static and dynamic balance in healthy community-dwelling older adults. Their results were mixed; Pilates training significantly improved static and dynamic balance, but the improvements were not different from the control group. A confounding factor in this study was the cross-over design (ie, the order of Pilates training or the control—no training). The cross-over included a 6-week washout period that was intended to allow a performance regression in the Pilates-trained group. Unexpectedly, the effects of Pilates on static balance appeared to be latent and persistent. For example, the range of mediolateral sway with eyes open decreased during the 5 weeks of Pilates training, but continued to decline during the control period (Fig 2A). The authors suggested that the latency could be explained by neural adaptations initiated during Pilates and then carried into daily living. The strongest effect of Pilates was on static balance under conditions of eyes closed and standing on foam (Fig 2D). In this most challenging static balance measure of the study, postural sway decreased with Pilates regardless of the order of the interventions. The dynamic balance outcomes were seen for the timed up and go and 4 square step test. There were trends for both measures to improve (become faster) in the group who had Pilates training first (Fig 3). Oddly, the group who crossed into the Pilates training did not have improvements in dynamic balance.

If Pilates training were a potent intervention for improving dynamic balance, the order of the interventions would be inconsequential. It is possible that the changes seen in the most challenging measure of static balance were seen because there are fewer encounters with this type of perturbation in healthy community-dwelling adults. Conversely, the small changes seen in the dynamic balance outcomes could reflect a smaller challenge to the functional ability of the healthy participants. There were no significant improvements in ankle or knee strength attributed to Pilates. Although this study was carefully constructed, questions remain about the value of Pilates training for improving balance in older adults.

C. M. Jankowski, PhD

Physical Activity and Physical Function in Older Adults: The 45 and Up Study
Yorston LC, Kolt GS, Rosenkranz RR, et al (Univ of Western Sydney, Penrith, New South Wales, Australia)
J Am Geriatr Soc 60:719-725, 2012

Objectives.—To determine the strength of the relationship between physical activity and physical function in older adults.

Design.—Cross-sectional.

Setting.—The 45 and Up Study baseline questionnaire, New South Wales, Australia.

Participants.—Ninety-one thousand three hundred seventy-five Australian men and women aged 65 and older from the 45 and Up Study.

TABLE 2.—Multivariable Logistic Regression Analysis: The Likelihood of Functional Limitation According to Variable (Physical Activity, Psychological Distress, Age, Sex, Body Mass Index, Educational Attainment, and Smoking History)

Variable	Functional Limitation, n (%)		Odds Ratio of Having a Functional Limitation (95% Confidence Interval)	
	None	Some	Raw	Adjusted*
Physical activity tertile				
Lowest[†]	9,127 (35.0)	17,061 (65.0)	1.00	1.00
Middle	15,010 (58.0)	10,865 (42.0)	0.39 (0.38–0.41)	0.48 (0.46–0.50)
Highest	17,688 (65.5)	9,313 (34.5)	0.28 (0.27–0.29)	0.36 (0.34–0.37)
Psychological distress				
Well[†]	36,351 (58.0)	26,302 (42.0)	1.00	1.00
Mild disorder	800 (24.3)	2,486 (75.7)	4.28 (3.94–4.66)	3.92 (3.57–4.30)
Moderate disorder	217 (17.1)	1,049 (82.9)	6.76 (5.78–7.89)	5.64 (4.78–6.65)
Severe disorder	238 (20.6)	916 (79.4)	5.15 (4.43–6.00)	4.19 (3.55–4.94)
Age				
65–74[†]	29,282 (63.5)	16,855 (36.5)	1.00	1.00
75–84	11,432 (41.9)	15,837 (58.1)	2.38 (2.30–2.46)	2.79 (2.68–2.90)
≥ 85	1,156 (20.3)	4,547 (79.7)	6.95 (6.41–7.53)	7.76 (7.11–8.46)
Sex				
Male[†]	24,763 (58.7)	17,444 (41.3)	1.00	1.00
Female	17,074 (46.3)	19,795 (53.7)	1.64 (1.59–1.69)	1.95 (1.88–2.03)
BMI				
Normal[†]	16,701 (59.8)	11,241 (40.2)	1.00	1.00
Underweight	495 (41.1)	709 (58.9)	2.05 (1.80–2.34)	1.35 (1.16–1.57)
Overweight	16,772 (56.0)	13,181 (44.0)	1.19 (1.14–1.23)	1.47 (1.41–1.53)
Obese	5,008 (36.2)	8,824 (63.8)	2.66 (2.54–2.78)	3.25 (3.09–3.42)
Education				
No certificate[†]	5,101 (41.6)	7,173 (58.4)	1.00	1.00
School or intermediate	9,905 (49.4)	10,162 (50.6)	0.71 (0.67–0.74)	0.83 (0.78–0.88)
Higher school or leaving certificate	3,875 (52.8)	9,469 (47.2)	0.63 (0.59–0.68)	0.77 (0.71–0.83)
Trade	5,563 (53.5)	4,837 (46.5)	0.60 (0.56–0.64)	0.90 (0.84–0.96)
Certificate or diploma	8,213 (57.7)	6,023 (42.3)	0.51 (0.48–0.54)	0.72 (0.68–0.77)
Degree+	8,503 (64.5)	4,673 (35.5)	0.38 (0.36–0.41)	0.58 (0.54–0.61)
Smoking history				
Nonsmoker[†]	24,234 (54.4)	20,327 (45.6)	1.00	1.00
Smoker	17,616 (51.0)	16,899 (49.0)	1.16 (1.12–1.20)	1.36 (1.31–1.42)

*Adjusted for physical activity, psychological distress, age, sex, education, smoking history, and body mass index (BMI).
[†]Reference.

Measurements.—Physical activity engagement (Active Australia Survey), physical function (Medical Outcomes Study Physical Functioning), psychological distress (Kessler-10), and self-reported age, smoking history, education, height, and weight were all measured.

Results.—Higher levels of physical activity were associated with better physical function in older adults (correlation coefficient = 0.166, $P < .001$). Participants engaging in higher levels of physical activity had progressively lower likelihoods of functional limitation (middle tertile: odds ratio (OR) = 0.39, 95% confidence interval (CI) = 0.38–0.41; highest tertile: OR = 0.28, 95% CI = 0.27–0.29). This relationship remained significant, but weakened slightly, when adjusted for age, sex, body mass index, smoking history, psychological distress, and educational attainment (middle tertile:

adjusted OR (AOR) = 0.48, 95% CI = 0.46–0.50; highest tertile: AOR = 0.36, 95% CI = 0.34–0.37).

Conclusion.—There is a significant, positive relationship between physical activity and physical function in older adults, with older adults who are more physically active being less likely to experience functional limitation than their more-sedentary counterparts. Level of engagement in physical activity is an important predictor of physical function in older adults (Table 2).

▶ The remarkable finding from this study is the strong influence of psychological distress on the relationship of physical activity (PA) and physical function. In this very large (62 290) Australian study of adults aged 65 years and older, performing some PA was associated with better physical function. The odds ratio of having a functional limitation was reduced by approximately 60% in the subpopulation that reported at least some PA as compared to no PA (Table 2). However, older adults who had any level of psychological distress had a 4-fold greater likelihood of a functional limitation compared to peers without distress. Moderate distress was associated with a nearly 7-fold increased likelihood of functional limitation. When adjusted for physical activity and additional covariates, these odds ratios were reduced slightly. To put the influence of psychological distress on physical function into context, the odds ratio of a physical limitation was approximately 7.0 in adults aged 85 years or older compared to peers aged 65 to 74 years. Advanced age had the greatest influence on the PA and physical function relationship, followed very closely by psychological distress.

These results suggest that strategies to maintain functional independence in older adults may be best targeted toward increasing PA in the "young" elderly and attempting to maintain PA through advanced aging. Equally important is to target older adults with psychological distress, even if reported as mild, for appropriate stress mitigation therapies and support to increase PA. The reader should bear in mind that in this study, PA, functional limitation, and psychological distress were self-reported using validated instruments. An example of the Kessler-10 psychological distress survey question is "In the past four weeks, about how often did you feel worn out for no good reasons?," which is scored on a 1 to 5 scale of increasing distress.

C. M. Jankowski, PhD

New records in aerobic power among octogenarian lifelong endurance athletes
Trappe S, Hayes E, Galpin A, et al (Ball State Univ, Muncie, IN; et al)
J Appl Physiol 114:3-10, 2013

We examined whole body aerobic capacity and myocellular markers of oxidative metabolism in lifelong endurance athletes [$n = 9$, 81 ± 1 yr, 68 ± 3 kg, body mass index (BMI) = 23 ± 1 kg/m^2] and age-matched, healthy, untrained men ($n = 6$; 82 ± 1 y, 77 ± 5 kg, BMI = 26 ± 1 kg/m^2). The endurance athletes were cross-country skiers, including a former

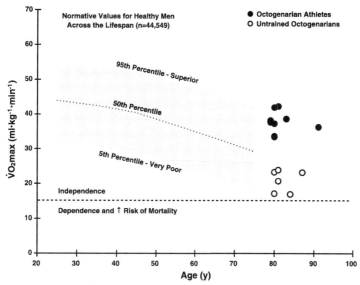

FIGURE 1.—Individual $\dot{V}o_{2max}$ data from the octogenarian lifelong endurance athletes and healthy untrained octogenarians. The dotted line represents the prognostic exercise capacity [5 metabolic equivalents (METs), $17.5 \text{ ml} \cdot \text{kg}^{-1} \cdot \text{min}^{-1}$] generally necessary for an independent lifestyle and associated with an increased risk for mortality as described by Meyers et al. (41). The normative values for healthy men across the life span ($n = 44,549$) were originally obtained from the Cooper Institute in Dallas, TX, and have been summarized by the American College of Sports Medicine (1). (Reprinted from Journal of Applied Physiology. Trappe S, Hayes E, Galpin A, et al. New records in aerobic power among octogenarian lifelong endurance athletes. *J Appl Physiol.* 2013;114:3-10, with permission from the American Physiological Society.)

Olympic champion and several national/regional champions, with a history of aerobic exercise and participation in endurance events throughout their lives. Each subject performed a maximal cycle test to assess aerobic capacity ($\dot{V}o_{2max}$). Subjects had a resting vastus lateralis muscle biopsy to assess oxidative enzymes (citrate synthase and βHAD) and molecular (mRNA) targets associated with mitochondrial biogenesis [peroxisome proliferator-activated receptor-γ coactivator 1α (PGC-1α) and mitochondrial transcription factor A (Tfam)]. The octogenarian athletes had a higher ($P < 0.05$) absolute (2.6 ± 0.1 vs. 1.6 ± 0.1 l/min) and relative (38 ± 1 vs. $21 \pm 1 \text{ ml} \cdot \text{kg}^{-1} \cdot \text{min}^{-1}$) $\dot{V}o_{2max}$, ventilation (79 ± 3 vs. 64 ± 7 l/min), heart rate (160 ± 5 vs. 146 ± 8 beats per minute), and final workload (182 ± 4 vs. 131 ± 14 W). Skeletal muscle oxidative enzymes were 54% (citrate synthase) and 42% (βHAD) higher ($P < 0.05$) in the octogenarian athletes. Likewise, basal PGC-1α and Tfam mRNA were 135% and 80% greater ($P < 0.05$) in the octogenarian athletes. To our knowledge, the $\dot{V}o_{2max}$ of the lifelong endurance athletes is the highest recorded in humans >80 yr of age and comparable to nonendurance trained men 40 years younger. The superior cardiovascular and skeletal muscle health profile of the octogenarian athletes provides a large functional reserve above the aerobic frailty threshold and is associated with lower risk for disability and mortality (Fig 1).

▶ I have long argued that an enhancement in the quality of life as an octogenarian is one of the strongest reasons for maintaining an active lifestyle.[1] Seniors are no longer able to lead an independent life if they have allowed their maximal oxygen intake to drop below a threshold of about 15 mL/[kg·min],[1-3] and maintenance of oxygen transport thus makes an important contribution to keeping an elderly person out of the confines of a nursing home. The data of Trappe et al show that lifelong cross-country skiing champions at an average age of 82 years still have an aerobic power of 38 ml/[kg·min], higher than that of many young and middle-age men. One 91-year-old still showed a value of 36 ml/[kg·min] (Fig 1). With a loss of perhaps 5 ml/[kg·min] per decade of life, and other factors being equal, this group of skiers could well maintain independence to the age of 128 years compared with 85 to 90 years in the untrained subjects. In the face of such data, claims that regular physical activity can increase the quality-adjusted lifespan by 10 to 20 years seem quite conservative. The group of skiers was still quite active, accumulating an accelerometer count averaging 8000 steps/day. Nevertheless, perhaps 2500 of these counts arose from incidental movements around the home, and the remaining 5500 counts would equate to only 4 km of walking per day, hardly an impossible task for an octogenarian. The maximal oxygen intake values in Fig 1 are higher than in some other reports on those who have maintained lifelong activity, and the skiers may have had unusually favorable genes. Nevertheless, Harridge et al[4] also found values averaging 27 mL/[kg·min] in active men older than 80 years. The message is clear—it is not necessary for seniors to accept as inevitable a decline of oxygen transport to the level at which their independence is threatened.

R. J. Shephard, MD (Lond), PhD, DPE

References

1. Shephard RJ. *Aging, Physical Activity and Health*. Champaign, IL: HumaN Kinetics; 1997.
2. Paterson DH, Stathokostas L. Physical activity, fitness and gender in relation to morbidity, survival, quality of life and independence in old age. In: Shephard RJ, ed. *Gender, Physical Activity and Aging*. Boca Raton, FL: CRC Press; 2002.
3. Myers J, Prakash M, Froelicher V, Do D, Partington S, Atwood JE. Exercise capacity and mortality among men referred for exercise testing. *N Engl J Med*. 2002;346:793-801.
4. Harridge S, Magnusson G, Saltin B. Life-long endurance-trained elderly men have high aerobic power, but have similar muscle strength to non-active elderly men. *Aging (Milano)*. 1997;9:80-87.

New records in aerobic power among octogenarian lifelong endurance athletes

Trappe S, Hayes E, Galpin A, et al (Ball State Univ, Muncie, IN; et al)
J Appl Physiol 114:3-10, 2013

We examined whole body aerobic capacity and myocellular markers of oxidative metabolism in lifelong endurance athletes [n = 9, 81 ± 1 yr, 68 ± 3 kg, body mass index (BMI) = 23 ± 1 kg/m^2] and age-matched, healthy, untrained men (n = 6; 82 ± 1 y, 77 ± 5 kg, BMI = 26 ± 1 kg/m^2). The endurance athletes were cross-country skiers, including a former Olympic champion and several national/regional champions, with a history of aerobic exercise and participation in endurance events throughout their lives. Each subject performed a maximal cycle test to assess aerobic capacity ($\dot{V}o_{2max}$). Subjects had a resting vastus lateralis muscle biopsy to assess oxidative enzymes (citrate synthase and βHAD) and molecular (mRNA) targets associated with mitochondrial biogenesis [peroxisome proliferator-activated receptor-γ coactivator 1α (PGC-1α) and mitochondrial transcription factor A (Tfam)]. The octogenarian athletes had a higher ($P < 0.05$) absolute (2.6 ± 0.1 vs. 1.6 ± 0.1 l/min) and relative (38 ± 1 vs.

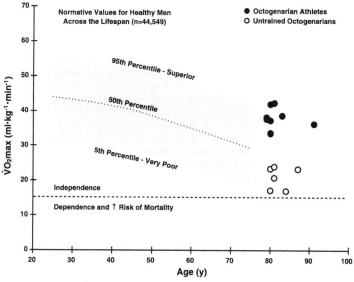

FIGURE 1.—Individual $\dot{V}o_{2max}$ data from the octogenarian lifelong endurance athletes and healthy untrained octogenarians. The dotted line represents the prognostic exercise capacity [5 metabolic equivalents (METs), 17.5 ml·kg^{-1}·min^{-1}] generally necessary for an independent lifestyle and associated with an increased risk for mortality as described by Meyers et al. (41). The normative values for healthy men across the life span (*n* = 44,549) were originally obtained from the Cooper Institute in Dallas, TX, and have been summarized by the American College of Sports Medicine (1). *Editor's Note*: Please refer to original journal article for full references. (Reprinted from Trappe S, Hayes E, Galpin A, et al. New records in aerobic power among octogenarian lifelong endurance athletes. *J Appl Physiol.* 2013;114:3-10, with permission from the American Physiological Society.)

$21 \pm 1 \text{ ml} \cdot \text{kg}^{-1} \cdot \text{min}^{-1}$) $\dot{V}o_{2max}$, ventilation (79 ± 3 vs. 64 ± 7 l/min), heart rate (160 ± 5 vs. 146 ± 8 beats per minute), and final workload (182 ± 4 vs. 131 ± 14 W). Skeletal muscle oxidative enzymes were 54% (citrate synthase) and 42% (βHAD) higher ($P < 0.05$) in the octogenarian athletes. Likewise, basal PGC-1α and Tfam mRNA were 135% and 80% greater ($P < 0.05$) in the octogenarian athletes. To our knowledge, the $\dot{V}o_{2max}$ of the lifelong endurance athletes is the highest recorded in humans >80 yr of age and comparable to nonendurance trained men 40 years younger. The superior cardiovascular and skeletal muscle health profile of the octogenarian athletes provides a large functional reserve above the aerobic frailty threshold and is associated with lower risk for disability and mortality (Fig 1).

▶ These are unique and compelling data, and as summarized in Fig 1, the cardiovascular fitness level of the octogenarian athletes was approximately double compared with the untrained octogenarians. This elevation in aerobic fitness in old age is more than likely the result of lifelong endurance exercise habits and favorable genetic traits. The high aerobic capacity of about 11 METs and related functional reserve among the octogenarian athletes places them at low risk for all-cause mortality. In contrast, untrained independent-living octogenarians have a low functional capacity of about 6 METS, close to the aerobic frailty threshold. Overall, these data support the concept that good aerobic fitness is an achievable goal even in old age.

D. C. Nieman, DrPH

New records in aerobic power among octogenarian lifelong endurance athletes

Trappe S, Hayes E, Galpin A, et al (Ball State Univ, Muncie, IN; et al)
J Appl Physiol 114:3-10, 2013

We examined whole body aerobic capacity and myocellular markers of oxidative metabolism in lifelong endurance athletes [$n = 9$, 81 ± 1 yr, 68 ± 3 kg, body mass index (BMI) $= 23 \pm 1$ kg/m^2] and age-matched, healthy, untrained men (n = 6; 82 ± 1 y, 77 ± 5 kg, BMI $= 26 \pm 1$ kg/m^2). The endurance athletes were cross-country skiers, including a former Olympic champion and several national/regional champions, with a history of aerobic exercise and participation in endurance events throughout their lives. Each subject performed a maximal cycle test to assess aerobic capacity ($\dot{V}o_{2max}$). Subjects had a resting vastus lateralis muscle biopsy to assess oxidative enzymes (citrate synthase and βHAD) and molecular (mRNA) targets associated with mitochondrial biogenesis [peroxisome proliferator-activated receptor-γ coactivator 1α (PGC-1α) and mitochondrial transcription factor A (Tfam)]. The octogenarian athletes had a higher ($P < 0.05$) absolute (2.6 ± 0.1 vs. $1.6 \pm 0.1 \cdot$ l/min) and relative (38 ± 1 vs. $21 \pm 1 \text{ ml} \cdot \text{kg}^{-1} \cdot \text{min}^{-1}$) $\dot{V}o_{2max}$, ventilation (79 ± 3 vs. 64 ± 7 l/min), heart rate (160 ± 5 vs. 146 ± 8 beats per minute), and final workload

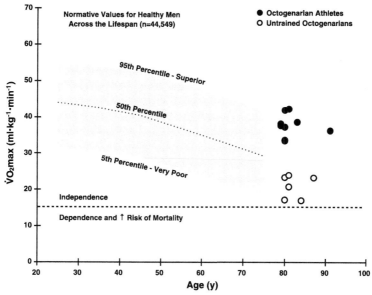

FIGURE 1.—Individual $\dot{V}o_{2max}$ data from the octogenarian lifelong endurance athletes and healthy untrained octogenarians. The dotted line represents the prognostic exercise capacity [5 metabolic equivalents (METs), $17.5\ ml\cdot kg^{-1}\cdot min^{-1}$] generally necessary for an independent lifestyle and associated with an increased risk for mortality as described by Meyers et al. (41). The normative values for healthy men across the life span ($n = 44{,}549$) were originally obtained from the Cooper Institute in Dallas, TX, and have been summarized by the American College of Sports Medicine (1). *Editor's Note*: Please refer to original journal article for full references. (Reprinted from Journal of Applied Physiology. Trappe S, Hayes E, Galpin A, et al. New records in aerobic power among octogenarian lifelong endurance athletes. *J Appl Physiol.* 2013;114:3-10, with permission from the American Physiological Society.)

(182 ± 4 vs. 131 ± 14 W). Skeletal muscle oxidative enzymes were 54% (citrate synthase) and 42% (βHAD) higher ($P < 0.05$) in the octogenarian athletes. Likewise, basal PGC-1α and Tfam mRNA were 135% and 80% greater ($P < 0.05$) in the octogenarian athletes. To our knowledge, the $\dot{V}o_{2max}$ of the lifelong endurance athletes is the highest recorded in humans > 80 yr of age and comparable to nonendurance trained men 40 years younger. The superior cardiovascular and skeletal muscle health profile of the octogenarian athletes provides a large functional reserve above the aerobic frailty threshold and is associated with lower risk for disability and mortality (Fig 1).

▶ The elite octogenarian athletes in this study demonstrated the high end of the cardiovascular spectrum of function. The $\dot{V}o_{2max}$ (absolute, relative to body weight, relative to lean mass) of the athletes was nearly double that of their untrained and healthy counterparts. Equally impressive were the differences in maximum ventilation and stroke volume (as measured by O_2 pulse). At the level of skeletal muscle, oxidative enzyme activity and the expression of mitochondrial genes were significantly greater in the athletes, signifying peripheral adaptations synchronized with their cardiorespiratory capacity. The maximum workload was approximately11 metabolic equivalents (METS) in the athletes and approximately

6 METS in the untrained men. The importance of this difference is best seen in Fig 1. At 5 METS, functional independence is compromised. The margin between 5 METS and maximum achievable workload is the functional reserve. By virtue of genetics, rigorous training in young adulthood, and sustained high-intensity and high-volume training in middle and old age (continuously for 50 years), the athletes had a broad functional reserve, whereas the untrained men hovered just greater than that 5-MET threshold. As the authors noted, the untrained men were impressive in their own right, completing more than 4000 steps/day and achieving maximal criteria on the cycle ergometer test. Yet, the untrained octogenarians had only a 1-MET functional reserve. The estimated age-related change in $\dot{V}o_{2max}$ in the elite athletes was approximately 7.5% per decade, consistent with previous estimates and longitudinal studies. These results point to the importance of building and protecting functional reserve earlier in adulthood to maintain reserve in advanced age. Lifelong physical activity and activity initiated later in life are necessary to build functional reserve and protect it in advanced aging.

C. M. Jankowski, PhD

Mortality in former Olympic athletes: retrospective cohort analysis

Zwiers R, Zantvoord FWA, Engelaer FM, et al (Leyden Academy on Vitality and Aging, Leiden, Netherlands; Leiden Univ Med Center, Netherlands)
BMJ 345:e7456, 2012

Objective.—To assess the mortality risk in subsequent years (adjusted for year of birth, nationality, and sex) of former Olympic athletes from disciplines with different levels of exercise intensity.

Design.—Retrospective cohort study.

Setting.—Former Olympic athletes.

Participants.—9889 athletes (with a known age at death) who participated in the Olympic Games between 1896 and 1936, representing 43 types of disciplines with different levels of cardiovascular, static, and dynamic intensity exercise; high or low risk of bodily collision; and different levels of physical contact.

Main Outcome Measure.—All cause mortality.

Results.—Hazard ratios for mortality among athletes from disciplines with moderate cardiovascular intensity (1.01, 95% confidence interval 0.96 to 1.07) or high cardiovascular intensity (0.98, 0.92 to 1.04) were similar to those in athletes from disciplines with low cardiovascular intensity. The underlying static and dynamic components in exercise intensity showed similar non-significant results. Increased mortality was seen among athletes from disciplines with a high risk of bodily collision (hazard ratio 1.11, 1.06 to 1.15) and with high levels of physical contact (1.16, 1.11 to 1.22). In a multivariate analysis, the effect of high cardiovascular intensity remained similar (hazard ratio 1.05, 0.89 to 1.25); the increased mortality associated with high physical contact persisted (hazard ratio 1.13, 1.06 to 1.21), but that for bodily collision became non-significant (1.03, 0.98 to 1.09) as a consequence of its close relation with physical contact.

TABLE 1.—Hazard Ratios of Mortality for Athletes in Disciplines with Different Intensities of Exercise

Intensity	Univariate Analysis* Hazard Ratio (95% CI)	P Value	Multivariate Analysis† Hazard Ratio (95% CI)	P Value
Cardiovascular:				
Low	Reference		Reference	
Moderate	1.01 (0.96 to 1.07)	0.71	1.04 (0.95 to 1.15)	0.40
High	0.98 (0.92 to 1.04)	0.46	1.05 (0.89 to 1.25)	0.58
Static:				
Low	Reference		Reference	
Moderate	0.94 (0.89 to 0.99)	0.02	0.93 (0.85 to 1.01)	0.09
High	0.99 (0.94 to 1.04)	0.62	0.95 (0.85 to 1.07)	0.40
Dynamic:				
Low	Reference		Reference	
Moderate	0.94 (0.89 to 0.99)	0.03	0.94 (0.87 to 1.01)	0.09
High	0.97 (0.92 to 1.02)	0.19	0.94 (0.83 to 1.06)	0.34

*Adjusted for sex, year of birth, and nationality.
†Additionally includes all types of exercise intensity (cardiovascular, static, and dynamic) in model.

Conclusions.—Among former Olympic athletes, engagement in disciplines with high intensity exercise did not bring a survival benefit compared with disciplines with low intensity exercise. Those who engaged in disciplines with high levels of physical contact had higher mortality than other Olympians later in life (Table 1).

▶ It has been recognized for many years that endurance athletes have several years of advantage of life expectancy relative to the general population.[1-3] Some have considered this as further proof of the health advantages of a very active lifestyle, but other factors including an ectomorphic body build, avoidance of cigarette smoking, and the wealth and status conferred by top athletic status undoubtedly contribute to their actuarial advantage. The article by Zwiers et al suggests that cardiovascular training makes only a minor contribution, because benefit is seen equally among participants in low-intensity sports such as cricket, curling, golf, and shooting (Fig 1 in the original article). The article also underlines that there are adverse risks in sports with a high risk of collision (11%) or physical contact (16%) relative to other competitors.

R. J. Shephard, MD (Lond), PhD, DPE

References

1. Karvonen MJ, Klemola H, Virkajärvi J, Kekkonen A. Longevity of endurance skiers. *Med Sci Sports.* 1974;6:49-51.
2. Sarna S, Kaprio J. Life expectancy of former elite athletes. *Sports Med.* 1994;17:149-151.
3. Clarke PM, Walter SJ, Hayen A, Mallon WJ, Heijmans J, Studdert DM. Survival of the fittest: retrospective cohort study of the longevity of Olympic medallists in the modern era. *BMJ.* 2012;345:e8308.

Enhanced Fitness: A Randomized Controlled Trial of the Effects of Home-Based Physical Activity Counseling on Glycemic Control in Older Adults with Prediabetes Mellitus

Morey MC, Pieper CF, Edelman DE, et al (Duke Univ, Durham, NC; et al)
J Am Geriatr Soc 60:1655-1662, 2012

Objectives.—To determine whether a home-based multicomponent physical activity counseling (PAC) intervention is effective in reducing glycemic measures in older outpatients with prediabetes mellitus.

Design.—Controlled clinical trial.

Setting.—Primary care clinics of the Durham Veterans Affairs (VA) Medical Center between September 29, 2008, and March 25, 2010.

Participants.—Three hundred two overweight (body mass index 25–45 kg/m^2), older (60–89) outpatients with impaired glucose tolerance (fasting blood glucose 100–125 mg/dL, glycosylated hemoglobin (HbA1c) <7%) randomly assigned to a PAC intervention group (n = 180) or a usual care control group (n = 122).

Intervention.—A 12-month, home-based multicomponent PAC program including one in-person baseline counseling session, regular telephone counseling, physician endorsement in clinic with monthly automated encouragement, and customized mailed materials. All study participants, including controls, received a consultation in a VA weight management program.

Measurements.—The primary outcome was a homeostasis model assessment of insulin resistance (HOMA-IR), calculated from fasting insulin and glucose levels at baseline and 3 and 12 months. HbA1c was the secondary indicator of glycemic control. Other secondary outcomes were anthropometric measures and self-reported physical activity, health-related quality of life, and physical function.

Results.—There were no significant differences between the PAC and control groups over time for any of the glycemic indicators. Both groups had small declines over time of approximately 6% in fasting blood glucose ($P < .001$), and other glycemic indicators remained stable. The declines in glucose were not sufficient to affect the change in HOMA-IR scores due to fluctuations in insulin over time. Endurance physical activity increased significantly in the PAC group ($P < .001$) and not in the usual care group.

Conclusion.—Home-based telephone counseling increased physical activity levels but was insufficient to improve glycemic indicators in older outpatients with prediabetes mellitus.

▶ In this study, a home-based exercise intervention supported by telephone counseling did not improve glycemic control in prediabetic older women and men (aged 60–89). Approximately 17% of the study population was older than 75 years old and about 96% were male. The goal of the exercise intervention was to increase physical activity, primarily walking, to 150 minutes per week. Lower extremity resistance training, using resistance bands, for 15 minutes 3 times per week, was also prescribed in keeping with current public health recommendations. The usual care (control) group comprised men who could choose to participate in the MOVE! Program developed by the Veterans Administration. About 30% of the usual care group chose the MOVE! counseling. The intervention and MOVE! Program included a baseline individual counseling session that included goal setting. The intervention group was provided with regular telephone counseling every 2 weeks for 6 weeks and then monthly for the remainder of the year. Physical activity by self-report doubled in the intervention group over the year and was stable in the usual care group. On average, the intervention group did not achieve the goal of 150 minutes of exercise per week. Accelerometers were worn by a subset of the intervention group subjects. Steps per day increased modestly, from 5241 at baseline to 5585 after 3 months and 5643 at the 12-month assessment (n = 48 at this time point). Low-cost interventions for lifestyle modifications to control chronic disease risk are increasingly attractive as health care costs rise and the target population grows. However, this study does not lend support to the efficacy of a home and telephone counseling approach to glycemic control in older adults, primarily male, who were prediabetic.

C. M. Jankowski, PhD

Physical activity and all-cause mortality in older women and men

Brown WJ, McLaughlin D, Leung J, et al (The Univ of Queensland, St Lucia, Australia; et al)
Br J Sports Med 46:664-668, 2012

Background.—Regular physical activity is associated with reduced risk of mortality in middle-aged adults; however, associations between physical activity and mortality in older people have been less well studied. The objective of this study was to compare relationships between physical activity and mortality in older women and men.

Methods.—The prospective cohort design involved 7080 women aged 70—75 years and 11 668 men aged 65—83 years at baseline, from two Australian cohorts — the Australian Longitudinal Study on Women's Health and the Health in Men Study. Self-reported low, moderate and vigorous intensity physical activity, socio-demographic, behavioural and health characteristics were assessed in relation to all-cause mortality from the National Death Index from 1996 to 2009; the median follow-up of 10.4 (women) and 11.5 (men) years.

Results.—There were 1807 (25.5%) and 4705 (40.3%) deaths in women and men, respectively. After adjustment for behavioural risk factors, demographic variables and self-reported health at baseline, there was an inverse dose — response relationship between physical activity and all-cause mortality. Compared with women and men who reported no activity, there were statistically significant lower hazard ratios for women who reported any activity and for men who reported activities equivalent to at least 300 metabolic equivalent. min/week. Risk reductions were 30—50% greater in women than in men in every physical activity category.

TABLE 2.—HRs* (and 95% CI) for All-Cause Mortality Before 1 October 2009, by Physical Activity at Baseline. The Left Columns Show Data From the Entire Sample, the Right Columns Show Data After Excluding Deaths in the First 2 Years of Follow-Up

Physical Activity (MET Min/Week) Number of Deaths	Entire Sample			Excluding Deaths in Years 1 and 2		
	Women 1807 HR (95% CI)	Men 4705 HR (95% CI)	Men:Women Ratio HR (95% CI)	Women 1656 HR (95% CI)	Men 4214 HR (95% CI)	Men:Women Ratio HR (95% CI)
None (0)						
Very low (1—< 300)	0.67 (0.58 to 0.76)	0.95 (0.83 to 1.08)	1.47 (1.29 to 1.66)	0.71 (0.62 to 0.82)	1.00 (0.87 to 1.14)	1.49 (1.31 to 1.71)
Low (300—<450)	0.59 (0.48 to 0.71)	0.86 (0.76 to 0.98)	1.32 (1.17 to 1.49)	0.60 (0.49 to 0.74)	0.86 (0.75 to 0.98)	1.27 (1.12 to 1.45)
Moderate (450—< 600)	0.56 (0.46 to 0.68)	0.88 (0.78 to 0.99)	1.35 (1.20 to 1.51)	0.59 (0.49 to 0.72)	0.90 (0.80 to 1.02)	1.35 (1.20 to 1.52)
Moderate-high (600—< 1050)	0.53 (0.45 to 0.62)	0.81 (0.74 to 0.89)	1.24 (1.14 to 1.35)	0.55 (0.47 to 0.65)	0.84 (0.77 to 0.92)	1.25 (1.15 to 1.37)
High (1050—< 1500)	0.60 (0.50 to 0.72)	0.78 (0.71 to 0.86)	1.21 (1.11 to 1.32)	0.63 (0.52 to 0.77)	0.82 (0.74 to 0.90)	1.22 (1.11 to 1.34)
Very high (≥ 1500)	0.52 (0.44 to 0.62)	0.73 (0.67 to 0.79)	1.12 (1.04 to 1.22)	0.56 (0.47 to 0.67)	0.75 (0.69 to 0.83)	1.13 (1.04 to 1.23)

MET, metabolic equivalent.
*Adjusted for age, marital status, education, body mass index, smoking, alcohol and chronic disease.

Conclusions.—Physical activity is inversely associated with all-cause mortality in older men and women. The relationship is stronger in women than in men, and there are benefits from even low levels of activity (Table 2).

▶ There is now little disagreement that regular moderately vigorous physical activity has a beneficial influence on the prognosis of middle-aged adults, after allowing for confounding influences. However, the situation is less clear in elderly patients. Several important questions arise in this age group, in particular, can benefit be obtained from much lower intensities of effort than those recommended in middle age,[1,2] and can vigorous activity sometimes worsen the prognosis? Existing studies of this question have tended to have a limited sample size, and it is thus helpful to have the present account of data from 2 large-scale prospective Australian studies covering a period of 10 to 11 years. The main weakness, as in most large-scale surveys, was the need to rely on self-reports, both to assess the individual's initial health and to make a 7-level categorization of habitual physical activity. It seems both surprising and doubtful that 12% of the women and 23% of the men in this population were claiming an activity level of more than 1500 metabolic equivalent (MET) minutes per week. Nevertheless, the hazard ratios suggest that benefit was associated with very small amounts of reported physical activity, particularly in women (the commonly recommended public health recommendation equates to 450 MET minutes per week).[3] Moreover, the data suggest only a small advantage from greater reported volumes of activity (Table 2). The data were adjusted for smoking status and body mass index; in the men (but not the women) this information was obtained by interview. The physical activity questionnaires also differed between men and women, which may explain the apparent sex difference in the benefits of physical activity. In terms of our primary questions, it seems that in the elderly, any activity is better than none, but there is some additional advantage in reaching or exceeding public health recommendations. A further important issue, not discussed, is the quality-adjusted life expectancy for the various activity categories.

R. J. Shephard, MD (Lond), PhD, DPE

References

1. Gregg EW, Cauley JA, Stone K, et al. Relationship of changes in physical activity and mortality among older women. *JAMA.* 2003;289:2379-2386.
2. Schooling CM, Lam TH, Li ZB, et al. Obesity, physical activity, and mortality in a prospective Chinese elderly cohort. *Arch Intern Med.* 2006;166:1498-1504.
3. Nelson ME, Rejeski WJ, Blair SN, et al. Physical activity and public health in older adults: recommendation from the American College of Sports Medicine and the American Heart Association. *Med Sci Sports Exerc.* 2007;39:1435-1445.

Inflammatory markers in skeletal muscle of older adults

Caldow MK, Cameron-Smith D, Levinger P, et al (Deakin Univ, Melbourne, Australia; La Trobe Univ, Melbourne, Australia; et al)
Eur J Appl Physiol 113:509-517, 2013

Older adults have an increase in circulating markers of inflammation. The current study examined whether there is an increase in the expression of inflammatory markers within the *vastus lateralis*, a major locomotive muscle, of older adults, and if so, whether the reduction in muscle strength and aerobic capacity in older adults is related to increased muscle inflammation. Skeletal muscle biopsies were taken from older adults ($n = 17$, 67 ± 1.6 years) and young individuals ($n = 16$, 24 ± 0.6 years) under resting and fasting conditions. Muscle was analyzed for mRNA levels of intracellular inflammatory molecules (MCP1, TNFα and IL-1β) and total cellular protein abundance of cytokines, chemokines and kinases (IL-6, IL-8, MCP1, TNFα, p65 (NF-κB), JNK1/2 and STAT3). MCP1 expression was significantly higher ($p < 0.05$; 50%, mRNA and 40%, protein) in elderly than younger participants, as was IL-8 (4%). No detectable difference in kinase protein expression was observed for STAT3, JNK or p65 (NF-κB), TNFα or IL-6. Muscle strength was lower in the elderly compared to the young group (1.55 ± 0.17 vs. 2.56 ± 0.13 Nm/kg, $p < 0.001$). The elderly group also had a significantly lower VO_{2peak} compared to the young group (24.9 ± 1.9 vs. 39.3 ± 1.9, $p < 0.001$), but muscle strength and VO_{2peak} were not correlated with the examined inflammatory markers. Older adults have increased MCP1 (mRNA and protein abundance) and IL-8 (protein abundance) and also reduced muscle strength and VO_{2peak}. However, the reduction in muscle strength and VO_{2peak} was not related to the increase in muscle inflammatory markers in this cohort.

▶ Inflammatory burden has been implicated in sarcopenia, muscle weakness, impaired physical function, and suppressed regenerative capacity of muscle cells in older adults. In this preliminary study, Caldow and colleagues compared inflammatory markers in skeletal muscle tissue of older and young adults. The snapshot of inflammatory burden within muscle (*vastus lateralis*) showed few age-related distinctions. MCP1 gene and protein expression and interleukin (IL)-8 protein expression were significantly elevated in tissue from older adults compared with the young. No age-group differences were found for pro-inflammatory cytokines (IL-6 and tumor necrosis factor-α) and transcription factors (JNK 1/2, p65 NF-kB, and STAT3) that regulate pro-inflammatory cytokines. The functions of MCP1 and IL-8 include the recruitment of inflammatory cells for muscle repair, regeneration, and adaptation. Blood MCP1 increases in an age-dependent manner, which suggests either greater inflammation or reduced efficiency of MCP1 in response to a given inflammatory state. As expected, the older adults in this study had lower maximal muscle strength and aerobic capacity compared with the young. Muscular strength and aerobic capacity were not significantly associated with any of the targeted inflammatory markers, except for a tendency for greater MCP1 mRNA to be associated with lower aerobic capacity. The older group included adults with chronic disease, such as diabetes mellitus and hypertension, but they were otherwise healthy and as physically active as the younger adults. The findings suggest that in nonfrail older adults in stable health, cytokine burden may be quite comparable to that in younger adults. This study joins a few others that examined inflammation at the tissue level in older adults but did not include plasma concentrations or expression of the targeted inflammatory mediators for a comparison of local and systemic factors.

C. M. Jankowski, PhD

Protein Supplementation Improves Physical Performance in Frail Elderly People: A Randomized, Double-Blind, Placebo-Controlled Trial

Tieland M, van de Rest O, Dirks ML, et al (Top Inst Food and Nutrition, Wageningen, The Netherlands; Wageningen Univ, The Netherlands; Maastricht Univ Med Centre, The Netherlands)
J Am Med Dir Assoc 13:720-726, 2012

Objectives.—Protein supplementation has been proposed as an effective dietary strategy to increase skeletal muscle mass and improve physical performance in frail elderly people. Our objective was to assess the impact of 24 weeks of dietary protein supplementation on muscle mass, strength, and physical performance in frail elderly people.

Design/Setting/Participants.—A total of 65 frail elderly subjects were included and randomly allocated to either daily protein or placebo supplementation (15 g protein at breakfast and lunch).

Measurements.—Skeletal muscle mass (DXA), muscle fiber size (muscle biopsy), strength (1-RM), and physical performance (SPPB) were assessed at baseline, and after 12 and 24 weeks of dietary intervention.

Results.—Skeletal muscle mass did not change in the protein- (from 45.8 ± 1.7 to 45.8 ± 1.7 kg) or placebosupplemented group (from 46.7 ± 1.7 to 46.6 ± 1.7 kg) following 24 weeks of intervention ($P > .05$). In accordance, type I and II muscle fiber size did not change over time ($P > .05$). Muscle strength increased significantly in both groups ($P < .01$), with leg extension strength tending to increase to a greater extent in the protein (57 ± 5 to 68 ± 5 kg) compared with the placebo group (57 ± 5 to 63 ± 5 kg) (treatment × time interaction effect: $P = .059$). Physical performance improved significantly from 8.9 ± 0.6 to 10.0 ± 0.6 points in the protein group and did not change in the placebo group (from 7.8 ± 0.6 to 7.9 ± 0.6 points) (treatment × time interaction effect: $P = .02$).

Conclusion.—Dietary protein supplementation improves physical performance, but does not increase skeletal muscle mass in frail elderly people.

▶ In this study, physical function improved significantly in sedentary, frail older (age 80 years) adults who consumed a protein supplement daily for 24 weeks. The participants met at least 3 of 5 frailty criteria: unintentional weight loss, muscle weakness, self-reported exhaustion, slow walking speed, and low physical activity. The supplement was a 250-mL beverage providing 150 mg of milk protein or matching nonprotein placebo taken at breakfast and lunch. The timing of the supplement was important because breakfast and lunch meals tend to have low protein content compared with the evening meal. The main physical function outcome was the change in the Short Physical Performance Battery (SPPB) score. The SPPB comprises tests of balance, gait speed, and chair rise ability. Scores range from 0 to 12 with 5 to 9 categorized as moderately frail and less than 5 as frail. Both groups had moderate frailty at baseline, but the protein group improved from pre- to nonfrail (8.9 ± 0.6 to 10.0 ± 0.6 points; placebo, 7.8 ± 0.6 to 7.9 ± 0.6 points). Compliance to the beverage was 95%, and dietary intake of protein in regular meals did not change during the study. The protein group received additional total daily protein rather than substituting meal protein for the supplement. This outcome could be attributed to providing the supplement at breakfast and lunch but not dinner. Lean mass did not change significantly in either group. The protein group had a borderline improvement in leg extension strength compared with placebo. The trends for increases in muscle strength in the protein group are consistent with improved physical function and suggest early neuromuscular adaptations.

C. M. Jankowski, PhD

Effect of Potassium Citrate on Bone Density, Microarchitecture, and Fracture Risk in Healthy Older Adults without Osteoporosis: A Randomized Controlled Trial

Jehle S, Hulter HN, Krapf R (Univ of Basel, Switzerland; Univ of California, San Francisco)
J Clin Endocrinol Metab 98:207-217, 2013

Context.—The acid load imposed by a modern diet may play an important role in the pathophysiology of osteoporosis.

Objective.—Our objective was to evaluate the skeletal efficacy and safety and the effect on fracture prediction of K-citrate to neutralize diet-induced acid loads.

Design and Setting.—We conducted a randomized, double-blind, placebo-controlled trial at a teaching hospital.

Subjects.—Subjects included 201 elderly (>65 yr old) healthy men and women (*t*-score of −0.6 at lumbar spine).

Intervention.—Intervention was 60 mEq of K-citrate daily or placebo by mouth. All subjects received calcium and vitamin D.

Outcome Measures.—The primary outcome was change in areal bone mineral density (aBMD) at the lumbar spine by dual-energy x-ray absorptiometry after 24 months. Secondary endpoints included changes in volumetric density and microarchitectural parameters by high-resolution peripheral quantitative computed tomography in both radii and both tibiae and fracture risk assessment by FRAX (Switzerland).

Results.—K-citrate increased aBMD at lumbar spine from baseline by 1.7 ± 1.5% [95% confidence interval (CI) = 1.0–2.3, $P < 0.001$] net of placebo after 24 months. High-resolution peripheral quantitative computed tomography-measured trabecular densities increased at nondominant tibia (1.3 ± 1.3%, CI = 0.7−1.9, $P < 0.001$) and nondominant radius (2.0 ± 2.0%, CI = 1.4−2.7, $P < 0.001$). At nondominant radius, trabecular bone volume/tissue volume increased by 0.9 ± 0.8%, (CI = 0.1−1.7), trabecular thickness by 1.5 ± 1.6% (CI = 0.7−2.3), and trabecular number by 1.9 ± 1.8% (CI = 0.7−3.1, for all, $P < 0.05$). K-citrate diminished fracture prediction score by FRAX significantly in both sexes.

Conclusions.—Among a group of healthy elderly persons without osteoporosis, treatment with K-citrate for 24 months resulted in a significant increase in aBMD and volumetric BMD at several sites tested, while also improving bone microarchitecture. Based on the effect on fracture prediction, an effect on future fractures by K-citrate is possible.

▶ In this study, potassium (K)-citrate was investigated as an alkalinizing treatment to offset the acidic state found in older adults resulting from a Western diet and age-related changes in renal function. A pathological connection between metabolic acidosis and bone mineral density (BMD) is supported by the inhibition of osteoblast function and increased osteoclast activity during metabolic acidosis. In women and men aged 69 years, Jehle and colleagues found that K-citrate (60 mEq/day) significantly increased areal BMD of the lumbar spine, femoral neck, and total body when compared with placebo. The number and density of trabeculae in the tibia and radius increased with K-citrate. Conversely, no significant changes were seen in cortical bone. The profile of circulating bone markers suggested a transient (up to 12 months) decrease in bone resorption and a latent (18 to 24 months) and sustained increase in bone formation. The changes in BMD lent to a decrease in fracture risk, as determined by FRAX, in the K-citrate–treated adults. Importantly, the effects of K-citrate were independent of sex and age within the 65- to 80-year range. All participants had normal BMD (average lumbar spine T-score of −0.6) at study entry, were nonvegetarian, and were provided with calcium carbonate (500 mg/day) and vitamin D3 (400 IU/day) supplements. The authors noted that the participants had relatively low acid production at study entry that may have diminished the effects of K-citrate to shift acid-base balance. In fact, the magnitude of increase in BMD was positively correlated with baseline urinary acid excretion. The dose-response for K-citrate and changes in bone quality, effects in older adults with established osteoporosis, and consequences of K-citrate withdrawal will be interesting developments in bone therapeutics.

C. M. Jankowski, PhD

Physical Activity Prevents Progression for Cognitive Impairment and Vascular Dementia: Results From the LADIS (Leukoaraiosis and Disability) Study

Verdelho A, on behalf of the LADIS Study (Univ of Lisbon, Portugal; et al)
Stroke 43:3331-3335, 2012

Background and Purpose.—We aimed to study if physical activity could interfere with progression for cognitive impairment and dementia in older people with white matter changes living independently.

Methods.—The LADIS (Leukoaraiosis and Disability) prospective multinational European study evaluates the impact of white matter changes on the transition of independent elderly subjects into disability. Subjects were evaluated yearly during 3 years with a comprehensive clinical protocol and cognitive assessment with classification of cognitive impairment and dementia according to usual clinical criteria. Physical activity was recorded during the clinical interview. MRI was performed at entry and at the end of the study.

Results.—Six hundred thirty-nine subjects were included (74.1 ± 5 years old, 55% women, 9.6 ± 3.8 years of schooling, 64% physically active). At the end of follow-up, 90 patients had dementia (vascular dementia, 54; Alzheimer disease with vascular component, 34; frontotemporal dementia, 2), and 147 had cognitive impairment not dementia. Using Cox regression analysis, physical activity reduced the risk of cognitive impairment (dementia and not dementia: $\beta = -0.45$, $P = 0.002$; hazard ratio, 0.64; 95% CI, 0.48–0.85), dementia ($\beta = -0.49$, $P = 0.043$; hazard ratio, 0.61; 95% CI, 0.38–0.98), and vascular dementia ($\beta = -0.86$, $P = 0.008$; hazard ratio, 0.42; 95% CI, 0.22–0.80), independent of age, education, white matter change severity, medial temporal atrophy, previous and incident stroke, and diabetes.

Conclusions.—Physical activity reduces the risk of cognitive impairment, mainly vascular dementia, in older people living independently.

▶ Physical activity can prevent the functional and cognitive decline that comes with aging, and the progression of dementia, including Alzheimer disease.[1-3] Potential reasons for this benefit may include improved cerebral blood flow, reduced vascular risk factors and enhanced endothelial function, and decreased secretion of stress hormones.[4] Data from this study support the hypothesis that older subjects with vascular risk factors and vascular cerebral damage benefit from regular physical activity.

D. C. Nieman, DrPH

References

1. Larson EB, Wang L, Bowen JD, et al. Exercise is associated with reduced risk for incident dementia among persons 65 years of age and older. *Ann Intern Med.* 2006;144:73-81.
2. Weuve J, Kang JH, Manson JE, Breteler MM, Ware JH, Grodstein F. Physical activity, including walking, and cognitive function in older women. *JAMA.* 2004; 292:1454-1461.

3. Rovio S, Kåreholt I, Helkala EL, et al. Leisure-time physical activity at midlife and the risk of dementia and Alzheimer's disease. *Lancet Neurol.* 2005;4:705-711.
4. Kramer AF, Colcombe SJ, McAuley E, Scalf PE, Erickson KI. Fitness, aging and neurocognitive function. *Neurobiol Aging.* 2005;26:124-127.

Relationship between Physical Activity and Brain Atrophy Progression

Yuki A, Lee S, Kim H, et al (Natl Ctr for Geriatrics and Gerontology, Obu city, Aichi Prefecture, Japan; Tokaigakuen Univ, Miyoshi, Aichi Prefecture, Japan; et al)
Med Sci Sports Exerc 44:2362-2368, 2012

Introduction.—Brain atrophy is associated with impairment in cognitive function and learning function. The aim of this study was to determine whether daily physical activity prevents age-related brain atrophy progression.

Methods.—The participants were 381 men and 393 women who had participated in both the baseline and the follow-up surveys (mean duration = 8.2 yr). Magnetic resonance imaging of the frontal and temporal lobes was performed at the time of the baseline and follow-up surveys. The daily physical activities and total energy expenditures of the participants were recorded at baseline with uniaxial accelerometry sensors. Multiple logistic regression models were fit to determine the association between activity energy expenditure, number of steps, and total energy expenditure variables and frontal and temporal lobe atrophy progression while controlling for possible confounders.

Results.—In male participants, the odds ratio of frontal lobe atrophy progression for the fifth quintile compared with the first quintile in activity energy expenditure was 3.408 (95% confidence interval = 1.205−9.643) and for the number of steps was 3.651 (95% confidence interval = 1.304−10.219). Men and women with low total energy expenditure were at risk for frontal lobe atrophy progression. There were no significant differences between temporal lobe atrophy progression and physical activity or total energy expenditure.

Conclusion.—The results indicate that physical activity and total energy expenditure are significant predictors of frontal lobe atrophy progression during an 8-yr period. Promoting participation in activities may be beneficial for attenuating age-related frontal lobe atrophy and for preventing dementia.

▶ Previous research showed that brain atrophy was associated with cognitive function impairment.[1] In this 8-year study of 774 community-living, middle-age, and elderly Japanese people, low levels of physical activity were significant predictors of the risk for frontal lobe brain atrophy. The authors concluded that promoting participation in physical activities may be beneficial in preventing dementia and attenuating age-related frontal lobe atrophy. Thirty minutes of moderate-to-vigorous intensity activity per day, equivalent to walking 5700 steps, was sufficient to reduce the risk of frontal lobe atrophy progression.

D. C. Nieman, DrPH

Reference

1. Killiany RJ, Gomez-Isla T, Moss M, et al. Use of structural magnetic resonance imaging to predict who will get Alzheimer's disease. *Ann Neurol.* 2000;47:430-439.

Physical Training Improves Motor Performance in People with Dementia: A Randomized Controlled Trial
Hauer K, Schwenk M, Zieschang T, et al (Univ of Heidelberg, Germany; et al)
J Am Geriatr Soc 60:8-15, 2012

Objectives.—To determine whether a specific, standardized training regimen can improve muscle strength and physical functioning in people with dementia.

Design.—Double-blinded, randomized, controlled trial with 3-month intervention and 3-month follow-up period in 2006 to 2009.

Setting.—Outpatient geriatric rehabilitation.

Participants.—Individuals with confirmed mild to moderate dementia, no severe somatic or psychological disease, and ability to walk 10 m. Most participants were still living independently with or without supportive care.

Intervention.—Supervised, progressive resistance and functional group training for 3 months specifically developed for people with dementia (intervention, n = 62) compared with a low-intensity motor placebo activity (control, n = 60).

Measurements.—Primary outcome measures were one-repetition maximum in a leg press device for maximal strength and duration of the five-chair-stand test for functional performance. Secondary outcome measures were assessed for a number of established parameters for maximal strength, physical function, and physical activity.

Results.—Training significantly improved both primary outcomes (percentage change from baseline: maximal strength, intervention group (IG): +51.5 ± 41.5 kg vs control group (CG): −1.0 ± 28.9 kg, $P < .001$; functional performance, IG: −25.9 ± 15.1 seconds vs CG: +11.3 ± 60.4 seconds, $P < .001$). Secondary analysis confirmed effects for all strength and functional parameters. Training gains were partly sustained during follow-up. Low baseline performance on motor tasks but not cognitive impairment predicted positive training response. Physical activity increased significantly during the intervention ($P < .001$).

Conclusion.—The intensive, dementia-adjusted training was feasible and substantially improved motor performance in frail, older people with dementia and may represent a model for structured rehabilitation or outpatient training.

▶ Hauer and colleagues have raised the quality bar for exercise intervention studies focused on adults with dementia. This is an important study for clinicians who are advising caregivers of adults with dementia and leaders of exercise classes for this population. The aim of the study was to determine if a patient-centered resistance and functional training intervention would improve physical function in adults with mild to moderate cognitive impairment. The participants were carefully screened for cognitive impairment, including standardized neuropsychological testing and a medical history of dementia. Half of the 112 participants had an Alzheimer's disease diagnosis, whereas the remainder had vascular or other types of dementia. More than 80% of the participants were living independently, partly with supportive care. The intervention included twice-weekly moderate intensity (70-80% 1RM) resistance training and functional training (eg, stair climbing, sit-to-stand repetitions). The control condition was twice-weekly supervised sessions of light exercise and ball games. The training adherence was more than 90% for the active training and control groups. Muscle strength and 5 chair stand test performance increased significantly in the intervention group after 3 months of training. Numerous secondary functional outcomes, including balance and gait, showed significant intervention effects as well. Both groups increased their level of physical activity, which is an important finding because dementia is associated with profound apathy, including apathy toward movement. In a 3-month follow-up to the intervention, strength and chair stand performance remained greater than the pre-intervention levels in the resistance trained group. As seen in studies of frail older adults, individuals with the lowest baseline performance had the greatest improvements in function and strength. It is important for the quality of life of individuals with mild to moderate dementia, and their caregivers, that functional performance is preserved and physical activity maintained. This study provides strong evidence that adults with dementia can accomplish resistance and functional training at a level that improves their strength and function.

C. M. Jankowski, PhD

Special Populations

Autonomic Function and Exercise Performance in Elite Athletes with Cervical Spinal Cord Injury

West CR, Romer LM, Krassioukov A (Univ of British Columbia, Vancouver, Canada; Brunel Univ, Uxbridge, UK)
Med Sci Sports Exerc 45:261-267, 2013

Introduction.—"Complete" cervical spinal cord injury (SCI) is commonly believed to cause the decentralization of spinal sympathetic circuits and a consequent inability to meet the hemodynamic demands of exercise. Recently, however, we have noticed that athletes with motor complete

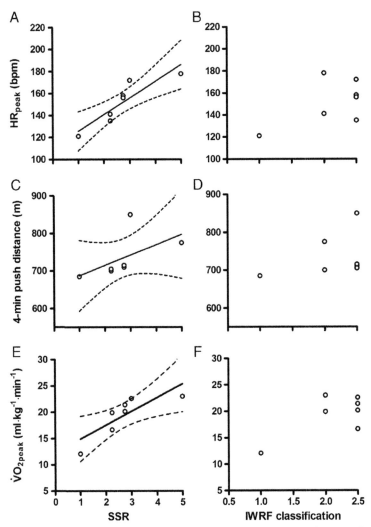

FIGURE 2.—Associations between sympathetic skin response (SSR), IWRF classification, and indices of exercise performance. Note that SSR was strongly correlated with all performance outcomes (panels A, C, and E), whereas IWRF classification was not (panels B, D, and F). Broken lines denote 95% CI. (Reprinted from West CR, Romer LM, Krassioukov A. Autonomic function and exercise performance in elite athletes with cervical spinal cord injury. *Med Sci Sports Exerc.* 2013;45:261-267, with permission from the American College of Sports Medicine.)

cervical SCI exhibit an exercise-induced tachycardia that appears to be at odds with the known effects of sympathetic decentralization.

Purpose.—This study aimed to determine the physiological basis of this response and, in doing so, to investigate associations between autonomic function, International Wheelchair Rugby Federation (IWRF) classification, and indices of exercise performance in highly trained athletes.

Methods.—Seven Paralympic wheelchair rugby players with motor complete cervical SCI were firstly classified according to IWRF classification, then assessed for autonomic function (sympathetic skin response [SSR]) and cardiovascular function (systolic blood pressure in response to sit-up tilt). Next, HR_{peak} and distance covered during a field-based maximal 4-min push were measured. Finally, peak oxygen uptake ($\dot{V}O_{2peak}$) and HR_{peak} during laboratory-based maximal incremental arm-crank exercise were measured.

Results.—All athletes demonstrated intact SSR (2.7 ± 1.2 responses from five stimulations), little or no change in systolic blood pressure in response to sit-up tilt (-22 ± 16 mm Hg), and exercise-induced tachycardia ($HR_{peak} = 152 \pm 20$ bpm). SSR was significantly correlated with HR_{peak} in the field, 4-min push distance, and $\dot{V}O_{2peak}$ (all $\rho \geq 0.946$), whereas current IWRF classification was not.

Conclusions.—All participants exhibited partial preservation of descending sympathetic control. We also found that the degree of remaining SSR, but not IWRF classification, was strongly correlated with indices of exercise performance. The findings suggest that the degree of remaining sympathetic control is an important determinant of exercise performance in athletes with cervical SCI (Fig 2).

▶ The matching of disability levels in competitors with spinal injuries is controversial, and some might judge an almost impossible task. This article draws attention to an issue not as yet considered: the ability to induce an increase of heart rate through the sympathetic nervous system. With a "complete" cervical injury, cardiac acceleration during exercise depends largely on a withdrawal of vagal tone. This leaves the heart beating at the intrinsic rate set by the sinoatrial node, about 100 beats/min,[1] with late supplementation by a "spillover" of epinephrine from the adrenals bringing the rate up to perhaps 130 beats/min.[2] In practice, rates often exceed this level, suggesting some residual sympathetic function, an issue not considered in current assessment schemes.[3] This study of 7 wheelchair rugby players with C6 or C7 lesions demonstrated evidence of residual sympathetic function in terms of the response to median nerve stimulation, and further noted that such residual function influenced aspects of performance such as the 4-minute push distance (Fig 2). The mean heart rate reached during the 4-minute push was 152 beats/min, and 1 subject reached a heart rate of 178. If these findings are confirmed in a larger study, it will be necessary to consider adding autonomic testing to the evaluation of wheelchair athletes.

R. J. Shephard, MD (Lond), PhD, DPE

References

1. Stinson EB, Griepp RB, Schroeder JS, Dong E Jr, Shumway NE. Hemodynamic observations one and two years after cardiac transplantation in man. *Circulation.* 1972;45:1183-1194.
2. Theisen D. Cardiovascular determinants of exercise capacity in the Paralympic athlete with spinal cord injury. *Exp Physiol.* 2012;97:319-324.
3. Mills PB, Krassioukov A. Autonomic function as a missing piece of the classification of Paralympic athletes with spinal cord injury. *Spinal Cord.* 2011;49:768-776.

Article Index

Chapter 1: Epidemiology, Prevention of Injuries, Lesions of Head and Neck

Chapter 2: Other Musculoskeletal Injuries

Chapter 3: Biomechanics, Muscle Strength and Training

Chapter 4: Physical Activity, Cardiorespiratory Physiology and Immune Function

Chapter 5: Metabolism and Obesity, Nutrition and Doping

Chapter 6: Cardiorespiratory Disorders

Chapter 7: Other Medical Conditions

Chapter 8: Environmental Factors

Chapter 9: Special Considerations: Children, Women, the Elderly, and Special Populations

Author Index

Printed and bound by CPI Group (UK) Ltd, Croydon, CR0 4YY

08/05/2025

01864755-0014